FUTURE OF EMERGENCY CARE

HOSPITAL-BASED EMERGENCY CARE
AT THE BREAKING POINT

Committee on the Future of Emergency Care
in the United States Health System

Board on Health Care Services

INSTITUTE OF MEDICINE
OF THE NATIONAL ACADEMIES

THE NATIONAL ACADEMIES PRESS
Washington, D.C.
www.nap.edu

THE NATIONAL ACADEMIES PRESS   500 Fifth Street, N.W.   Washington, DC 20001

NOTICE: The project that is the subject of this report was approved by the Governing Board of the National Research Council, whose members are drawn from the councils of the National Academy of Sciences, the National Academy of Engineering, and the Institute of Medicine. The members of the committee responsible for the report were chosen for their special competences and with regard for appropriate balance.

This study was supported by Contract No. 282-99-0045 between the National Academy of Sciences and the U.S. Department of Health and Human Services' Agency for Healthcare Research and Quality (AHRQ); Contract No. B03-06 between the National Academy of Sciences and the Josiah Macy, Jr. Foundation; and Contract No. HHSH25056047 between the National Academy of Sciences and the U.S. Department of Health and Human Services' Health Resources and Services Administration (HRSA) and Centers for Disease Control and Prevention (CDC), and the U.S. Department of Transportation's National Highway Traffic Safety Administration (NHTSA). Any opinions, findings, conclusions, or recommendations expressed in this publication are those of the author(s) and do not necessarily reflect the view of the organizations or agencies that provided support for this project.

Library of Congress Cataloging-in-Publication Data

Hospital-based emergency care : at the breaking point / Committee on the Future of Emergency Care in the United States Health System, Board on Health Care Services.
    p. ; cm. — (Future of emergency care series)
  Includes bibliographical references and index.
  ISBN-13: 978-0-309-10173-8 (hardback)
  ISBN-10: 0-309-10173-5 (hardback)
  1. Hospitals—Emergency services. 2. Emergency medical services. I. Institute of Medicine (U.S.). Committee on the Future of Emergency Care in the United States Health System. II. Series.
  [DNLM: 1. Emergency Service, Hospital—United States. 2. Health Care Reform—United States. WX 215 H8261 2007]
  RA975.5.E5H67723 2007
  362.11—dc22

                                          2007000079

"Knowing is not enough; we must apply.
Willing is not enough; we must do."
— Goethe

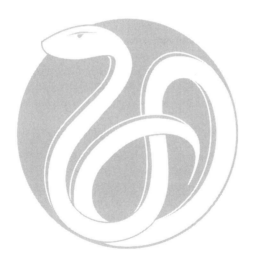

INSTITUTE OF MEDICINE
OF THE NATIONAL ACADEMIES

Advising the Nation. Improving Health.

THE NATIONAL ACADEMIES
Advisers to the Nation on Science, Engineering, and Medicine

The **National Academy of Sciences** is a private, nonprofit, self-perpetuating society of distinguished scholars engaged in scientific and engineering research, dedicated to the furtherance of science and technology and to their use for the general welfare. Upon the authority of the charter granted to it by the Congress in 1863, the Academy has a mandate that requires it to advise the federal government on scientific and technical matters. Dr. Ralph J. Cicerone is president of the National Academy of Sciences.

The **National Academy of Engineering** was established in 1964, under the charter of the National Academy of Sciences, as a parallel organization of outstanding engineers. It is autonomous in its administration and in the selection of its members, sharing with the National Academy of Sciences the responsibility for advising the federal government. The National Academy of Engineering also sponsors engineering programs aimed at meeting national needs, encourages education and research, and recognizes the superior achievements of engineers. Dr. Wm. A. Wulf is president of the National Academy of Engineering.

The **Institute of Medicine** was established in 1970 by the National Academy of Sciences to secure the services of eminent members of appropriate professions in the examination of policy matters pertaining to the health of the public. The Institute acts under the responsibility given to the National Academy of Sciences by its congressional charter to be an adviser to the federal government and, upon its own initiative, to identify issues of medical care, research, and education. Dr. Harvey V. Fineberg is president of the Institute of Medicine.

The **National Research Council** was organized by the National Academy of Sciences in 1916 to associate the broad community of science and technology with the Academy's purposes of furthering knowledge and advising the federal government. Functioning in accordance with general policies determined by the Academy, the Council has become the principal operating agency of both the National Academy of Sciences and the National Academy of Engineering in providing services to the government, the public, and the scientific and engineering communities. The Council is administered jointly by both Academies and the Institute of Medicine. Dr. Ralph J. Cicerone and Dr. Wm. A. Wulf are chair and vice chair, respectively, of the National Research Council.

www.national-academies.org

PETER M. LAYDE, Professor and Interim Director, Health Policy Institute and Co-Director, Injury Research Center, Medical College of Wisconsin, Milwaukee

EUGENE LITVAK, Professor of Health Care and Operations Management Director, Program for Management of Variability in Health Care Delivery, Boston University Health Policy Institute, Massachusetts

RICHARD A. ORR, Associate Director, Cardiac Intensive Care Unit, Medical Director, Children's Hospital Transport Team of Pittsburgh and Professor, University of Pittsburgh School of Medicine, Children's Hospital of Pittsburgh, Pennsylvania

JERRY L. OVERTON, Executive Director, Richmond Ambulance Authority, Virginia

JOHN E. PRESCOTT, Dean, West Virginia University School of Medicine, Morgantown

NELS D. SANDDAL, President, Critical Illness and Trauma Foundation, Bozeman, Montana

C. WILLIAM SCHWAB, Professor of Surgery, Chief, Division of Traumatology and Surgical Critical Care, Department of Surgery, University of Pennsylvania Medical Center, Philadelphia

MARK D. SMITH, President and CEO, California Healthcare Foundation, Oakland

DAVID N. SUNDWALL, Executive Director, Utah Department of Health, Salt Lake City

BENJAMIN WHEATLEY, Program Officer
ANISHA S. DHARSHI, Research Associate
SHEILA J. MADHANI, Program Officer
CANDACE TRENUM, Senior Program Assistant

Reviewers

This report has been reviewed in draft form by individuals chosen for their diverse perspectives and technical expertise, in accordance with procedures approved by the National Research Council's Report Review Committee. The purpose of this independent review is to provide candid and critical comments that will assist the institution in making its published report as sound as possible and to ensure that the report meets institutional standards for objectivity, evidence, and responsiveness to the study charge. The review comments and draft manuscript remain confidential to protect the integrity of the deliberative process. We wish to thank the following individuals for their review of this report:

E. JOHN GALLAGHER, Department of Emergency Medicine, Albert Einstein College of Medicine, Montefiore Medical Center, Bronx, New York

KRISTINE M. GEBBIE, Center for Health Policy, Columbia University School of Nursing, New York, New York

LEWIS R. GOLDFRANK, Department of Emergency Medicine, New York University School of Medicine, New York University Medical Center and Bellevue Hospital Center, New York

JERRIS R. HEDGES, School of Medicine, Oregon Health & Science University, Portland

GARY JOHNSON, Department of Family Medicine, University of Nevada School of Medicine, Reno

D. RANDY KUYKENDALL, Emergency Medical and Trauma Services
  Section, Health Facilities & Emergency Medical Services Division,
  Colorado Department of Public Health & Environment, Colorado
  Springs
RONALD V. MAIER, Department of Surgery, Harborview Medical
  Center, Seattle, Washington
MITCHELL T. RABKIN, Harvard Medical School, Beth Israel Deaconess
  Medical Center, Boston, Massachusetts
SARA ROSENBAUM, Department of Health Policy, School of Public
  Health and Health Services, The George Washington University Medical
  Center, Washington, District of Columbia
ALEX B. VALADKA, Department of Neurological Surgery, University of
  Texas Medical School at Houston

Although the reviewers listed above have provided many constructive comments and suggestions, they were not asked to endorse the conclusions or recommendations nor did they see the final draft of the report before its release. The review of this report was overseen by **Enriqueta C. Bond,** Burroughs Wellcome Fund, and **Don E. Detmer,** American Medical Informatics Association. Appointed by the National Research Council and the Institute of Medicine, they were responsible for making certain that an independent examination of this report was carried out in accordance with institutional procedures and that all review comments were carefully considered. Responsibility for the final content of this report rests entirely with the authoring committee and the institution.

Foreword

The state of emergency care affects every American. When illness or injury strikes, Americans count on the emergency care system to respond with timely and high-quality care. Yet today, the emergency and trauma care that Americans receive can fall short of what they expect and deserve.

Emergency care is a window on health care, revealing both what is right and what is wrong with the care delivery system. Americans increasingly rely on hospital emergency departments because of the skilled specialists and advanced technologies they offer. At the same time, the increasing use of the emergency care system represents failures of the larger health care system—the growing numbers of uninsured Americans, the limited alternatives available in many communities, and the inadequate preventive care and chronic care management received by many. The resulting demands on the system can degrade the quality of emergency care and hinder the ability to provide urgent and lifesaving care to seriously ill and injured patients wherever and whenever they need it.

The Committee on the Future of Emergency Care in the United States Health System, ably chaired by Gail Warden, set out to examine the emergency care system in the United States; explore its strengths, limitations, and future challenges; describe a desired vision of the emergency care system; and recommend strategies required to achieve that vision. Their efforts build on past contributions of the National Academies, including the landmark National Research Council report *Accidental Death and Disability: The Neglected Disease of Modern Society* in 1966, *Injury in America: A Continuing Public Health Problem* in 1985, and *Emergency Medical Services for Children* in 1993.

The committee's task in the present study was to examine the full scope of emergency care, from 9-1-1 and medical dispatch to hospital-based emergency and trauma care. The three reports produced by the committee—*Hospital-Based Emergency Care: At the Breaking Point, Emergency Medical Services at the Crossroads,* and *Emergency Care for Children: Growing Pains*—provide three different perspectives on the emergency care system. The series as a whole unites the often fragmented prehospital and hospital-based systems under a common vision for the future of emergency care.

As the committee prepared its reports, federal and state policy makers were turning their attention to the possibility of an avian influenza pandemic. Americans are asking whether we as a nation are prepared for such an event. The emergency care system is on the front lines of surveillance and treatment. The more secure and stable our emergency care system is, the better prepared we will be to handle any possible outbreak. In this light, the recommendations presented in these reports take on increased urgency. The guidance they offer can assist all of the stakeholders in emergency care—the public, policy makers, providers, and educators—to chart the future of emergency care in the United States.

Harvey V. Fineberg, M.D., Ph.D.
President, Institute of Medicine
June 2006

Preface

Emergency care has made important advances in recent decades: emergency 9-1-1 service now links virtually all ill and injured Americans to immediate medical response; organized trauma systems transport patients to advanced, life-saving care within minutes; and advances in resuscitation and lifesaving procedures yield outcomes unheard of just two decades ago. Yet just under the surface, a growing national crisis in emergency care is brewing. Emergency departments (EDs) are frequently overloaded, with patients sometimes lining hallways and waiting hours and even days to be admitted to inpatient beds. Ambulance diversion, in which overcrowded EDs close their doors to incoming ambulances, has become a common, even daily problem in many cities. Patients with severe trauma or illness are often brought to the ED only to find that the specialists needed to treat them are unavailable. The transport of patients to available emergency care facilities is often fragmented and disorganized, and the quality of emergency medical services (EMS) is highly inconsistent from one town, city, or region to the next. In some areas, the system's task of dealing with emergencies is compounded by an additional task: providing nonemergent care for many of the 45 million uninsured Americans. Furthermore, the system is ill prepared to handle large-scale emergencies, whether a natural disaster, an influenza pandemic, or an act of terrorism.

This crisis is multifaceted and impacts every aspect of emergency care—from prehospital EMS to hospital-based emergency and trauma care. The American public places its faith in the ability of the emergency care system to respond appropriately whenever and wherever a serious illness or injury occurs. But while the public is largely unaware of the crisis, it is real and growing.

The Institute of Medicine's Committee on the Future of Emergency Care in the United States Health System was convened in September 2003 to examine the emergency care system in the United States, to create a vision for the future of the system, and to make recommendations for helping the nation achieve that vision. The committee's findings and recommendations are presented in the three reports in the *Future of Emergency Care* series:

- *Hospital-Based Emergency Care: At the Breaking Point* explores the changing role of the hospital ED and describes the national epidemic of overcrowded EDs and trauma centers. The range of issues addressed includes uncompensated emergency and trauma care, the availability of specialists, medical liability exposure, management of patient flow, hospital disaster preparedness, and support for emergency and trauma research.
- *Emergency Medical Services at the Crossroads* describes the development of EMS over the last four decades and the fragmented system that exists today. It explores a range of issues that affect the delivery of prehospital EMS, including communications systems; coordination of the regional flow of patients to hospitals and trauma centers; reimbursement of EMS services; national training and credentialing standards; innovations in triage, treatment, and transport; integration of all components of EMS into disaster preparedness, planning, and response actions; and the lack of clinical evidence to support much of the care that is delivered.
- *Emergency Care for Children: Growing Pains* describes the special challenges of emergency care for children and considers the progress that has been made in this area in the 20 years since the establishment of the federal Emergency Medical Services for Children (EMS-C) program. It addresses how issues affecting the emergency care system generally have an even greater impact on the outcomes of critically ill and injured children. The topics addressed include the state of pediatric readiness, pediatric training and standards of care in emergency care, pediatric medication issues, disaster preparedness for children, and pediatric research and data collection.

THE IMPORTANCE AND SCOPE OF EMERGENCY CARE

Each year in the United States approximately 114 million visits to EDs occur, and 16 million of these patients arrive by ambulance. In 2002, 43 percent of all hospital admissions in the United States entered through the ED. The emergency care system deals with an extraordinary range of patients, from febrile infants, to business executives with chest pain, to elderly patients who have fallen.

EDs are an impressive public health success story in terms of access to care. Americans of all walks of life know where the nearest ED is and understand that it is available 24 hours a day, 7 days a week. Trauma systems also represent an impressive achievement. They are a critical component of the emergency care system since approximately 35 percent of ED visits are injury-related, and injuries are the number one killer of people between the ages of 1 and 44. Yet the development of trauma systems has been inconsistent across states and regions.

In addition to its traditional role of providing urgent and lifesaving care, the emergency care system has become the "safety net of the safety net," providing primary care services to millions of Americans who are uninsured or otherwise lack access to other community services. Hospital EDs and trauma centers are the only providers required by federal law to accept, evaluate, and stabilize all who present for care, regardless of their ability to pay. An unintended but predictable consequence of this legal duty is a system that is overloaded and underfunded to carry out its mission. This situation can hinder access to emergency care for insured and uninsured alike, and compromise the quality of care provided to all. Further, EDs have become the preferred setting for many patients and an important adjunct to community physicians' practices. Indeed, the recent growth in ED use has been driven by patients with private health insurance. In addition to these responsibilities, emergency care providers have been tasked with the enormous challenge of preparing for a wide range of emergencies, from bioterrorism to natural disasters and pandemic disease. While balancing all of these tasks is difficult for every organization providing emergency care, it is an even greater challenge for small, rural providers with limited resources.

Improved Emergency Medical Services: A Public Health Imperative

Since the Institute of Medicine (IOM) embarked on this study, concern about a possible avian influenza pandemic has led to worldwide assessment of preparedness for such an event. Reflecting this concern, a national summit on pandemic influenza preparedness was convened by Department of Health and Human Services Secretary Michael O. Leavitt on December 5, 2005, in Washington, D.C., and has been followed by statewide summits throughout the country. At these meetings, many of the deficiencies noted by the IOM's Committee on the Future of Emergency Care in the United States Health System have been identified as weaknesses in the nation's ability to respond to large-scale emergency situations, whether disease outbreaks, naturally occurring disasters, or

continued

acts of terrorism. During any such event, local hospitals and emergency departments will be on the front lines. Yet of the millions of dollars going into preparedness efforts, a tiny fraction has made its way to medical preparedness, and much of that has focused on one of the least likely threats—bioterrorism. The result is that few hospital and EMS professionals have had even minimal disaster preparedness training; even fewer have access to personal protective equipment; hospitals, many already stretched to the limit, lack the ability to absorb any significant surge in casualties; and supplies of critical hospital equipment, such as decontamination showers, negative pressure rooms, ventilators, and intensive care unit beds, are wholly inadequate. A system struggling to meet the day-to-day needs of the public will not have the capacity to deal with a sustained surge of patients.

FRAMEWORK FOR THIS STUDY

This year marks the fortieth anniversary of the publication of the landmark National Academy of Sciences/National Research Council report *Accidental Death and Disability: The Neglected Disease of Modern Society*. That report described an epidemic of automobile-related and other injuries, and harshly criticized the deplorable state of trauma care nationwide. The report prompted a public outcry, and stimulated a flood of public and private initiatives to enhance highway safety and improve the medical response to injuries. Efforts included the development of trauma and prehospital EMS systems, creation of the specialty in emergency medicine, and establishment of federal programs to enhance the emergency care infrastructure and build a research base. To many, the 1966 report marked the birth of the modern emergency care system.

Since then, the National Academies and the Institute of Medicine (IOM) have produced a variety of reports examining various aspects of the emergency care system. The 1985 report *Injury in America* called for expanded research into the epidemiology and treatment of injury, and led to the development of the National Center for Injury Prevention and Control within the Centers for Disease Control and Prevention. The 1993 report *Emergency Medical Services for Children* exposed the limited capacity of the emergency care system to address the needs of children, and contributed to the expansion of the EMS-C program within the Department of Health and Human Services. It has been 10 years, however, since the IOM examined any aspect of emergency care in depth. Furthermore, no National Academies report has ever examined the full range of issues surrounding emergency care in the United States.

That is what this committee set out to do. The objectives of the study were to (1) examine the emergency care system in the United States; (2) explore its strengths, limitations, and future challenges; (3) describe a desired vision for the system; and (4) recommend strategies for achieving this vision.

STUDY DESIGN

The IOM Committee on the Future of Emergency Care in the United States Health System was formed in September 2003. In May 2004, the committee was expanded to comprise a main committee of 25 members and three subcommittees. A total of 40 main and subcommittee members, representing a broad range of expertise in health care and public policy, participated in the study. Between 2003 and 2006, the main committee and subcommittees met 19 times; heard public testimony from nearly 60 speakers; commissioned 11 research papers; conducted site visits; and gathered information from hundreds of experts, stakeholder groups, and interested individuals.

The magnitude of the effort reflects the scope and complexity of emergency care itself, which encompasses a broad continuum of services that includes prevention and bystander care; emergency calls to 9-1-1; dispatch of emergency personnel to the scene of injury or illness; triage, treatment, and transport of patients by ambulance and air medical services; hospital-based emergency and trauma care; subspecialty care by on-call specialists; and subsequent inpatient care. Emergency care's complexity can also be traced to the multiple locations, diverse professionals, and cultural differences that span this continuum of services. EMS, for example, is unlike any other field of medicine—over one-third of its professional workforce consists of volunteers. Further, EMS has one foot in the public safety realm and one foot in medical care, with nearly half of all such services being housed within fire departments. Hospital-based emergency care is also delivered by an extraordinarily diverse staff—emergency physicians, trauma surgeons, critical care specialists, and the many surgical and medical subspecialists who provide services on an on-call basis, as well as specially trained nurses, pharmacists, physician assistants, nurse practitioners, and others.

The division into a main committee and three subcommittees made it possible to break down this enormous effort into several discrete components. At the same time, the committee sought to examine emergency care as a comprehensive system, recognizing the interdependency of its component parts. To this end, the study process was highly integrated. The main committee and three subcommittees were designed to provide for substantial overlap, interaction, and cross-fertilization of expertise. The committee concluded that nothing will change without cooperative and visionary leadership at many levels and a concerted national effort among the principal stakeholders—federal, state, and local officials; hospital leadership; physicians, nurses, and other clinicians; and the public.

The committee hopes that the reports in the *Future of Emergency Care* series will stimulate increased attention to and reform of the emergency care system in the United States. I wish to express my appreciation to the members of the committee and subcommittees and the many panelists who provided input at the meetings held for this study, and to the IOM staff for their time, effort, and commitment to the development of these important reports.

Gail L. Warden
Chair

Acknowledgments

The *Future of Emergency Care* series benefited from the contributions of many individuals and organizations. The committee and Institute of Medicine (IOM) staff take this opportunity to recognize and thank those who helped in the development of the reports in the series.

A large number of individuals assembled materials that helped the committee develop the evidence base for its analyses. The committee appreciates the contributions of experts from a variety of organizations and disciplines who gave presentations during committee meetings or authored papers that provided information incorporated into the series of reports. The full list of presenters is provided in Appendix C. Authors of commissioned papers are listed in Appendix D.

Committee members and IOM staff conducted a number of site visits throughout the course of the study to gain a better understanding of certain aspects of the emergency care system. We appreciate the willingness of staff from the following organizations to meet with us and respond to questions: Beth Israel Deaconess Medical Center, Boston Medical Center, Children's National Medical Center, Grady Memorial Hospital, Johns Hopkins Hospital, Maryland Institute for EMS Services Systems, Maryland State Police Aviation Division, Richmond Ambulance Association, and Washington Hospital Center.

We would also like to express appreciation to the many individuals who shared their expertise and resources on a wide range of issues: Karen Benson-Huck, Linda Fagnani, Carol Haraden, Lenworth Jacobs, Tom Judge, Nadine Levick, Ellen MacKenzie, Dawn Mancuso, Rick Murray, Ed

Racht, Dom Ruscio, Carol Spizziri, Caroline Steinberg, Rosemary Stevens, Peter Vicellio, and Mike Williams.

This study received funding from the Josiah Macy, Jr. Foundation, the National Highway Traffic Safety Administration (NHTSA), and three agencies within the Department of Health and Human Services: the Agency for Healthcare Research and Quality (AHRQ), the Centers for Disease Control and Prevention (CDC), and the Health Resources and Services Administration (HRSA). We would like to thank the staff from those organizations who provided us with information, documents, and insights throughout the project, including Drew Dawson, Laurie Flaherty, Susan McHenry, Gamunu Wijetunge, and David Bryson of NHTSA; Dan Kavanaugh, Christina Turgel, and David Heppel of HRSA; Robin Weinick and Pam Owens of AHRQ; Rick Hunt and Bob Bailey from CDC's National Center for Injury Prevention and Control; and many other helpful members of the staffs of those organizations.

Important research and writing contributions were made by Molly Hicks of Keene Mill Consulting, LLC. Karen Boyd, a Christine Mirzayan Science and Technology Fellow of the National Academies, and two student interns, Carla Bezold and Neesha Desai, developed background papers. Also, our thanks to Rona Briere, who edited the reports, and to Alisa Decatur, who prepared them for publication.

Contents

HOSPITAL-BASED EMERGENCY CARE

Summary

Hospital-based emergency and trauma care is critically important to the health and well-being of Americans. In 2003, nearly 114 million visits were made to hospital emergency departments (EDs)—more than one for every three people in the United States. About one-quarter of those visits were due to unintentional injuries, the leading cause of death for people aged 1 through 44. While most Americans encounter the ED only rarely, they count on it to be there when they need it.

Over the last several decades, the role of hospital-based emergency and trauma care has evolved. EDs continue to focus on their traditional mission of providing urgent and lifesaving care, but have taken on additional responsibilities to meet the needs of communities, providers, and patients. Today, their complex role also encompasses safety net care for uninsured patients, public health surveillance, disaster preparedness, and serving as an adjunct to community physician practices. In some rural communities, the hospital ED may be the main source of health care for a widely dispersed population. While the demands on emergency and trauma care have grown dramatically, however, the capacity of the system has not kept pace. Balancing these roles in the face of increasing patient volume and limited resources has become increasingly challenging. The situation is creating a widening gap between the quality of emergency care Americans expect and the quality they actually receive.

STUDY CHARGE

The Institute of Medicine's (IOM) Committee on the Future of Emergency Care in the United States Health System was formed in September

2003 to examine the emergency care system in the United States; explore its strengths, limitations, and future challenges; describe a desired vision of the system; and recommend strategies for achieving that vision. The committee was also tasked with taking a focused look at the state of pediatric emergency care, prehospital emergency care, and hospital-based emergency and trauma care. This is the third of three reports presenting the committee's findings and recommendations in these three areas. Summarized below are the committee's findings and recommendations for meeting the challenge of high demand for emergency care and achieving the vision of a 21st-century emergency care system.

THE CHALLENGE OF HIGH DEMAND AND INADEQUATE SYSTEM CAPACITY

Between 1993 and 2003, the population of the United States grew by 12 percent, hospital admissions increased by 13 percent, and ED visits rose by more than 2 million per year from 90.3 to 113.9 million—a 26 percent increase (see Figure ES-1). Not only is ED volume increasing, but patients coming to the ED are older and sicker and require more complex and time-consuming workups and treatments. Moreover, during this same period, the United States experienced a net loss of 703 hospitals, 198,000 hospital beds, and 425 hospital EDs, mainly in response to cost-cutting measures

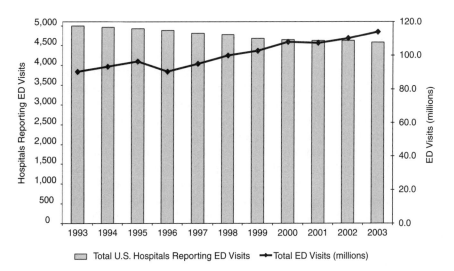

FIGURE ES-1 Hospital emergency departments versus numbers of visits.
SOURCE: AHA, 2005b; McCaig and Burt, 2005.

and lower reimbursements by managed care, Medicare, and other payers. By 2001, 60 percent of hospitals were operating at or over capacity.

The high demand for hospital-based emergency and trauma care reflects several trends. First, EDs have become one of the nation's principal sources of care for patients with limited access to other providers, including the 45 million uninsured Americans. Indeed, the Emergency Medical Treatment and Active Labor Act of 1986 prevents hospitals from restricting access for uninsured patients by requiring hospitals to provide a medical screening examination to all patients and to stabilize or transfer patients as needed. With limited access to community-based primary and specialty care, many turn to the emergency system when in medical need, often for conditions that have worsened because of a lack of regular primary care.

Medicaid beneficiaries also turn to the ED. In fact, Medicaid enrollees visit the ED at a higher rate than any other category of patient (81 visits per 100 enrollees)—double the rate of the uninsured population and nearly four times that of privately insured patients. Although Medicaid enrollees are insured, the low rates of provider reimbursement in many states limit the number of office-based practitioners who are willing to accept them as patients.

In addition, the ED often serves as primary care provider, a role for which it is not optimally designed. Rather, the ED is designed for rapid, high-intensity responses to acute injuries and illnesses. Physicians in the ED face constant interruptions and distractions, and typically lack access to the patient's full medical records. Because nonemergency patients are usually low triage priorities, they often experience extremely long wait times as they are passed over for more urgent cases.

Costs are another concern. When an ED is not busy, the cost of treating an additional nonemergency patient is probably quite low. But while the literature on this issue is mixed, a number of studies suggest that nonemergency care in the ED is more costly than that in alternative settings. Indeed, ED charges for minor problems have been estimated to be two to five times higher than those of a typical office visit. When the ED is at full capacity, treating additional patients who could be cared for in a different environment means fewer resources—physicians, nurses, ancillary personnel, equipment, and time and space—available to respond to emergency cases.

By law, the front door of the ED is always open. When a hospital's inpatient beds are full, as is frequently the case, ED providers cannot transfer the most severely ill and injured patients to an inpatient unit. As a result, ED patients who require hospitalization begin to back up in the ED. The aggregate result of this imbalance between public demand and hospital capacity is an epidemic of overcrowded EDs, frequent "boarding" of patients waiting for inpatient beds, and ambulance diversion:

• **Overcrowding**—ED overcrowding is a nationwide phenomenon, affecting rural and urban areas alike. In one study, 91 percent of EDs responding to a national survey reported overcrowding as a problem; almost 40 percent reported that overcrowding occurred daily. Overcrowding induces stress in providers and patients, and can lead to errors and impaired overall quality of care.

• **Boarding**—A consequence of crowded EDs is the practice of boarding—holding a patient who needs to be admitted in the ED until an inpatient bed becomes available. It is not unusual for patients in a busy hospital ED to be boarded for 48 hours or more. In a nationwide survey of nearly 90 EDs across the country, conducted on a typical Monday evening, 73 percent of hospitals reported boarding two or more patients. Boarding not only compromises the patient's hospital experience, but also adds to an already stressful work environment for physicians and nurses and enhances the potential for errors, delays in treatment, and diminished quality of care.

• **Ambulance diversion**—Another consequence of crowding is ambulance diversion—when EDs become saturated to the point that patient safety is compromised, ambulances are diverted to alternative hospitals. Once a safety valve to be used in extreme situations, this has now become a commonplace event. A recent study reported that 501,000 ambulances were diverted in 2003, an average of 1 per minute. According to the American Hospital Association, nearly half of all hospitals, and close to 70 percent of urban hospitals, reported time on diversion in 2004. Ambulance diversion can lead to catastrophic delays in treatment for seriously ill or injured patients. It also frequently leads to treatment in facilities with inadequate expertise and resources appropriate to the patient's severity of illness, placing the patient at significant risk.

FINDINGS AND RECOMMENDATIONS

This section presents the committee's key findings and recommendations for meeting the challenge of increased demand and inadequate capacity and improving the quality of hospital-based emergency and trauma care. These findings and recommendations address the need to enhance operational efficiency, the use of information technology, the burden of uncompensated care, inadequate disaster preparedness, the emergency care workforce, and the need for research in emergency care.

Enhanced Operational Efficiency

Hospital EDs and trauma centers have little control over external forces that contribute to crowding, such as increasing numbers of uninsured or the growing severity of patients' conditions. There is, however, a great deal they can do to manage the impact of these forces. Innovations in industrial engineering that have swept through other sectors of the economy, from banking to air travel to manufacturing, have failed to take hold in health care delivery—a sector of the economy that now consumes 16 percent of the nation's gross domestic product and is growing at twice the rate of inflation.

Tools derived from engineering and operations research have been directed successfully at the problem of hospital efficiency in general and ED crowding in particular. A wide range of tools have been developed and tested for addressing patient flow—defined as the movement of patients through the hospital system—generally with good success. Efficient patient flow can increase the volume of patients treated and discharged and minimize delays at each point in the delivery process while improving the quality of care. For example, while controlled studies have yet to be conducted, a growing body of experience suggests that using queuing theory to smooth the peaks and valleys of patient admissions can eliminate bottlenecks, reduce crowding, improve patient care, and reduce costs. The committee recommends that **hospital chief executive officers adopt enterprisewide operations management and related strategies to improve the quality and efficiency of emergency care (4.2).**[1]

A particularly promising technique for managing patient flow is the use of clinical decision units (CDUs), also known as observation units. The technique was developed as a means of monitoring patients with chest pain who had a low to intermediate probability of acute myocardial infarction (AMI). By observing patients for up to 23 hours, ED staff were able to rule out many patients at risk of AMI while using fewer resources than would have been consumed if these same patients had been admitted to the intensive care unit (ICU) or an inpatient telemetry unit. Today, the Centers for Medicare and Medicaid Services (CMS) reimburses CDU stays for only three conditions: chest pain, asthma, and congestive heart failure. Because of the demonstrated success of CDUs, the committee recommends that **the Centers for Medicare and Medicaid Services remove current restrictions on the medical conditions that are eligible for separate clinical decision unit payment (4.1).**

Incentives to Reduce Crowding and Boarding

While hospitals can use many approaches to reduce crowding and boarding, there are limited financial incentives for them to do so. Hospitals

---

[1]The committee's recommendations are numbered according to the chapter of the main report in which they appear. Thus, for example, recommendation 2.1 is the first recommendation in Chapter 2.

are not reimbursed for differences in costs that are often associated with admissions from the ED. Further, hospitals do not face significant negative financial consequences for operating crowded EDs. In 2004, following a July 2002 alert that tied treatment delays to more than 50 hospital deaths, the Joint Commission on Accreditation of Healthcare Organizations (JCAHO) instituted new guidelines that would have required accredited hospitals to take serious steps to reduce crowding, boarding, and diversion. Under industry pressure, however, these requirements were withdrawn and replaced with a weaker standard. The committee recommends that **the Joint Commission on Accreditation of Healthcare Organizations reinstate strong standards designed to sharply reduce and ultimately eliminate emergency department crowding, boarding, and diversion (4.4).** Furthermore, because the practices of boarding and diversion are so antithetical to quality medical care, the strongest possible measures should be taken to eliminate them. The committee recommends that **hospitals end the practices of boarding patients in the emergency department and ambulance diversion, except in the most extreme cases, such as a community mass casualty event. The Centers for Medicare and Medicaid Services should convene a working group that includes experts in emergency care, inpatient critical care, hospital operations management, nursing, and other relevant disciplines to develop boarding and diversion standards, as well as guidelines, measures, and incentives for implementation, monitoring, and enforcement of these standards (4.5).**

Leadership in Improving Hospital Efficiency

Beyond the use of incentives, the committee looks to hospital executives, including both chief executive officers (CEOs) and midlevel managers, to provide visionary leadership in promoting the use of patient flow and operations management approaches to improve hospital efficiency. Hospital leaders should be open to learning from the experiences of industries outside of health care, and should be bold and creative in applying these and other new ideas. To foster the development of hospital leadership in improving hospital efficiency, the committee recommends that **training in operations management and related approaches be promoted by professional associations; accrediting organizations, such as the Joint Commission on Accreditation of Healthcare Organizations and the National Committee for Quality Assurance; and educational institutions that provide training in clinical, health care management, and public health disciplines (4.3).**

Use of Information Technology

Opportunities to improve patient flow, operational efficiency, and quality of care can be enhanced by appropriate information technologies.

Hospitals, however, lag behind other industries in the use of information technologies, particularly those used to support process management.

Information technologies have broad application to hospitals and health systems, but their use involves unique needs and approaches in emergency care. Information is critically important for rapid decision making in emergency and trauma care. But emergency physicians are all too often deprived of critical patient information; indeed, it has been said that EDs operate on information "fumes." The following information technologies could significantly enhance emergency care: (1) dashboard systems that track and coordinate patient flow, (2) communications systems that enable ED physicians to link to patients' records or providers, (3) clinical decision-support programs that improve decision making, (4) documentation systems for collecting and storing patient data, (5) computerized training and information retrieval, and (6) systems to facilitate public health surveillance. Given their demonstrated effectiveness in the emergency care setting, the committee recommends that **hospitals adopt robust information and communications systems to improve the safety and quality of emergency care and enhance hospital efficiency (5.1)**. The committee recognizes that the appropriate prioritization of and investment in these approaches will vary based on each institution's resources and needs.

The Burden of Uncompensated Care

In most hospitals, if reimbursements fail to cover ED and trauma costs, these costs are subsidized by admissions that originate in the ED. But uncompensated care can be an extreme burden at hospitals that have large numbers of uninsured patients. Many hospital ED and trauma center closures are attributed to financial losses associated with emergency and trauma care. Public hospitals and tertiary medical centers bear a large share of this burden, as surrounding community hospitals often transfer their most complex, high-risk patients to the large safety net hospitals for specialized care. Often, the condition of these patients has deteriorated considerably since their arrival at the referring hospital. Hospitals receive Disproportionate Share Hospital (DSH) payments from both Medicare and Medicaid to compensate for these losses, but these payments are inadequate for hospitals with large safety net populations. As a result, the emergency and trauma care safety net system is at risk in many regions. To ensure the continued viability of a critical public safety function, the committee recommends that **Congress establish dedicated funding, separate from Disproportionate Share Hospital payments, to reimburse hospitals that provide significant amounts of uncompensated emergency and trauma care for the financial losses incurred by providing those services (2.1)**.

The committee believes that accurate determination of the optimal amount of funding to allocate for this purpose, which could run into the hundreds of millions of dollars, is beyond its expertise, but that the government must begin to address this issue immediately. The committee therefore recommends that **Congress initially appropriate $50 million for the purpose, to be administered by the Centers for Medicare and Medicaid Services (2.1a).** The Centers for Medicare and Medicaid Services should establish a working group to determine the allocation of these funds, which should be targeted to providers and localities at greatest risk; the working group should then determine funding needs for subsequent years (2.1b).

Inadequate Disaster Preparedness

On September 10, 2001, the cover story of *U.S. News and World Report* described an emergency care system in critical condition as a result of demands far in excess of its capacity. While the article focused on the day-to-day problems of diversion and boarding, the events of the following day brought home a frightening realization to many: If we cannot take care of our emergency patients on a normal day, how will we manage a large-scale disaster? More than 4 years after the terrorist attacks of 2001, Hurricane Katrina revealed how far we have is to go in this regard. While Katrina was unusual in its size and scope, the capacity of the emergency care system to respond effectively even to smaller disasters is very much in question.

Surge Capacity

Hospitals in many large cities are operating at or near full capacity. A multiple-car highway crash can create havoc in an ED. Few hospitals have the capacity to handle a major mass casualty event. One reason for this lack of capacity is the small amount of funding for bioterrorism and other emergency threats that has gone directly to hospitals. For example, hospital grants from the Health Resources and Services Administration's Bioterrorism Hospital Preparedness Program in 2002 were typically between $5,000 and $10,000—insufficient to equip even one critical care room.

Training

Training for ED workers in disaster preparedness is also deficient. In 2003, hospital training varied widely among staff: 92 percent of hospitals trained their nursing staff in responding to at least one type of threat, but residents and interns received any such training at only 49 percent of hospitals (although this represented an improvement over the situation prior to the terrorist attacks of 2001).

Protection of Hospitals and Staff

Protecting hospitals and their staff from biological or chemical events poses extraordinary challenges. The outbreak of severe acute respiratory syndrome (SARS) in Toronto in 2003 revealed the difficulties associated with containing even a small outbreak—particularly when health professionals themselves become both victims and spreaders of disease. One of the most important tools in such an event is negative pressure rooms that prevent the spread of airborne pathogens. Unfortunately, the number of such rooms is limited, and they are generally restricted to a handful of tertiary hospitals in each major population center. The committee believes that this lack of adequate negative pressure suites is a critical vulnerability of the current system, and that the existing capacity could be quickly overwhelmed by either a terrorist event or a major outbreak of avian influenza or some other airborne disease, posing an extreme danger to hospital workers and patients.

Staff must also be protected through appropriate personal protective equipment. Current training and equipment in this regard are inadequate. In 2005, the Occupational Safety and Health Administration developed guidelines for use of personal protective equipment, but more needs to be done.

Approaches to Improve Disaster Preparedness

To address the above concerns about surge capacity, training, and protection of hospitals and staff, the committee recommends that **Congress significantly increase total preparedness funding in fiscal year 2007 for hospital emergency preparedness in the following areas: strengthening and sustaining trauma care systems; enhancing emergency department, trauma center, and inpatient surge capacity; improving emergency medical services' response to explosives; designing evidence-based training programs; enhancing the availability of decontamination showers, standby intensive care unit capacity, negative pressure rooms, and appropriate personal protective equipment; and conducting international collaborative research on the civilian consequences of conventional weapons terrorism (7.3).**

In addition, to further address the need for competency in disaster medicine across disciplines, the committee recommends that **all institutions responsible for the training, continuing education, and credentialing and certification of professionals involved in emergency care (including medicine, nursing, emergency medical services, allied health, public health, and hospital administration) incorporate disaster preparedness training into their curricula and competency criteria (7.2).**

The Emergency Care Workforce

Emergency care is delivered in an inherently challenging environment, often requiring providers to make life-and-death decisions with little time and information. Emergency care providers wage battles on many fronts, including scheduling diagnostic tests; obtaining timely laboratory results and drugs; getting patients admitted to the hospital; finding specialists willing to come in during the middle of the night; and finding psychiatric centers, skilled nursing facilities, or specialists who are willing to accept referrals. ED staff often confront violence and deal with an array of social problems that confound their attempts to heal their patients. As a result, providers on the front lines of emergency care are increasingly exhausted, stressed out, and frustrated by the deteriorating state of emergency care and the safety net it supports.

On-Call Specialists

One of the most troubling trends is the increasing difficulty of finding specialists to take emergency call. Providing emergency call has become unattractive to many specialists in critical fields such as neurosurgery and orthopedics. Specialists have difficulty collecting payment for on-call services, in part because many emergency and trauma patients are uninsured; nearly 80 percent of specialists in one survey had difficulty obtaining payment for such services. Liability concerns also discourage many specialists from taking emergency call. Procedures performed on emergency patients are inherently risky and expose specialists to an increased likelihood of litigation. Patients are often sicker, and emergency procedures are frequently performed in the middle of the night or on weekends, when the hospital's staffing and capabilities are not at their peak. A national survey of neurosurgeons found that 36 percent had been sued by patients seen through the ED. These factors drive premiums for physicians who take emergency call well above those for physicians who do not. The problem has been exacerbated by recently revised guidelines under the Emergency Medical Treatment and Active Labor Act that make it easier for on-call physicians to limit their emergency practices.

Hospitals are using a number of different strategies to stabilize the services of on-call physicians. One promising approach is to regionalize the services of certain on-call specialties so that every hospital need not maintain on-call services for every specialty. Such regionalization would rationalize the limited supply of specialists by ensuring coverage at key tertiary and secondary locations based on actual need, replacing the current haphazard approach that is based on many factors other than need. For example, one county is developing a communitywide cooperative that will contract collectively for the services of certain specialists. The committee recommends that **hospitals, physician organizations, and public health agencies collaborate to regionalize critical specialty care on-call services (6.1)**.

Exposure of Emergency Providers to Medical Malpractice Claims

As noted above, physicians providing emergency and trauma care face extraordinary exposure to medical malpractice claims—far greater than those not providing such care. Safety net providers are especially affected by the liability problem: as on-call panels diminish at community hospitals, these hospitals increasingly export their sickest patients to the large safety net hospitals, which have no choice but to accept them. The result is even higher concentrations of uninsured, high-risk patients. Protections must be instituted so that emergency providers and EDs do not become the dumping ground for the liability crisis. Although the public is largely unaware of the situation, this crisis has already seriously eroded the capacity of emergency and trauma care across many cities. Therefore, the committee recommends that **Congress appoint a commission to examine the impact of medical malpractice lawsuits on the declining availability of providers in high-risk emergency and trauma care specialties, and to recommend appropriate state and federal actions to mitigate the adverse impact of these lawsuits and ensure quality of care (6.2)**.

The Rural Workforce

Rural EDs face persistent shortages of emergency and trauma physicians, as well as on-call specialists. With such shortages likely to continue, it is important to find alternative ways of enhancing emergency services in rural areas. One approach is to increase collaboration between rural hospitals and regional academic health centers to foster training, resource sharing, and coordination of care. The committee recommends that **states link rural hospitals with academic health centers to enhance opportunities for professional consultation, telemedicine, patient referral and transport, and continuing professional education (6.6)**.

Need for Emergency Care Research

Although emergency medicine and trauma surgery are relatively young specialties, researchers have made important contributions to both basic science and clinical practice that have dramatically improved emergency care and have resulted in significant advances in general medicine. Examples are assessment and management of cardiac arrest, including the development and refinement of guidelines for cardiopulmonary resuscitation (CPR), the pharmacology of resuscitation, understanding and treatment of hemorrhagic shock, and electrocardiogram (EKG) analysis of ventricular fibrillation. Because emergency care and trauma care are young fields, however, they are not strongly represented in the political infrastructure of the National Institutes of Health (NIH), its various institutes, and its study sections. As a result, scant resources are allocated to advance the science of such care, and few training grants are offered to develop researchers who want to focus on emergency care. For example, only .05 percent of NIH training grants awarded to medical schools goes to departments of emergency medicine—an average of only $51.66 per graduating resident. In contrast, internal medicine receives approximately $5,000.00 per graduating resident.

The current uncoordinated approach to organizing and funding emergency and trauma care has been inadequate. There are well-defined emergency and trauma care research questions that would benefit from a coordinated and well-funded research strategy. Therefore, the committee recommends that **the Secretary of the Department of Health and Human Services conduct a study to examine the gaps and opportunities in emergency and trauma care research, and recommend a strategy for the optimal organization and funding of the research effort (8.2).**

> This study should include consideration of training of new investigators, development of multicenter research networks, funding of General Clinical Research Centers that specifically include an emergency and trauma care component, involvement of emergency and trauma care researchers in the grant review and research advisory processes, and improved research coordination through a dedicated center or institute (8.2a).

> Congress and federal agencies involved in emergency and trauma care research (including the Department of Transportation, the Department of Health and Human Services, the Department of Homeland Security, and the Department of Defense) should implement the study's recommendations (8.2b).

ACHIEVING THE VISION OF A 21ST-CENTURY EMERGENCY CARE SYSTEM

Hospital-based emergency and trauma care is part of an interdependent system of emergency services; thus optimizing such care requires improvements in both hospital-based care and the larger system. To that end, the committee developed a vision for the future of emergency care that centers around three goals: coordination, regionalization, and accountability. Many elements of this vision have been advocated previously; however, progress toward achieving these elements has been derailed by deeply entrenched parochial interests and cultural attitudes, as well as funding cutbacks and practical impediments to change. Concerted, cooperative efforts at all levels of government—federal, state, regional, local—and the private sector are necessary to finally break through and achieve this vision.

Coordination

One of the most long-standing problems with the emergency care system is that services are fragmented. Prehospital emergency medical services (EMS), hospitals, trauma centers, and public health have traditionally worked in silos. For example, public safety and EMS agencies often lack common radio frequencies and protocols for communicating with each other during emergencies. Similarly, emergency care providers lack access to patient medical histories that could be useful in decision making.

Ensuring that each patient is directed to the most appropriate setting, including a level I trauma center when necessary, requires that many elements within the regional system—community hospitals, trauma centers, and particularly prehospital EMS—coordinate the regional flow of patients effectively. In addition to improving patient care, coordinating the regional flow of patients is a critical tool in reducing overcrowding in EDs.

Unfortunately, only a handful of systems around the country coordinate transport effectively at the regional level. Short of formally instituting diversion, there is typically little information sharing between hospitals and EMS regarding overloaded EDs and trauma centers and the availability of ED beds, operating suites, equipment, trauma surgeons, and critical specialists—information that could be used to balance the load among EDs and trauma centers regionwide. Too often a hospital's location places it in a logistical situation in which it is overloaded with emergencies and trauma cases while an ED several blocks away may be working at a comfortable 50 percent capacity. There is little incentive for ambulances to drive by a hospital to take patients to a facility that is less crowded.

The benefits to patients of better regional coordination have been demonstrated. The technologies needed to facilitate such coordination exist, and police and fire departments are ahead in this regard. The main impediment appears to be entrenched interests and a lack of vision to motivate change in the current system.

The committee envisions a system in which all patients receive well-planned and coordinated emergency care services. Dispatch, EMS, ED providers, public safety, and public health should be fully interconnected and united in an effort to ensure that each patient receives the most appropriate care, at the optimal location, with the minimum delay. From the standpoint of patients, delivery of emergency care services should be seamless.

Regionalization

Because not all hospitals within a community have the personnel and resources to support the delivery of high-level emergency care, critically ill and injured patients should be directed specifically to those facilities with such capabilities. That is the goal of regionalization. There is substantial evidence that the use of regionalization of services to direct such patients to designated hospitals with greater experience and resources improves outcomes and reduces costs across a range of high-risk conditions and procedures. Thus the committee supports further regionalization of emergency care services. However, use of this approach requires that prehospital providers, as well as patients and caregivers, be clear on which facilities have the necessary resources. Just as trauma centers are categorized according to their capabilities (i.e., level I–level IV/V), a standard national approach to the categorization of EDs that reflects their capabilities is needed so the categories will be clearly understood by providers and the public across all states and regions of the country. To that end, the committee recommends that **the Department of Health and Human Services and the National Highway Traffic Safety Administration, in partnership with professional organizations, convene a panel of individuals with multidisciplinary expertise to develop an evidence-based categorization system for emergency medical services, emergency departments, and trauma centers based on adult and pediatric service capabilities (3.1).**

This information, in turn, could be used to develop protocols that would guide EMS providers in the transport of patients and improve the regional coordination of patient flow. These protocols should be based on current and emerging evidence about the appropriate models for transport given the patient's condition and location, and should include protocols that, given appropriate information about the status of facilities, direct patients to less crowded local EDs rather than to the highest-level center. Therefore, the committee also recommends that **the National Highway Traffic Safety Administration, in partnership with professional organizations, convene a panel of individuals with multidisciplinary expertise to develop evidence-based model prehospital care protocols for the treatment, triage, and transport of patients (3.2).**

Accountability

Without accountability, participants in the emergency care system need not accept responsibility for failures and can avoid making changes to improve the delivery of care. Accountability has failed to take hold in emergency care to date because responsibility is dispersed across many different components of the system, so it is difficult even for policy makers to determine where system breakdowns occur and how they can subsequently be addressed.

To build accountability into the system, the committee recommends that **the Department of Health and Human Services convene a panel of individuals with emergency and trauma care expertise to develop evidence-based indicators of emergency and trauma care system performance (3.3).** Because of the need for an independent, national process with the broad participation of every component of emergency care, the federal government should play a lead role in promoting and funding the development of these performance indicators. The indicators developed should include structure and process measures, but evolve toward outcome measures over time. These performance measures should be nationally standardized so that statewide and national comparisons can be made. Measures should evaluate the performance of individual providers within the system, as well as that of the system as a whole. Measures should also be sensitive to the interdependence among the components of the system; for example, EMS response times may be related to EDs going on diversion.

Using the measures developed through such a national, evidence-based, multidisciplinary effort, performance data should be collected at regular intervals from all hospitals and EMS agencies in a community. Public dissemination of performance data is crucial to driving the needed changes in the delivery of emergency care services. Dissemination could take various forms, including public report cards, annual reports, and state public health reports. Because of the potential sensitivity of performance data, the data should initially be reported in the aggregate rather than at the level of the individual provider. Individual providers should have full access to their own data so they can understand and improve their performance, as well as contribute to the overall system. Over time, individual provider information should become an important part of the public information on the system. These performance measures should ultimately become the basis for pay-for-performance initiatives as those reimbursement techniques mature.

Achieving the Vision

States and regions face a variety of different situations, including the level of development of trauma systems; the effectiveness of state EMS offices and regional EMS councils; and the degree of coordination among fire departments, EMS, hospitals, trauma centers, and emergency management. Thus no single approach to enhancing emergency care systems will achieve the goals outlined above. A number of different avenues should be explored and evaluated to determine what types of systems are best able to achieve the three goals. The committee therefore recommends that **Congress establish a demonstration program, administered by the Health Resources** and Services Administration, to promote coordinated, regionalized, and accountable emergency care systems throughout the country, and appropriate $88 million over 5 years to this program (3.5). Grants should be targeted at states, which could develop projects at the state, regional, or local level; cross-state collaborative proposals would also be encouraged. Over time, and over a number of controlled initiatives, such a process should lead to important insights about what strategies work under different conditions. These insights would provide best-practice models that could be widely adopted to advance the nation toward the committee's vision for efficient, high-quality emergency and trauma care.

Supporting System Integration

Reducing fragmentation at the state and local levels will require federal leadership and support. Today, however, the federal agencies that support and regulate emergency services mirror the fragmentation of emergency services at the state and local levels. Prehospital EMS, hospital-based emergency care, trauma care, injury prevention and control, and medical disaster preparedness are scattered across numerous agencies within the Department of Health and Human Services, the U.S. Department of Transportation, and the Department of Homeland Security.

Strong federal leadership for emergency and trauma care is at the heart of the committee's vision for the future, and continued fragmentation of responsibility at the federal level is unacceptable. A lead federal agency could better move the emergency and trauma care system toward improved integration; unify decision making, including funding decisions; and represent all emergency and trauma care patients, providers, and settings, including prehospital EMS (both ground and air), hospital-based emergency and trauma care, pediatric emergency and trauma care, rural emergency and trauma care, and medical disaster preparedness. The committee therefore recommends that **Congress establish a lead agency for emergency and trauma care within 2 years of this report. The lead agency should be housed in the Department of Health and Human Services, and should have primary programmatic responsibility for the full continuum of emergency medical services and emergency and trauma care for adults and children, including medical 9-1-1 and emergency medical dispatch, prehospital emergency medical services (both ground and air), hospital-based emergency and trauma care, and medical-related disaster preparedness. Congress should establish a working group to make recommendations regarding the structure, funding, and responsibilities of the new agency, and develop and monitor the transition. The working group should have representation from federal and state agencies and professional disciplines involved in emergency and trauma care (3.6).**

1

Introduction

Memorial Hospital Emergency Department
Tuesday, 3:00 PM

Memorial Hospital, a large, urban medical center and level I trauma center, has an emergency department (ED) designed to hold 40 acute patients. It is operating well over capacity, with more than 80 patients actively undergoing care, 30 of whom lie on wheeled stretchers in hallways. Of these 80 patients, 24 are waiting to be admitted to inpatient beds; 4 have been waiting 7–10 hours, 1 for 20 hours, and 1 for over 24 hours. The hospital has been on EMS diversion for 5 hours, but with other nearby hospitals also on diversion, it is still receiving a steady stream of patients. Doctors and nurses used to the high stress of emergency care are maintaining relative order, although they have been operating at full tilt for most of the shift. The risk of errors from fatigue, stress, and hurry grows steadily higher. An EMS crew that has been waiting to offload a patient into the busy ED for more than 35 minutes stands by impatiently. The waiting room is crowded with more than 50 people—34 patients, family, and friends—including children, adults, and elderly. Some are in pain, at least one is bleeding, while others appear to have cold or flu symptoms.

A call from the dispatch center notifies the ED that five patients will soon arrive from a car crash on the nearby interstate, with injuries of varying severity. One is coming by helicopter, and the trauma team is mobilized. The ED director does her best to clear additional space in the ED. More nursing staff are requested, but none are available; the evening supervisor has been trying to call in personnel for the past 4 hours. The level of activity in the ED is growing visibly, and the amount of attention being provided to each patient is minimal. Several patients in the waiting room give up and leave before being seen by a physician, and two patients who are undergoing treatment in the ED sign out against the medical advice of staff.

To make matters worse, a nearby hospital requests transfer of a complex neurological and orthopedic case to Memorial. The patient is stable, but his condition may deteriorate without immediate intervention. Memorial is normally well equipped to handle such patients, but the neurological and orthopedic specialists on call to the hospital are already busy with other cases in the operating room.

As the night wears on, the volume of patients gradually declines. Although the ED has been pushed to the limit at times, a meltdown has been averted by the efforts of the staff. Nonetheless, despite the best efforts of the emergency care professionals—from emergency medical technicians to emergency doctors and nurses and on-call specialists—the quality of health care delivered by the emergency care system on this night was less than it could and should have been.

Hospital-based emergency and trauma care is critically important to the health and well-being of Americans. In 2003, nearly 114 million visits were made to hospital EDs, more than one for every three people in the United States. About one-quarter of those visits were due to unintentional injuries, the leading cause of death for people aged 1 through 44; indeed, traumatic injury has surpassed heart disease as the most expensive category of medical treatment, resulting in $71.6 billion dollars in expenditures per year (AHRQ, 2006). While most Americans encounter the ED only rarely, they count on it to be there when they need it.

Over the last several decades, the role of hospital-based emergency and trauma care has evolved substantially. EDs continue to focus on their traditional mission of providing urgent and lifesaving care, but have taken on additional responsibilities to meet the needs of communities, providers, and patients. EDs have become a key component of the health care safety net, providing a considerable volume of care to uninsured patients and Medicaid beneficiaries who often cannot access health services elsewhere. EDs are also an important public health partner, responsible for alerting public health agencies to possible threats in the community and sometimes counseling patients on prevention or self-care. Moreover, EDs play a central role in preparing their communities for disasters, and have become an important adjunct to community physicians' practices. While the demands on emergency and trauma care have grown dramatically, however, the capacity of the system has not kept pace. Balancing these roles in the face of increasing patient volume and limited resources has become increasingly challenging.

A GROWING NATIONAL CRISIS

Hospital EDs have become frequently crowded environments, with patients sometimes lining hallways and waiting hours and even days to be admitted to inpatient beds (Asplin et al., 2003). Ambulance diversion, once rare, is now a common if not daily event in many major cities, and can lead to catastrophic consequences for patients (GAO, 2001; Schafermeyer and Asplin, 2003). Specialists needed to treat emergency and trauma patients are increasingly difficult to find; the result is longer waits and at times, distant transport of critically ill or injured patients for specialty care. The emergency system itself appears to be crumbling in major cities. In Los Angeles, for example, 8 hospital EDs have closed since 2003, bringing the total closed countywide to over 60 in the last decade (see Box 1-1) (Robes, 2005).

These trends are symptomatic of a growing national crisis in emergency care. This crisis is multifaceted and impacts every aspect of emergency care—from prehospital EMS to hospital-based emergency and trauma care. Of the many challenges confronting hospital-based emergency and trauma care today, the following stand out for their complexity, gravity, and urgency:

• **Demand outpacing capacity**—Between 1993 and 2003, ED visits increased from 90.3 to 113.9 million, a 26 percent increase. During this same period, the United States experienced a net loss of 425 hospital EDs. The problem of excess demand is exacerbated by the above-noted role of the ED as one of the nation's principal sources of care for patients with limited access to other providers, including the 45 million uninsured Americans. The result of this growing imbalance between demand and capacity is a nationwide epidemic of ED overcrowding, boarding, and ambulance diversion.
• **ED crowding**—Crowding is the most obvious manifestation of the imbalance between ED demand and capacity. It occurs when patient volume backs up in the ED: many patients come in the front door, but not enough can be admitted to the hospital in a timely manner to make room for more incoming patients. As admitted patients back up in the ED, crowding be-

BOX 1-1
Meltdown of Emergency Care:
Emergency Department Closures in Los Angeles County

Los Angeles (L.A.) County, the largest county in the nation, is home to more than 10 million people (L.A. County Online, 2005). It also leads the nation in shuttered EDs. Between 1980 and 2000, 20 percent of the county's EDs closed (Sussman, 2000); since 2003, eight more hospital EDs and one trauma center have closed. At the same time, the number of patients seeking care at EDs has soared, so the facilities that remain are being forced to absorb an overwhelmingly large patient load. These hospitals are in an increasingly tenuous financial position (Robes, 2005).

While some ED closures may be justified by the changing needs of communities, the ED closures in L.A. County have led to serious consequences for patient care. The demand for emergency care at the EDs that remain is so high that waiting times can reach 8 to 12 hours (South Bay's ERs are in a State of Emergency, 2005). Additionally, L.A. County hospitals went on diversion an average of 23 percent of the time in 2004, meaning they closed their doors to patients arriving by ambulance almost one-quarter of the time. Paramedics in L.A. County report that the closure of EDs, coupled with frequent ED diversion, is forcing them to drive farther and farther to find a hospital that is able to care for a sick or injured patient. Longer transport times translate into delays in patients' receiving definitive care. But even once paramedics arrive at an open ED with a patient, one in eight trips involves an additional delay (Hymon, 2003). Because EDs are so crowded with patients, paramedics often must wait hours for the transported patient to be admitted to the ED. While the paramedics wait with the transported patient, they are unable to respond to other emergency calls.

comes severe. ED overcrowding blocks access to emergency care, induces stress in providers and patients alike, and can lead to errors and impaired quality of care.

- **Boarding**—A consequence of crowded EDs is the practice of boarding—holding a patient who needs to be admitted in the ED until an inpatient bed becomes available. In a nationwide survey of nearly 90 EDs across the country, conducted on a typical Monday evening, 73 percent of hospitals reported boarding two or more admitted patients. Boarding not only is frustrating and at times hazardous for the patient, but also adds to an already stressful work environment for physicians and nurses and enhances the potential for errors, delays in treatment, and diminished quality of care.
- **Ambulance diversion**—When EDs become saturated to the point that

Even the most severely injured patients are affected by problems within the system. The L.A. Fire Department, which oversees EMS, has a departmentwide mandate that requires a maximum transport time of 30 minutes for trauma patients. However, it is difficult for paramedics to find an open trauma center within a 30-minute radius, so at times they deliver patients to non–trauma centers (regular EDs that are less well equipped to handle serious injuries). These types of situations occur almost every weekend in L.A. (California Healthline, 2004).

The closure of L.A. County EDs and trauma centers can be attributed to financial pressures on hospitals, due particularly to the large volume of care they provide to uninsured patients. In fact, one in three ED patients in L.A. County is uninsured (Felch, 2004). Historically, about two-thirds of uninsured patients were served by the four county-run hospitals, while private hospitals cared for the remaining third. In 2003, however, because of cost concerns, the county changed its policies to limit the ability of private hospitals to transfer patients to the county hospitals. In the 14 months following the policy change, the number of uninsured doubled at some private hospitals and tripled at others (Felch, 2004).

In 2002, L.A. County voters overwhelmingly approved (73 to 27 percent) a modest tax on building improvements to fund emergency services, trauma care, and bioterrorism preparedness efforts countywide. This was the first voter-approved increase in the property tax since the 1970s. The measure passed after a $1.5 million media campaign that warned voters of a system collapse unless the tax was approved. Advertisements for the measure showing feverish paramedics driving around the city looking for a hospital with available beds struck a cord with voters (L.A. County Online, 2005). The measure, although a step in the right direction, has been described as "a $170-million answer to a $700 million problem" (Trauma Tax Falls Short, 2004). More ED closures are expected in the county.

patient safety is compromised, inbound ambulances may be diverted to alternative hospitals. Once a safety valve to be used in extreme situations, ambulance diversion has now become a commonplace event. A recent federal study reported that 501,000 ambulances were diverted in 2003, an average of 1 per minute. According to the American Hospital Association, nearly half of all hospitals, and close to 70 percent of urban hospitals, reported time on diversion in 2004. Ambulance diversions can lead to catastrophic delays in treatment for seriously ill or injured patients.

• Uncompensated care—Hospital EDs are required by federal law to provide emergency care to all in need without regard for the patient's ability to pay. No federal funding is allocated to offset the costs of this care. Uncompensated emergency and trauma care services can impose an extreme financial burden on hospitals that see large numbers of uninsured patients. Substantial financial losses and ED and trauma center closures have been attributed to uncompensated emergency and trauma care.

• **Inefficient use of resources**—Innovations in industrial engineering that have swept through other sectors of the economy, from banking to airlines to manufacturing, have failed to take hold in health care delivery. Tools and information technologies adapted from other industries could be used effectively to address the bottlenecks that occur in the flow of patients throughout the hospital and result in ED crowding. But hospitals have been slow to adopt these measures.

• **Inadequate surge capacity**—Many hospitals are already operating at or over capacity. Because major hospital EDs are already crowded with patients and may even be boarding large numbers of inpatients, there is little or no surge capacity to absorb a large influx of patients from a significant mass casualty event. Furthermore, supplies of specialized equipment, such as personal protective equipment, negative pressure rooms, and ventilators, are inadequate to meet the demands of a major disaster or an epidemic.

• **Inadequate protection for staff**—Hospital workers confront a host of daily hazards, from bloodborne and airborne pathogens to violent patients. Inadequate steps have been taken to protect hospital assets and staff in routine situations, let alone in the event of an infectious disease outbreak or a chemical or biological attack.

• **Inadequate supply of on-call specialists**—One of the most troubling aspects of the current emergency and trauma care system is the lack of available specialists to provide on-call services to hospital EDs and trauma centers. This is particularly true for highly skilled specialties such as neurosurgery, interventional cardiology, and orthopedic surgery.

• **Medical liability**—Emergency and trauma care providers, including hospitals, emergency and trauma physicians, and on-call specialists, face extraordinary liability exposure, leading many to limit the scope of their practice or stop assuming ED call.

• **Fragmented systems**—Emergency care systems are highly fragmented. Emergency medical services (EMS) agencies, hospitals, trauma centers, public safety services (e.g., police and fire), and public health agencies often lack effective communications and fail to coordinate well across the continuum of emergency care. Coordinating the regional flow of patients is critical to ensuring that each patient is directed to the most appropriate setting for care, yet few systems nationwide have effective coordination between EMS and hospital EDs and trauma centers.

• **Lack of performance measurement and accountability**—There is no standardized measurement or reporting of the performance of emergency and trauma care providers and systems. As a result, few people have any real understanding of the quality of care they can expect to receive from their local emergency providers.

• **Inadequate research funding and infrastructure**—Because emergency care is a relatively young field, it lacks a strong and stable research base within the National Institutes of Health and other agencies. Despite the importance of emergency and trauma care, research funding in the field lags well behind that in other fields.

IMPACT ON QUALITY AND PATIENT SAFETY

Quality and safety have been driving concerns of emergency care leaders for decades, and notable achievements in quality have been made. Improved care of patients with acute myocardial infarction, stroke, pneumonia, and sepsis are notable examples (Barron et al., 1999; Adams et al., 2002; Dellinger et al., 2004). Nonetheless, the numerous problems identified in this chapter have an impact on the quality and safety of the care provided by the system. The depth of this impact is difficult to determine. One way to assess the overall quality of the emergency care system is to consider the six quality aims defined by the Institute of Medicine (IOM) in *Crossing the Quality Chasm: A New Health System for the 21st Century* (IOM, 2001): care should be safe, effective, patient-centered, timely, efficient, and equitable (see Box 1-2). While the evidence base is limited, there are strong indications that the current emergency care system fails the American public in significant ways.

Safe

EDs are often high-risk, high-stress environments fraught with opportunities for error (Leape et al., 1991; Chisholm et al., 2000; Goldberg et al., 2002; Cosby, 2003; Weiss et al., 2004; Chamberlain et al., 2004; Selbst et al., 2004). A landmark study of hospitalized patients found that although the ED was the site of only 3 percent of adverse events, it was the site of 70 percent of those events attributed to negligence (Leape et al., 1991). Additional studies looking at hospital admissions and malpractice claims have also found the ED to be the site of a significant number of errors resulting in adverse events (Thomas et al., 2000). Two of the most common types of errors in the ED are failure to diagnose a patient properly (Leape et al., 1991; Weingart et al., 2000; Cosby, 2003; Thomas et al., 2004; White et al., 2004) and medication errors (IOM, 2006; Leape et al., 1991).

Errors in the ED are caused by multiple factors. ED staff are frequently interrupted in the course of their duties to attend to other patients or issues (Chisholm et al., 2001); are required to see a broad case mix of patients;

BOX 1-2
The Six Quality Aims of the Institute of Medicine's
***Quality Chasm* Report**

Health care should be:

Safe—avoiding injuries to patients from the care that is intended to help them.

Effective—providing services based on scientific knowledge to all who could benefit and refraining from providing services to those not likely to benefit.

Patient-centered—providing care that is respectful of and responsive to individual patient preferences, needs, and values and ensuring that patient values guide all clinical decisions.

Timely—reducing waits and sometimes harmful delays for both those who receive and those who give care.

Efficient—avoiding waste, including waste of equipment, supplies, ideas, and energy.

Equitable—providing care that does not vary in quality because of personal characteristics such as gender, ethnicity, geographic location, and socioeconomic status.

SOURCE: IOM, 2001, Pp. 5–6.

---

and must often make rapid clinical decisions, frequently without the benefit of medical histories or diagnostic tests (Selbst et al., 2004). Failures of communication or teamwork are significant problems in the ED, and in some cases have been shown to be direct contributors to adverse medical outcomes (Risser et al., 1999; White et al., 2004). The routine distractions of an ED are dramatically compounded when conditions are crowded. Problems include patients boarded in hallways for long periods; long waiting times; patients who decide to leave without being seen; others who demand to sign out against medical advice; and delays in diagnostic imaging, laboratory results, drug administration, and consultative support by on-call specialists.

Effective

In contrast to the surprisingly limited evidence base for a number of clinical practices that are widely used in the prehospital arena, hospital-based emergency care is substantially evidence based. In major tertiary hospitals, emergency and trauma care brings together the best of American medicine—highly trained, interdisciplinary teams of dedicated specialists armed with advanced medical technology. Beyond these large tertiary centers, however, the effectiveness of the system is less certain. Many community hospitals, especially in rural areas, do not have board-certified emergency physicians on staff. Many lack key specialists to back up their ED physicians. Furthermore, as discussed earlier, hospital EDs are often required to provide an enormous amount of primary care that would likely be provided better in other settings. Because ED physicians may not have access to the patient's medical record, they cannot easily address primary care issues that go beyond the patient's chief complaint. They have little or no opportunity for follow-up contact with patients, chronic care management, assurance of patient adherence to treatment, and coordination of care across providers and patient care settings.

Patient-Centered

EDs are designed to maximize visibility rather than to preserve patient privacy. At best they can hardly be considered patient-centered. A crowded ED, with its packed waiting rooms, long waiting times, and patients boarding in hallways, is even less so. Physicians and nurses find it nearly impossible to have a private conversation with a patient in such conditions. Injured or highly contagious patients may be placed in close proximity to children and individuals with only minor health problems who are using the ED for primary care.

Hospitals have begun to address these issues in a variety of ways. Some have established fast-track areas to deal with patients who are not truly emergency cases. Hospitals have also set up specialized areas, such as psychiatric and pediatric EDs within or adjacent to the main ED. Other approaches to making ED care more patient-centered include using bedside registration rather than making patients register first; sending physicians to the waiting room to see patients with simple problems, thus averting the need for long waits for an ED exam room; expediting inpatient admissions to clear crowded ED hallways; and treating pain more aggressively.

Timely

EDs are designed to provide timely care for unscheduled emergencies; nevertheless, timeliness of care in the ED is a growing concern. As noted, many patients experience long wait times before being seen, especially if they have a problem that is not immediately life-threatening, and the boarding of admitted patients who are waiting for an available inpatient bed has become commonplace. Long ED wait times can result in protracted pain and suffering and delays in diagnosis and treatment (Derlet et al., 2001; Derlet, 2002; James et al., 2005), and can lead some patients to leave without being seen

(Quinn et al., 2003) or to sign out against medical advice. Cognizant of these problems, ED staff and hospital administrators are attempting a variety of strategies to address them. Nevertheless, the problems persist.

Efficient

The health sector in general and emergency and trauma care services in particular lag behind other industries in adopting engineering principles and information technologies that can improve process management, lower costs, and enhance quality. Although EDs are quite efficient in some respects (they have diagnostic testing readily available and can complete in hours an in-depth evaluation that might otherwise require several days), they are highly dependent on hospital operations for efficient operation. When a hospital is full or its ancillary services are slow, ED crowding, inpatient boarding, and ambulance diversion are almost inevitable. These are system failures that could be addressed through better overall management of hospital operations. There are other dimensions of inefficiency in emergency care as well. For example, the increasing amount of primary care delivered in EDs has important cost and quality implications, and may detract from the ED's primary mission of providing emergency and lifesaving care. Further, the high degree of liability exposure in emergency and trauma care can lead to defensive medicine—the use of diagnostic tests and treatment measures primarily for the purpose of averting malpractice lawsuits (Lawthers et al., 1992; Berenson et al., 2003; Katz et al., 2005; Studdert et al., 2005).

Equitable

Disparities in the health care received by Americans on the basis of race and ethnicity were thoroughly documented in the IOM report *Unequal Treatment: Confronting Racial and Ethnic Disparities in Health Care* (IOM, 2003). Results of a small number of studies suggest that disparities may exist in access to emergency care and the treatment received. For example, there is evidence of variability in treatment, wait times, and insurance authorizations based on patients' race and ethnicity (Lowe and Bindman, 1994; Todd et al., 2000; Bazarian et al., 2003; Richardson et al., 2003; James et al., 2005), although other researchers have reported that for a given level of severity of illness, the decision to admit an ED patient to the hospital does not appear to be influenced by the patient's race, ethnicity, or payer status (Kellermann and Haley, 2003; Oster and Bindman, 2003). ED crowding, patient boarding, and ambulance diversion tend to be associated with large, urban medical centers, and thus have a disproportionate effect on racial and ethnic minorities that tend to dwell in the inner cities. Nonetheless, emergency care is arguably one of the more equitable settings in medicine, largely because of the Emergency Medical Treatment and Active Labor Act, which has created a broad mandate to serve all, regardless of ability to pay.

PURPOSE OF THIS STUDY

While the problems discussed in this report are not new, they have largely been overlooked until now. Within the last several years, the complex problems facing the emergency care system have erupted into public view. Negative stories have increasingly appeared in the media regarding slow EMS response, ambulance diversions, trauma center closures, the medical malpractice crisis, ground and air crashes occurring during patient transport, and the frequent lack of on-call specialist coverage. The events of September 11, 2001, and more recent disasters, such as the train bombings in Madrid and Hurricane Katrina, have sharpened the public's awareness of these issues.

The sponsors of this study—the Health Resources and Services Administration (HRSA), Emergency Medical Services for Children (EMS-C) program; the National Highway Traffic Safety Administration; the Agency for Healthcare Research and Quality; the Centers for Disease Control and Prevention, Center for Injury Prevention and Control; and the Josiah Macy, Jr. Foundation—requested that the IOM undertake a study aimed at assessing the current emergency care system, identifying its strengths and weaknesses, developing a comprehensive vision for the future of emergency care, and providing a blueprint for achieving that vision. The study was designed to encompass all of the key components of emergency care—prehospital EMS, hospital-based emergency care, trauma care, and injury prevention and control—in an integrated effort. The complete statement of task for the study committee is shown in Box 1-3.

This study builds on a large body of previous work, some conducted by the National Academies and some by other organizations. The landmark report *Accidental Death and Disability: The Neglected Disease of Modern Society* (NAS and NRC, 1966) first focused attention on the inadequacy of emergency and trauma care in the United States. This was followed by *Injury in America: A Continuing Public Health Problem* (NRC and IOM, 1985), which called for expanded research into the epidemiology and treatment of injury, and *Reducing the Burden of Injury* (IOM, 1999), which called for the development of a broad program for injury research, prevention, and control. The report *Emergency Medical Services for Children* (IOM, 1993) described the limited capacity of the developing emergency care system to address the special needs of children, and called for strong state and federal support for enhancements to emergency care education and training, infrastructure, research, and funding targeting the needs of children.

Other reports have touched on important specific aspects of emergency

---

BOX 1-3
Statement of Task for This Study

The objectives of this study are to: (1) examine the emergency care system in the United States; (2) explore its strengths, limitations, and future challenges; (3) describe a desired vision of the emergency care system; and (4) recommend strategies required to achieve that vision. In this context, the Subcommittee on Hospital-Based Emergency Care will identify and address a wide range of issues, including:

• the role and impact of the emergency department within the larger hospital and health care system;
• the interaction between the emergency department and inpatient and ancillary services, such as lab, pharmacy, and imaging;
• patient flow and information technology;
• workforce issues across multiple disciplines, including emergency physicians, nurses, and other members of the care team;
• the impact of technological innovations on emergency care;
• patient safety and the quality and efficiency of emergency care services;
• the legal and regulatory framework for emergency care, including the Emergency Medical Treatment and Active Labor Act (EMTALA), liability issues, and reimbursement; disaster preparedness, surge capacity, and surveillance;
• basic, clinical, and health services research relevant to emergency care; and
• special challenges of emergency care in rural settings.

---

care. A report of the Josiah Macy, Jr. Foundation, *The Role of Emergency Medicine in the Future of American Medical Care* (Josiah Macy, Jr. Foundation, 1995) examined the young specialty of emergency medicine and explored a vision for the future development of emergency medical practice, research, and care delivery. The IOM report *A Shared Destiny: Community Effects of Uninsurance* described the importance of the emergency care system to the national public health safety net and the enormous burden placed on hospitals by the growing uninsured population (IOM, 2004). *To Err Is Human: Building a Safer Health System* (IOM, 2000) and *Crossing the Quality Chasm: A New Health System for the 21st Century* (IOM, 2001) drew attention to the critical quality problems in health care, to which emergency care contributes significantly, and provided an important framework for assessing the performance of the emergency care system—the six quality aims reviewed above. *Building a Better Delivery System: A New*

Engineering/Health Care Partnership identified engineering and operations management tools from other industries that could be adapted to health care settings, assessed barriers to their adoption, and highlighted research opportunities for engineering applications to improve the health care delivery system (IOM, 2005).

In addition, a series of *Emergency Medical Services Agenda for the Future* reports sponsored by major federal agencies has addressed key issues. The original *Emergency Medical Services Agenda for the Future* (NHTSA, 1996), published in 1996, described a vision for an integrated emergency care system of the future, while a companion report, *Emergency Medical Services Agenda for the Future: Implementation Guide* (NHTSA, 1998) outlined specific steps for achieving that vision. Detailed assessments were then provided in *Emergency Medical Services Education Agenda for the Future: A Systems Approach* (NHTSA, 2000), *National EMS Research Agenda* (NHTSA, 2001a), *Rural and Frontier Emergency Medical Services Agenda for the Future* (NHTSA, 2003), *Trauma System Agenda for the Future* (NHTSA, 2001b), and *CDC Acute Injury Care Research Agenda: Guiding Research for the Future* (CDC National Center for Injury Control and Prevention, 2005).

As important as these preceding efforts have been, progress in implementing needed reforms has been slow, and much work remains to be done. Deeply entrenched parochial interests have impeded progress, and today the field is as fragmented as ever. Accountability remains dispersed, and there is little public understanding of either the importance or the profound limitations of emergency and trauma care.

STUDY SCOPE

The scope of this study is broad, like the field of emergency care itself. It encompasses the full range of activities associated with emergency care, including first aid and cardiopulmonary resuscitation (CPR) rendered by bystanders; 9-1-1 and dispatch; emergency medical response and treatment at the scene; transport of patients via ambulance or air medical service; emergency assessment and treatment at the hospital ED or trauma center; critical care services in the operating room, the intensive care unit, or other inpatient departments; interfacility transport of patients; treatment in specialized facilities such as burn, stroke, and cardiac centers, as well as children's hospitals; and access to follow-up in community-based referral sites, such as primary care practices, skilled nursing facilities, psychiatric hospitals, and substance abuse clinics.

Emergency care is unique in the health field because it operates at the intersection of medical care, public health, and public safety. Consequently, the study views emergency care from all three perspectives. In addition to exploring the traditional role of the emergency care system as provider of urgent and lifesaving care, the study considers the system's roles in public health—including surveillance to detect injury trends and disease outbreaks—and as a critical component of the public safety net. Also addressed are the multiple interactions between emergency care and community providers: urgent care that can substitute for ED services, use of the emergency care system as an adjunct to physician practices, and the role of preventive services and chronic care management that can reduce the need for emergency services. The study further considers emergency care's public safety role and its intersection with police, fire, and emergency management services. Finally, emergency care is examined within a systems framework: how the many components of the system, such as EDs, EMS, community providers, and on-call specialists, work together—or frequently fail to work together—to achieve a level of performance for the system as a whole.

STUDY APPROACH

The committee was structured to balance the desire for an integrated, systems approach to the study with an interest in placing focused attention on hospital-based, EMS, and pediatric emergency care issues. The result was a main committee and three subcommittees representing the latter three focus areas (see Figure 1-1).

The main committee guided the overall study process and separately addressed a set of overarching systemwide issues. The three subcommittees examined the unique challenges associated with hospital-based emergency and trauma care, prehospital EMS, and the provision of emergency services to children. The membership of the main committee and subcommittees overlapped—the 11-member pediatric subcommittee, for example, included

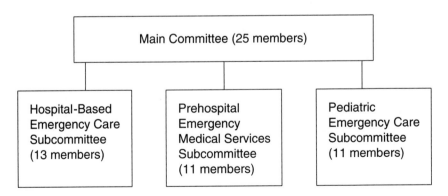

FIGURE 1-1 Committee and subcommittee structure.

5 members from the main committee. Subcommittees met both separately—reporting their discussions and findings to the main committee—and in a combined session with the main committee. A total of 40 individuals[1] served across all four committees (see Appendix A). Biographical information on each committee member is contained in Appendix B.

The committee and subcommittees held 17 meetings from February 2004 through October 2005, heard testimony from a wide range of experts (see Appendix C), and commissioned 11 technical papers (see Appendix D). Staff and committee members met with a variety of stakeholders and interested individuals, conducted study visits, and participated in public meetings sponsored by stakeholder groups and the study sponsors.

A NOTE ABOUT TERMINOLOGY

There is substantial confusion about terminology in emergency care. To ensure clarity and consistency, this study uses the following terminology throughout. *Emergency medical services*, or EMS, denotes prehospital emergency medical services, such as 9-1-1 and dispatch, emergency medical response, field triage and stabilization, and transport by ambulance or helicopter to a hospital and between facilities. *EMS system* refers to the organized delivery system for EMS within a specified geographic area—local, regional, state, or national—as indicated by the context.

Emergency care is defined more broadly than EMS and encompasses the full continuum of services involved in emergency medical care, including EMS, hospital-based emergency and trauma care, on-call specialty care, bystander care, and injury prevention and control. *Emergency care system* refers to the organized delivery system for emergency care within a specified geographic area. It is important to note that the committee's definitions of emergency care and emergency care system may be narrower than other definitions, such as those used by the federal Emergency Medical Services for Children program, which also encompass injury prevention and rehabilitation services.

Trauma care is the care received by a victim of trauma in any setting, while a *trauma center* is a hospital specifically designated to provide trauma care. Some trauma care is provided in settings other than a trauma center. *Trauma system* refers to the organized delivery system for trauma care at the local, regional, state, or national level. Trauma care is an essential component of emergency care. *Primary care* and *ambulatory care* are often mentioned in the context of the expanding role of the ED. Such care is usually described as the first point of care for patients except in emergencies.

---

[1]One committee member resigned from the original 41-member body during the course of the study.

It is typically office- or clinic-based medical care that includes diagnosis, treatment, prevention, and ongoing care management, and can include the establishment of patient–physician relationships and continuity of care over time. Ambulatory care is all care that is provided outside the hospital. Primary care is a subset of ambulatory care; however, the two are used somewhat interchangeably throughout the report to indicate the type of care that is typically given outside of the hospital but is increasingly being delivered in EDs.

For the purposes of this report, the terms *children* and *pediatric* denote infants, children, and adolescents through age 18. To avoid confusion, the terms *emergency medical services for children* and *EMS-C* denote the HRSA program itself.

ORGANIZATION OF THE REPORT

This report—one of a series of three—summarizes the committee's findings and recommendations regarding hospital-based emergency care:

- Chapter 2 describes the evolution of emergency and trauma care and the multiple roles currently served by the emergency care system—from care for those in urgent need to primary care for the uninsured, public health surveillance, and preparation for disasters.
- Chapter 3 defines the committee's broad vision for an emergency care system that is coordinated, regionalized, and accountable.
- Chapter 4 considers the efficiency of emergency and trauma care in the context of other industries, and explores applications of engineering techniques that could be used to improve the efficiency and quality of emergency services.
- Chapter 5 takes a focused look at the array of new information and clinical technologies that have the potential to transform medicine and emergency care over the next two decades, and offers guidance on how to prioritize these technologies to enhance emergency care most cost-effectively.
- Chapter 6 addresses workforce issues and focuses on one of the most serious problems confronting emergency and trauma care today—the shortage of specialists available to take emergency call. It also addresses the neglected problem of provider safety and the need for better protection from the day-to-day hazards encountered in emergency care, a theme echoed in the next chapter in the context of biological and chemical threats.
- Chapter 7 deals with disaster preparedness and the current lack of hospital capacity to address normal surges in ED visits, much less a major mass casualty event.
- Chapter 8 describes the significant achievements of emergency and trauma care research and the vast range of opportunities for expanding

the evidence base in basic, clinical, and health systems–oriented research. It also considers the meager funding that supports this critically important enterprise.

• Appendix A contains a chart of all committee and subcommittee members.

• Appendix B contains biographical information for members of the main committee and the Subcommittee on Hospital-Based Emergency Care.

• Appendix C lists the presentations that were made during public sessions of the committee meetings.

• Appendix D lists the research papers commissioned by the committee.

• Appendix E provides additional statistical information about ED utilization, supplementing that in Chapter 2.

• Appendix F also supplements Chapter 2 by providing a description of the historical development of the emergency and trauma care fields.

• Appendix G summarizes the recommendations from all three reports in the *Future of Emergency Care* series in a table that indicates the entity with primary responsibility for implementing each recommendation.

REFERENCES

Adams R, Acker J, Alberts M, Andrews L, Atkinson R, Fenelon K, Furlan A, Girgus M, Horton K, Hughes R, Koroshetz W, Latchaw R, Magnis E, Mayberg M, Pancioli A, Robertson RM, Shephard T, Smith R, Smith SC Jr, Smith S, Stranne SK, Kenton EJ III, Bashe G, Chavez A, Goldstein L, Hodosh R, Keitel C, Kelly-Hayes M, Leonard A, Morgenstern L, Wood JO. 2002. Recommendations for improving the quality of care through stroke centers and systems: An examination of stroke center identification options. Multidisciplinary consensus recommendations from the Advisory Working Group on Stroke Center Identification Options of the American Stroke Association. *Stroke* 33(1):e1–e7.

AHRQ (Agency for Healthcare Research and Quality). 2006. *Costs of Treating Trauma Disorders Now Comparable to Medical Expenses for Heart Disease.* [Online]. Available: http://www.ahrq.gov/news/nn/nn012506.htm [accessed May 16, 2006].

Asplin BR, Magid DJ, Rhodes KV, Solberg LI, Lurie N, Camargo CA Jr. 2003. A conceptual model of emergency department crowding. *Annals of Emergency Medicine* 42(2):173–180.

Barron HV, Rundle A, Gurwitz J, Tiefenbrunn A. 1999. Reperfusion therapy for acute myocardial infarction: Observations from the national registry of myocardial infarction 2. *Cardiology in Review* 7(3):156–160.

Bazarian JJ, Pope C, McClung J, Cheng YT, Flesher W. 2003. Ethnic and racial disparities in emergency department care for mild traumatic brain injury. *Academic Emergency Medicine* 10(11):1209–1217.

Berenson RA, Kuo S, May JH. 2003. Medical malpractice liability crisis meets markets: Stress in unexpected places. *Issue Brief (Center for Studying Health System Change)* (68):1–7.

California Healthline. 2004. *Emergency Department, Trauma Unit Closures Increasing Patient Wait Times in Los Angeles County.* [Online]. Available: http://www.californiahealthline.org/index.cfm?action=dsplItem&itemid=107158 [accessed January 5, 2006].

CDC (Centers for Disease Control and Prevention) National Center for Injury Control and Prevention. 2005. *CDC Acute Injury Care Research Agenda: Guiding Research for the Future.* Atlanta, GA: CDC.

Chamberlain J, Slonim A, Joseph J. 2004. Reducing errors and promoting safety in pediatric emergency care. *Ambulatory Pediatrics* 4(1):55–63.

Chisholm CD, Collison EK, Nelson DR, Cordell WH. 2000. Emergency department workplace interruptions: Are emergency physicians "interrupt-driven" and "multitasking"? *Academic Emergency Medicine* 7(11):1239–1243.

Chisholm CD, Dornfeld AM, Nelson DR, Cordell WH. 2001. Work interrupted: A comparison of workplace interruptions in emergency departments and primary care offices. *Annals of Emergency Medicine* 38(2):146–151.

Cosby KS. 2003. A framework for classifying factors that contribute to error in the emergency department. *Annals of Emergency Medicine* 42(6):815–823.

Dellinger RP, Carlet JM, Masur H, Gerlach H, Calandra T, Cohen J, Gea-Banacloche J, Keh D, Marshall JC, Parker MM, Ramsay G, Zimmerman JL, Vincent JL, Levy MM, Surviving Sepsis Campaign Management Guidelines Committee. 2004. Surviving sepsis campaign guidelines for management of severe sepsis and septic shock. *Critical Care Medicine* 32(3):858–873.

Derlet RW. 2002. Overcrowding in emergency departments: Increased demand and decreased capacity. *Annals of Emergency Medicine* 39(4):430–432.

Derlet R, Richards J, Kravitz R. 2001. Frequent overcrowding in U.S. emergency departments. *Academic Emergency Medicine* 8(2):151–155.

Felch J. 2004, August 24. Domino effect feared from closures of emergency rooms. *Los Angeles Times.* P. A1.

GAO (U.S. Government Accountability Office). 2001. *Emergency Care: EMTALA Implementation and Enforcement Issues.* Washington, DC: U.S. Government Printing Office.

Goldberg R, Kuhn G, Andrew L, Thomas H. 2002. Coping with medical mistakes and errors in judgment. *Annals of Emergency Medicine* 39(3):287–292.

Hymon S. 2003, December 19. Study cites paramedic response delay crews are often unable to take urgent calls because they are waiting for patients to be admitted to an ER. *Los Angeles Times.* P. B3.

IOM (Institute of Medicine). 1993. *Emergency Medical Services for Children.* Washington, DC: National Academy Press.

IOM. 1999. *Reducing the Burden of Injury.* Washington, DC: National Academy Press.

IOM. 2000. *To Err Is Human: Building a Safer Health System.* Washington, DC: National Academy Press.

IOM. 2001. *Crossing the Quality Chasm: A New Health System for the 21st Century.* Washington, DC: National Academy Press.

IOM. 2003. *Unequal Treatment: Confronting Racial and Ethnic Disparities in Health Care.* Washington, DC: The National Academies Press.

IOM. 2004. *A Shared Destiny: Community Effects of Uninsurance.* Washington, DC: The National Academies Press.

IOM. 2005. *Building a Better Delivery System: A New Engineering/Health Care Partnership.* Washington, DC: The National Academies Press.

IOM. 2006. *Preventing Medication Errors.* Washington, DC: The National Academies Press.

James CA, Bourgeois FT, Shannon MW. 2005. Association of race/ethnicity with emergency department wait times. *Pediatrics* 115(3):e310–e315.

Josiah Macy, Jr. Foundation. 1995. *The Role of Emergency Medicine in the Future of American Medical Care.* New York, NY: Josiah Macy, Jr. Foundation.

Katz DA, Williams GC, Brown RL, Aufderheide TP, Bogner M, Rahko PS, Selker HP. 2005. Emergency physicians' fear of malpractice in evaluating patients with possible acute cardiac ischemia. *Annals of Emergency Medicine* 46(6):525–533.

Kellermann AL, Haley LH. 2003. Hospital emergency departments: Where the doctor is always "in." *Medical Care* 41(2):195–197.

L.A. County Online. 2005. *General Info: Overview.* [Online]. Available: http://lacounty.info/overview.htm [accessed February 1, 2006].

Lawthers AG, Localio AR, Laird NM, Lipsitz S, Hebert L, Brennan TA. 1992. Physicians' perceptions of the risk of being sued. *Journal of Health Politics, Policy and Law* 17(3):463–482.

Leape L, Brennan TA, Laird N, Lawthers AG, Localio AR, Barnes BA, Hebert L, Newhouse JP, Weiler PC, Hiatt H. 1991. The nature of adverse events in hospitalized patients: Results of the Harvard medical practice study. *New England Journal of Medicine* 324:377–384.

Lowe RA, Bindman AB. 1994. The ED and triage of nonurgent patients. *Annals of Emergency Medicine* 24(5):990–992.

NAS, NRC (National Academy of Sciences, National Research Council). 1966. *Accidental Death and Disability: The Neglected Disease of Modern Society.* Washington, DC: National Academy of Sciences.

NHTSA (National Highway Traffic Safety Administration). 1996. *Emergency Medical Services Agenda for the Future* (U.S. Department of Transportation, HS 808441). Washington, DC: U.S. Government Printing Office.

NHTSA. 1998. *Emergency Medical Services Agenda for the Future: Implementation Guide.* Washington, DC: U.S. Department of Transportation.

NHTSA. 2000. *Emergency Medical Services Education Agenda for the Future: A Systems Approach.* Washington, DC: U.S. Department of Transportation.

NHTSA. 2001a. *National EMS Research Agenda.* Washington, DC: U.S. Department of Transportation.

NHTSA. 2001b. *Trauma System Agenda for the Future.* Washington, DC: U.S. Department of Transportation.

NHTSA. 2003. *Rural and Frontier Emergency Medical Services Agenda for the Future.* Washington, DC: NHTSA.

NRC, IOM (National Research Council, Institute of Medicine). 1985. *Injury in America: A Continuing Public Health Problem.* Washington, DC: National Academy Press.

Oster A, Bindman AB. 2003. Emergency department visits for ambulatory care sensitive conditions: Insights into preventable hospitalizations. *Medical Care* 41(2):198–207.

Quinn JV, Polevoi SK, Kramer NR, Callaham ML. 2003. Factors associated with patients who leave without being seen. *Academic Emergency Medicine* 10(5):523–524.

Richardson LD, Babcock Irvin C, Tamayo-Sarver JH. 2003. Racial and ethnic disparities in the clinical practice of emergency medicine. *Academic Emergency Medicine* 10(11):1184–1188.

Risser DT, Rice MM, Salisbury ML, Simon R, Jay GD, Berns SD. 1999. The potential for improved teamwork to reduce medical errors in the emergency department. The MedTeams Research Consortium. *Annals of Emergency Medicine* 34(3):373–383.

Robes K. 2005. Medical center may close ER: Rising cost of uninsured patient care part of the problem. *Long Beach Press Telegram.*

Schafermeyer RW, Asplin BR. 2003. Hospital and emergency department crowding in the United States. *Emergency Medicine (Fremantle, W.A.)* 15(1):22–27.

Selbst SM, Levine S, Mull C, Bradford K, Friedman M. 2004. Preventing medical errors in pediatric emergency medicine. *Pediatric Emergency Care* 20(10):702–709.

South Bay's ERs Are in a State of Emergency. 2005, February 6. *South Bay Daily Breeze.*

Studdert DM, Mello MM, Sage WM, DesRoches CM, Peugh J, Zapert K, Brennan TA. 2005. Defensive medicine among high-risk specialist physicians in a volatile malpractice environment. *Journal of the American Medical Association* 293(21):2609–2617.

Sussman D. 2000, May 25. Emergency shutdown: ER closures place patient care in jeopardy. *Nurse Week.com.* [Online]. Available: http://www.nurseweek.com/features/00-05/er.html [accessed January 16, 2006].

Thomas EJ, Studdert DM, Burstin HR, Orav EJ, Zeena T, Williams EJ, Howard KM, Weiler PC, Brennan TA. 2000. Incidence and types of adverse events and negligent care in Utah and Colorado. *Medical Care* 38(3):261–271.

Thomas M, Morton R, Mackway-Jones K. 2004. Identifying and comparing risks in emergency medicine. *Emergency Medicine Journal* 21(4):469–472.

Todd K, Deaton C, D'Adamo A, Goe L. 2000. Ethnicity and analgesic practice. *Annals of Emergency Medicine* 35(1):11–16.

Trauma Tax Falls Short. 2004, August 27. *Los Angeles Times.* P. B12.

Weingart SN, Wilson RM, Gibberd RW, Harrison B. 2000. Epidemiology of medical error. *British Medical Journal* 320(7237):774–777.

Weiss SJ, Derlet R, Arndahl J, Ernst AA, Richards J, Fernandez-Frackelton M, Schwab R, Stair TO, Vicellio P, Levy D, Brautigan M, Johnson A, Nick TG. 2004. Estimating the degree of emergency department overcrowding in academic medical centers: Results of the national ED overcrowding study (NEDOCs). *Academic Emergency Medicine* 11(1):38–50.

White AA, Wright SW, Blanco R, Lemonds B, Sisco J, Bledsoe S, Irwin C, Isenhour J, Pichert JW. 2004. Cause-and-effect analysis of risk management files to assess patient care in the emergency department. *Academic Emergency Medicine* 11(10):1035–1041.

2

The Evolving Role of Hospital-Based Emergency Care

The emergence of the modern emergency department (ED) is a surprisingly recent development. Prior to the 1960s, emergency rooms were often poorly equipped, understaffed, unsupervised, and largely ignored. In many hospitals, the emergency room was a single room staffed by nurses and physicians with little or no training in the treatment of injuries. It was also common to use foreign medical school graduates in this capacity (Rosen, 1995). In teaching hospitals, the emergency areas were staffed by junior house officers, and faculty supervision was limited (Rosen, 1995). One young medical student in the 1950s described emergency rooms as "dismal places, staffed by doctors who could not keep a job—alcoholics and drifters" (University of Michigan, 2003, p. 50).

Over four decades, the hospital ED has been transformed into a highly effective setting for urgent and lifesaving care, as well as a core provider of ambulatory care in many communities. An extraordinary range of capabilities converge in the ED—highly trained emergency providers, the latest imaging and therapeutic technologies, and on-call specialists in almost every field—all available 24 hours a day, 7 days a week.

The appeal of the modern ED is undeniable—it is in some ways all things to all people. To the uninsured, it is a refuge. To the community physician, it is a valuable practice asset. To the patient, it is convenient, one-stop shopping. To the hospital itself, it is an escape valve for strained inpatient capacity. The demands being placed on emergency care, however, are overwhelming the system, and the result is a growing national crisis. The decrement in emergency care capacity and quality, however, is almost invisible to those outside the system. Few people have regular contact with the emergency care system, but when serious illness or injury strikes, the system they expect to be there may fail them, with catastrophic results. This chapter explains the increasing demands being placed on hospital-based emergency care, describes the nature of the crisis, and explores how it impacts individuals day to day.

IMBALANCE BETWEEN DEMAND AND CAPACITY

In the decade between 1993 and 2003, the United States experienced a net loss of 703 hospitals, an 11 percent decline. The number of inpatient beds fell by 198,000, or 17 percent, and the number of hospitals with EDs declined by 425, a 9 percent decrease (AHA, 2005b). This sharp decline in capacity was largely in response to cost-cutting measures and lower reimbursements by managed care, Medicare, and other payers (discussed below), as well as shorter lengths of stay and reduced admissions due to evolving clinical models of care.

During this same period, the population of the United States grew by 12 percent and hospital admissions by 13 percent. Between 1993 and 2003, ED visits rose from 90.3 to 113.9 million, a 26 percent increase, representing an average of more than 2 million additional visits per year (see Figure 2-1) (McCaig and Burt, 2005). The outcome of these intersecting trends of

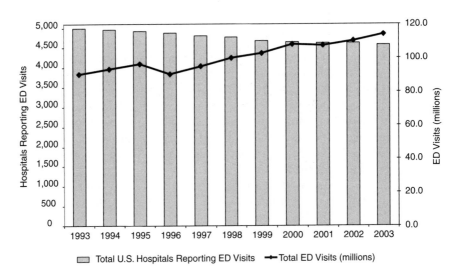

FIGURE 2-1 Hospital EDs versus ED visits.
SOURCES: AHA, 2005b; McCaig and Burt, 2005.

falling capacity and rising use was inevitable. By 2001, 60 percent of U.S. hospitals reported that they were operating at or over capacity (The Lewin Group, 2002).

Not only is ED volume increasing, but patients are presenting with more serious or complex illnesses. The U.S. population is aging, and thanks to advances in the treatment of HIV, cancer, and kidney and heart disease, many people live with significant comorbidities and chronic illnesses (Derlet and Richards, 2000; Bazzoli et al., 2003). These patients require more complex and time-consuming workups and treatments.

By law, the ED's front door is always open, and there is growing public demand for its services. Among the normal flow of patients into the ED, some require hospitalization, some are treated and released, some are transferred, and a few die while in the ED. Nationwide, about 13.9 percent of ED patients were admitted to the hospital in 2003 (McCaig and Burt, 2005); this figure represents about 43 percent of all hospital patients in 2002 (Merrill and Elixhauser, 2005). But when a hospital's inpatient beds are full, the result is a bottleneck to admitting the most severely ill and injured from the ED. As a result, patients who require hospitalization begin to back up in the ED (Andrulis et al., 1991; Asplin et al., 2003). The most common cause of this bottleneck is the inability to admit critically ill patients because all of the hospital's intensive care unit (ICU) beds are filled (GAO, 2003). When delays in accessing inpatient beds become excessive, these patients are commonly referred to as "boarders" because they are technically inpatients but cannot leave the ED. "Boarder" is a misnomer, however, because it implies that these patients require little care. In fact, ED boarders often represent the sickest patients and the most complex cases in the ED—which is why they require hospitalization. And since these patients cannot be moved upstairs, the ED staff must provide ongoing care while simultaneously evaluating and stabilizing incoming ED patients. High levels of hospital occupancy not only create ED "boarders" but also can dramatically worsen ED crowding if community physicians who are unable to secure a bed for their scheduled admissions start sending patients through the ED instead. In either case, the normal congestion in the ED is increased. The problem is depicted in Figure 2-2.

The result of this imbalance is an epidemic of overcrowded EDs, frequent boarding of patients waiting for inpatient beds, diversion of ambulances, and patients who leave without being seen or leave against medical advice (Kellermann, 1991).

Overcrowding

ED overcrowding is a nationwide phenomenon, affecting urban and rural areas alike (Richardson et al., 2002). In one study, 91 percent of EDs

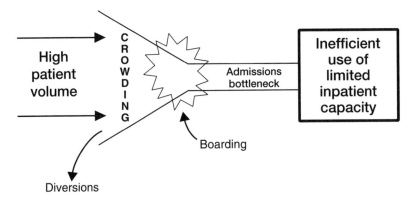

FIGURE 2-2 Consequences of the imbalance between ED patient volume and inpatient capacity.

responding to a national survey reported overcrowding as a problem; almost 40 percent reported that overcrowding occurred daily (Derlet et al., 2001). Another study, using data from the National Emergency Department Overcrowding Study, found that academic medical center EDs were crowded on average 35 percent of the time. This study developed a common set of criteria for identifying crowding across hospitals based on several common elements: all ED beds full, people in hallways, diversion at some time, waiting room full, doctors rushed, and wait times to be treated of greater than 1 hour (Weiss et al., 2004; Bradley, 2005).

Overcrowding can adversely impact the quality of care in the ED and trauma centers. It can also lead to dangerous delays in treatment in the ED and cause delays in emergency medical services (EMS) transport (Schull et al., 2003, 2004).

Boarding

The most common cause of ED crowding is the boarding of admitted patients in the ED. A Government Accountability Office (GAO) study found that in 2001, 90 percent of hospitals boarded patients for at least 2 hours, and about 20 percent of hospitals reported an average boarding time of 8 hours (GAO, 2003). It is not unusual for patients in a busy hospital to board for up to 24 or even 48 hours. In a point-in-time survey of nearly 90 hospital EDs across the country, 73 percent of hospitals reported boarding two or more patients on a typical Monday evening (ACEP, 2003a). The potential for errors, life-threatening delays in treatment, and diminished overall quality of care is enormous in these situations (Andrulis et al., 1991; Conn, 1993; Litvak et al., 2001; Needleman et al., 2002; Schull et al., 2004).

Ambulance Diversions

Another indication of the degree of ED crowding is the frequency of ambulances being diverted to alternative hospitals—a now common, if not daily, event in many major cities. According to the American Hospital Association (AHA), nearly half of all hospitals (46 percent), 68 percent of teaching hospitals, and 69 percent of urban hospitals reported time on diversion in 2004 (AHA, 2005b). A GAO study found that 69 percent of hospitals went on diversion at least once in 2001 (GAO, 2003). A Massachusetts Department of Public Health survey indicated that 67 of 76 hospitals responding to the survey "either diverted or employed special procedures" during one week in February 2001 to meet the demands on the ED (Massachusetts Department of Public Health, 2001). A report using data from the 2003 National Hospital Ambulatory Medical Care Survey indicated that 501,000 ambulances were diverted in 2003 (Burt et al., 2006).

To date, data on the health outcomes associated with diversion are limited. A 2002 study by the Joint Commission for Accreditation of Healthcare Organizations (JCAHO) revealed that over half of all ED events described as sentinel were caused by delayed treatment (Delays in Treatment, 2002). According to an AHA survey, hospitals reporting 20 percent or greater time spent on diversion had longer wait times for treatment by a physician, longer average lengths of stay in ED treatment, longer wait times for transfer from the ED to an acute or critical care bed, and longer wait times for transfer from the ED to a psychiatric bed (The Lewin Group, 2002). A study of trauma patients in Houston found that the numbers of deaths among these patients were consistently greater than average on days with high levels of diversion, but the differences were not statistically significant (Begley et al., 2004). In Canada, reports of a patient's death while en route to an open hospital because his local ED was on diversion raised questions about the legality of ambulance diversion (Walker, 2002).

Ambulance diversions indicate a lack of ability to handle surges in the need for emergency care. If operating at a normal level forces ambulances to be diverted on a regular basis, it may be expected that in the event of a terrorist attack, natural disaster, or other severe and widespread medical emergency, the emergency system would be unprepared for the volume and severity of ED visits (Moroney, 2002).

Patients Who Leave Without Being Seen

In 2003, about 1.9 million ED patients left without being seen by a physician or other emergency care provider; this figure represents 1.7 percent of all ED patients, versus 1.1 percent in 1993 (McCaig and Burt, 2005). While the majority of these patients had low acuity levels, that was not always the case. Studies have shown that some of these patients were in need of immediate medical attention (Baker et al., 1991; Fernandes et al., 1997). One study revealed that those who left without being seen were twice as likely to report pain or a worsening of their problem as those who were seen. Another study found that 27 percent of those who left without being seen returned to an ED, and 4 percent required subsequent hospitalization (Bindman et al., 1991).

Crowding and wait times are important predictors of patients leaving the ED without being seen (Fernandes et al., 1994; Hobbs et al., 2000). One study found that the numbers of such patients increase as ED utilization rises above capacity (Quinn et al., 2003). In addition to patients who leave without being seen, another study found that about 1.2 million or 1 percent of all ED patients leave "against medical advice," in other words, once assessment or treatment has begun, but before it has been completed (McCaig and Burt, 2005).

THE EMERGENCY DEPARTMENT AS A CORE COMPONENT OF COMMUNITY AMBULATORY CARE

The "Safety Net of the Safety Net"

Hospital EDs are the provider of last resort for millions of patients who are uninsured or lack adequate access to care from community providers. The number of uninsured in the United States is now estimated to exceed 45 million and continues to climb (DeNavas-Walt et al., 2005); the number is expected to reach 51.2–53.7 million by 2006 (Simmons and Goldberg, 2003). Some suggest that an additional 29 million Americans are underinsured, lacking sufficient coverage for essential medical care (O'Brien et al., 1999).

The Institute of Medicine (IOM) report *America's Health Care Safety Net: Intact but Endangered* called attention to the growing threats to the nation's health care safety net—increasing numbers of uninsured; erosion of direct and indirect subsidies to providers, including Medicaid Disproportionate Share Hospital (DSH) payments and cost-based reimbursement to Federally Qualified Health Centers (FQHCs); and the continuing growth of Medicaid managed care, which lowers payments and diverts patients from core safety net providers (IOM, 2000). The IOM's six-part *Insuring Health* series comprehensively examined the consequences of uninsurance in the United States. *A Shared Destiny: Community Effects of Uninsurance*, one of the reports in that series, demonstrated the impact of uninsurance on the demand for safety net services and in particular the burden this places on an overextended emergency care system (IOM, 2003). Many of these uninsured patients have no regular source of care and fail to realize the benefits associated with having a primary care provider. An earlier IOM Report, *Primary Care: America's Health in a New Era*, examined the features of primary care—including integration of medical services; coordination of physical, mental, emotional, and social concerns; and sustained clinician–patient relationships—and documented the decrements in quality of care and health that result from inadequate public access to primary care (IOM, 1996). With limited access to community-based alternatives to the emergency system—public clinics, specialists, psychiatric facilities, and other services—many of these people turn to the emergency care system when in medical need, often for conditions that have worsened because of a lack of primary care.

Because the emergency care system is the only component of the nation's safety net that must provide care to everyone, regardless of insurance coverage or ability to pay, hospitals have no alternative but to try to absorb these patients as best as they can. Community-based services, when faced with high demand, can restrict access. Community health centers typically operate only during business hours, maintain long waiting lists, and may lack significant specialty and diagnostic services that are required to fully address their patients' needs. EDs, by contrast, have no such options—they are mandated to serve all who come. Without the ED to fall back on, other community safety net services would be equally overwhelmed. Thus, the emergency care system truly has become the "safety net of the safety net."

Use of the ED for Nonurgent Care

Just over half of ED visits in 2003 were categorized as emergent or urgent, translating into a need for care within 15 minutes to 1 hour of arrival at the ED, while about 33 percent of visits were categorized as semiurgent or nonurgent, requiring attention within 1 hour or 24 hours, respectively (McCaig and Burt, 2004) (see Figure 2-3). Defining ED care as nonurgent or medically unnecessary is controversial because the terms are difficult to define and may vary depending on who is defining them. Is necessity determined by the patient's signs and symptoms at the time of arrival, or by the diagnosis at the time of hospital admission or discharge from the ED? A patient with chest pain would certainly consider this a proper reason to seek ED care, but a patient discharged with a diagnosis of heartburn might be judged by his insurer to have made an inappropriate ED visit. How likely is it that a physician, patient, and insurer will agree on the level of urgency of any given case? Around these gray areas, however, most would agree that there are patients who could be treated as well or better in a different setting if this care were available.

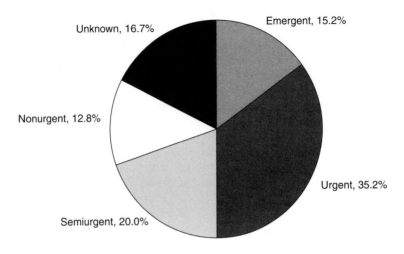

FIGURE 2-3 Percent distribution of ED visits by the immediacy with which patients should be seen, 2003.
SOURCE: McCaig and Burt, 2005.

Other components of the health care system that serve large safety net populations have received substantial government support. For example, community health centers are funded by a federal grant program under Section 330 of the Public Health Service Act and are administered by the Health Resources and Services Administration (HRSA). They received more than $1.7 billion in federal funding in 2005 and served an estimated 14 million patients. In fiscal year 2002, President Bush proposed a 5-year, $780 million initiative to increase the number of community health center sites throughout the nation in order to reach an additional 6.1 million patients by the end of 2006. By the end of 2005, 428 new sites had been established, and many more had increased their medical capacity (HRSA Bureau of Primary Health Care, 2006).

A recent report of the Centers for Disease Control and Prevention (CDC) revealed that EDs represent an important component of the ambulatory care system (12.7 percent of all visits) (Schappert and Burt, 2006). The proportion is much higher in many rural and urban communities where the local ED is the principal provider. Despite its importance in providing ambulatory care and the legal requirement to accept all patients regardless of insurance coverage or ability to pay, hospital emergency care receives little direct federal support.

Why Nonurgent Patients Use the ED

Research has identified several important determinants of nonurgent utilization of the ED. These include financial barriers to and limited availability of alternative sources of care, referrals to the ED by community physicians, and patients' preference for the ED over other alternatives.

Financial barriers Studies have shown that a significant number of patients use the ED for nonurgent matters because of financial barriers. While often unable to access private physician practices, uninsured patients do have access to public health clinics operated by local and county health departments, including FQHCs. But these clinics are limited in number and geographic distribution. In addition, they may have limited hours, long waits, and queues for new patients. Unlike EDs, they are neither typically open around the clock nor required by law to accept all who come. They may also have limited services. For example, many provide primary care services but lack the resources to provide specialty care and diagnostic services. Results of a recent study suggest that expanding primary care capacity may actually increase demand for ED care (Cunningham and May, 2003). According to the authors, patients with access to primary care are more likely to seek specialty care and diagnostic services.

Although Medicaid beneficiaries have a source of payment for medical care, the rates of reimbursement are so low that the number of office-based practitioners who are willing to accept such patients is low (The Medicaid Access Study Group, 1994). One study (Oster and Bindman, 2003) found that uninsured and Medicaid patients have higher rates of ED utilization and are less likely to have a follow-up visit scheduled with a regular physician. In another study, research assistants posing as Medicaid patients attempted to secure appointments with clinics and physician practices. Fully 56 percent of these providers declined to give an appointment, and the most prevalent reason given was "not accepting Medicaid patients." When asked for an alternative, most either offered none or advised the caller to "go to an emergency room" (The Medicaid Access Study Group, 1994). Similar barriers to follow-up care exist as well, even after an ED visit for a serious health problem (Asplin et al., 2005). Research assistants posing as ED patients telephoned physician offices and clinics to schedule an urgent follow-up visit for a serious problem diagnosed in the ED (pneumonia, severe hypertension, or suspected ectopic pregnancy). When callers stated that they had private insurance coverage, they were almost twice as likely to get an appointment as the same callers when they stated that they were covered by Medicaid, and about 2.5 times more likely to get an appointment than when they stated a willingness to pay $20 up front and arrange for complete payment later. Of note, nearly 98 percent of clinics specifically inquired about the caller's ability to pay, but only 28 percent inquired about the caller's health.

One consequence of Medicaid patients' lack of access to primary care is greater reliance on the ED. Medicaid recipients use the ED more than any other group, and their rate of utilization is increasing—81 visits per 100 persons in 2003, versus 65.4 per 100 the year before. This is double the rate of the uninsured population (41.4 percent) and nearly four times that of privately insured patients (21.5 percent) (McCaig and Burt, 2005). All but privately insured individuals also increased their utilization rates from the year before (McCaig and Burt, 2004, 2005). Numerous studies have also found that Medicaid patients disproportionately use the ED for non-urgent conditions, often relying on the ED as their primary source of care (Cunningham et al., 1995; Liu et al., 1999; Sarver et al., 2002; Irvin et al., 2003b). This phenomenon appears to be due largely to a lack of access to care in other settings.

Limited availability of alternative sources of care   Even in the absence of financial barriers, patients may use the ED because of limited access to alternative sources of care. Having a usual source of care can deter utilization of the ED for nonurgent purposes (Petersen et al., 1998), but even patients with a usual source of care frequently use the ED after hours when clinics and physician offices are closed. Recent trends in utilization indicate that insured patients, who are less likely to face financial barriers, are using the ED in larger numbers (Cunningham and May, 2003). The most common reason "walk-in" patients seek care in the ED is because they are experiencing painful or worrisome symptoms that they believe require immediate evaluation and treatment (Young et al., 1996).

The ED as an adjunct to physician practices   There is evidence that physicians and clinics are increasingly using the ED as an adjunct to their practices, referring patients there for a variety of reasons, including their own convenience after regular hours, reluctance to take on complicated cases, the need for diagnostic tests that they cannot perform in the office, and liability concerns (Berenson et al., 2003; Studdert et al., 2005). In a three-site study in Phoenix, Arizona, researchers found that while two-thirds of patients had not contacted a health professional prior to their ED visit, 80 percent of those who had done so had been referred to the ED (St. Luke's Health Initiative, 2004). The Medicaid Access Study Group found that a majority of clinics that declined to see Medicaid patients with minor problems failed to offer any advice about alternatives. The second most common option was to tell the caller to seek care in an ED. A national study of ambulatory use of hospital EDs revealed that 19 percent of "walk-in" patients had been instructed to seek care in the ED by a health care provider (Young et al.,

1996). This phenomenon, sometimes called "physician deflection," is likely to accelerate in the future because primary care offices will be unable to keep pace with the technological advances required to address complex patient needs. Office physicians may consider potentially acute patients to be safer in the ED, and therefore refer such patients directly to the ED even if appointments are available. In addition, referral to the ED has sometimes become the only way to refer patients to certain specialists, who refuse Medicaid patients in many cases. Chronic disease management, medication management, counseling, and case management resources, on the other hand, are aspects of care that primary and specialty care ambulatory practices should be able to provide as an alternative to the ED.

Patient preference   Patients are increasingly using the ED for the convenience of obtaining timely resolution of health care problems (Young et al., 1996; Guttman et al., 2003). Some patients use the ED if they feel they need immediate attention but cannot see their primary care provider within 24 hours (Stratmann and Ullman, 1975; Andren and Rosenqvist, 1985). Patients who try to reach their physician by phone in the evening or on weekends may have difficulty getting through or may be instructed to use the ED. Patients whose primary care providers have extended evening or weekend office hours have been found to have lower rates of ED utilization (Lowe et al., 2003).

Patients may also prefer the ED if they believe it is the best place to obtain access to specialized equipment (Roth, 1971; Smith and McNamara, 1988; Brown and Goel, 1994). Increasingly, admitting physicians are insisting that EDs complete highly detailed workups before they will admit a patient to the hospital. This may explain in part the increasing use of diagnostics such as magnetic resonance imaging (MRI) and computer-assisted tomography (CAT) scans in the ED—up 103 percent from 1992–1999 according to CDC. Some patients may also view the ED as a convenient site for one-stop shopping for medical care. Even with a wait of 2 or more hours, patients can have all of their needs met in a single visit to the ED, and possibly avoid a much longer total time spent seeking care and obtaining diagnostic testing from multiple providers.

Concerns About Nonurgent Utilization

The delivery of nonurgent care in the ED is of concern for three reasons. First, the primary care delivered in the ED may be of lower quality than that in other settings. The ED is designed for rapid, high-intensity response to acute injuries and illnesses. It is fast-paced and requires intensive concentration of resources for short durations. Such an environment is ill suited to the provision of primary and preventive care (Derlet and Richards, 2000).

Physicians in the ED typically do not have a relationship with the patient, often lack complete patient medical records, face constant interruptions and distractions, and have no means of patient follow-up. Further, because they have low triage priority, these patients have extremely long wait times—sometimes 6 hours or more.

Second, nonurgent ED utilization may be less cost-effective than care provided in other settings. EDs and trauma centers are expected to provide a full array of services around the clock, and the fixed costs associated with maintaining this readiness can be substantial. On the other hand, this standby capacity is likely to result in low marginal costs, making it efficient to provide nonurgent care in the ED, at least during slack periods. The literature is mixed on this issue. Some studies support the notion that nonurgent care costs in the emergency setting may be substantially higher than those in a primary care setting (Fleming and Jones, 1983; White-Means and Thornton, 1995). Greater costs in the former setting may result from the frequent lack of patient records and the inability to construct a patient history, which result in a high frequency of full workups (Murphy et al., 1996). ED charges for services for minor problems have been estimated to be two to five times higher than those incurred in a typical office visit (Kusserow, 1992; Baker and Baker, 1994), resulting in $5–7 billion in excess charges in 1993 (Baker and Baker, 1994). While studies probably overestimate these excess costs, they are nevertheless substantial. Bamezai and colleagues (2005) used data on all California hospitals with EDs from 1990 to 1998 to calculate average outpatient ED costs ranging from $116 to $130 for nontrauma EDs and $171 to $215 for trauma EDs, depending on volume. In contrast, Williams (1996) studied a sample of six hospitals in Michigan and found that average and marginal costs of ED visits were quite low, especially for those classified as nonurgent—perhaps below the cost of a typical physician visit. However, if hospitals build additional high-cost ED capacity as a result of the increased use of the ED for nonurgent care, the true cost of providing such care in the ED will be much higher than the marginal or average cost of treatment.

Third, nonurgent utilization may detract from the ED's primary mission of providing emergency and lifesaving care. Regardless of their efficiency on average, EDs do not have unlimited resources. When the ED becomes saturated with patients who could be cared for in a different environment, fewer resources, including physicians, nurses, ancillary personnel, equipment, time, and space, are available to respond to emergency cases.

Identifying Nonurgent Visits

Identifying nonurgent visits is not a simple matter. The inability of patients to distinguish accurately between emergent/urgent and nonurgent conditions has been documented (Lowe and Bindman, 1997). Patients may overestimate the urgency of their condition—in one study, 82 percent of nonurgent patients considered their condition to be urgent (Gill and Riley, 1996). On the other hand, many nonurgent patients understand that their condition is not urgent; they use the ED for a variety reasons outlined above, knowing that they can receive nonurgent care. In a case study of over 400 individuals using the ED, researchers found that more than one-third described their condition as other than an emergency (Guttman et al., 2003).

An even more important question is how many urgent patients under-estimate the urgency of their condition, a miscalculation that could delay care and have catastrophic consequences. A survey of patients across 56 hospital EDs nationwide found that 5 percent of patients who viewed their condition as nonurgent were subsequently admitted to the hospital (Young et al., 1996). In another study, using National Hospital Ambulatory Medical Care Survey (NHAMCS) data from 1992–1996, 4 percent of nonurgent patients were subsequently hospitalized (Liu et al., 1999). These studies probably underestimated the magnitude of the problem as they did not account for patients who never show up at the ED because they underestimate the urgency of their condition. Further, indirect evidence of patients underestimating the urgency of their condition is provided by the failure to call 9-1-1 in cases of heart attacks and other life-threatening emergencies (NHAAP Coordinating Committee, 2004), although other factors, such as feelings of embarrassment and loss of control, also play a role in the failure to call EMS.

The bottom line is that attempts to eliminate nonurgent visits should not discourage patients from seeking help at the ED, in particular when their condition lies in the gray area where the distinction between life-threatening emergencies and nonurgent acute episodes is blurred. It is important for patients to be able to choose the ED if they are uncertain about where on this spectrum their particular condition falls.

Scheduled Versus Unscheduled Visits

A useful way to conceptualize the utilization of ED services is to consider them within the broad context of all health care services within a community. Services can be categorized according to whether they are scheduled or unscheduled. Scheduled services are those that are predictable and planned; they include regular doctor visits and scheduled surgeries, for example. Unscheduled services are those that are unpredictable and irregular because of unexpected injuries or illnesses, such as a heart attack, trauma from a car crash, or a sports injury (Asplin et al., 2003).

Scheduled and unscheduled visits are illustrated in Figures 2-4a and

50

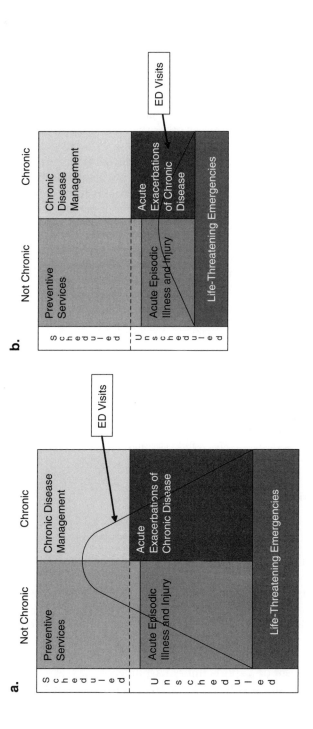

FIGURE 2-4a Current distribution of all care visits.

FIGURE 2-4b Ideal distribution of all health care visits.

2-4b. In each figure, the area of the entire box represents all health care visits. The blocks on the right side represent services that are related to preexisting chronic conditions, for example, asthma or congestive heart failure, while those on the left side are not related to a chronic condition. The top two blocks represent visits for primary care services such as preventive care and management of chronic conditions, which are largely scheduled in nature. The middle two blocks represent visits that are typically unscheduled, including those for acute exacerbations of chronic disease, such as a severe episode of asthma, and acute episodic illness and injury, which may include a case of the flu or a sports injury. (Note that a small proportion of preventive services is included in unscheduled visits.) The bottom block represents life-threatening emergencies, such as heart attacks and serious traumatic injuries.

The ED is one of many sites in the health care delivery system that might provide the types of services in the top four blocks, while the bottom block is, ideally, the exclusive domain of EDs and trauma centers. The area beneath the dashed line indicates care that is provided within the ED. The vast majority of scheduled care will occur outside of the ED at provider locations throughout the community, such as physician offices, diagnostic facilities, and hospital inpatient facilities. Likewise, sites outside of the ED will deliver a large proportion of unscheduled care for both acute episodic illness and injury and acute exacerbations of chronic disease. The relative size of each block within the figures, along with the location of the line depicting the ED's role, will vary depending on a number of factors. Aday and Anderson (1974) proposed a model of community access to medical care that categorizes these as predisposing factors, such as the health status of the community and the amount of preventive care that is provided, and enabling factors, which increase or reduce barriers to access such as insurance coverage and the supply of physicians and other services.

Figure 2-4a represents a hypothetical distribution of medical services between EDs and other providers that is typical of many communities today. Preventive services and chronic disease management are provided mainly outside the ED, while acute illnesses and exacerbations of chronic disease are often treated in the ED. One can envision variations of Figure 2-4a based on differences among communities or groups of patients. For example, suburban and rural community hospitals are likely to look quite different from urban safety net hospitals; the latter have been shown to have 25 percent more nonurgent cases and 10 percent more patients presenting with emergent conditions that are treatable by primary care (Burt and Arispe, 2004).

The relative dimensions of the blocks in the figures are also likely to vary over the 24-hour cycle. There is evidence, for example, that a significant portion of the nonurgent care that is provided in the ED, including visits associated with chronic care management and acute exacerbations of chronic disease, takes place during evenings and weekends, when alternative providers are not available.

Communities with strong access to preventive care and chronic disease management services outside the ED may have less demand for such care in the ED. More important, by improving health and reducing the frequency of acute episodes, it may be possible to reduce the proportion of unscheduled care in the community. Improved preventive care may also reduce the need for chronic disease management itself. These effects are shown in Figure 2-4b as a smaller row representing unscheduled care, a smaller column representing chronic care visits, and the dashed line indicating a smaller amount of care delivered in the ED. Better access to chronic care management and preventive care may also reduce the amount of care for life-threatening emergencies, also indicated in Figure 2-4b by the reduced size of the bottom block. For example, communities that do a better job of managing asthma care will have fewer and less severe acute asthma attacks among the population.

This picture is complicated somewhat by Cunningham and Hadley's (2004) observation that increased access to community clinics resulted in greater use of the ED, presumably because enhanced primary care heightened the demand for a limited supply of specialized and diagnostic care. The above discussion also ignores a potentially important long-term effect of prevention and chronic disease management—that increasing life spans may result in a growth in the amount of medical care demanded overall.

Other versions of Figures 2-4a and 2-4b might include a "nightmare scenario" combining the anticipated burden of chronic disease due to the aging of the baby boomers with a system that continued to manage chronic disease in a disorganized and uncoordinated fashion. In this scenario, the entire area of the figures would be larger, and the amount of care provided in the ED, especially for acute exacerbations of chronic disease, would be extremely high.

REIMBURSEMENT FOR EMERGENCY AND TRAUMA CARE

Substantial evidence demonstrates that reimbursement to safety net hospitals is inadequate to cover the costs of emergency and trauma care. Of the 114 million ED visits in 2003, 36 percent of patients had private insurance, 21 percent were enrolled in Medicaid or the State Children's Health Insurance Program (SCHIP), and 16 percent were covered by Medicare (see Figure 2-5). The payer mix varies widely across hospitals, however, and differences in that mix can have a substantial impact on a hospital's financial condition. Some hospitals treat a large number of uninsured patients, many of whom are unable to pay for their care. To address this gap, the Centers

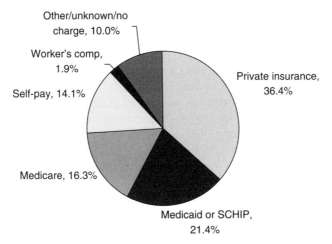

FIGURE 2-5 Payment sources for ED visits, 2003.
SOURCE: McCaig and Burt, 2005.

for Medicare and Medicaid Services (CMS) provides DSH payments to these hospitals, as well as payments for treating undocumented aliens. A number of states also provide additional support to emergency and trauma care systems through general revenues or special taxes.

The Uninsured, or Self-Pay

As discussed earlier, the uninsured use the ED at a significant rate: they made about 41.4 visits per 100 individuals in 2003, and they represented 14.1 percent of all ED utilization in 2003 (McCaig and Burt, 2005). A recent study documented that ED use by uninsured patients is increasing (Cunningham and Hadley, 2004). The rate of reimbursement for services provided to these patients is difficult to quantify but is known to be quite low, and these patients account for a large proportion of the losses associated with hospital ED and trauma care.

Medicaid

Medicaid payment methods vary by state. The most common method is fee-for-service, which is used in 23 states. Second most common is a cost-based reimbursement system. A prospective payment system similar to that of Medicare (Kaiser Commission on Medicaid and the Uninsured, 2003) is used by some states, and many states use a combination of methods.

Medicaid payments are supplemented by DSH payments to offset losses for hospitals with high levels of uncompensated care. These payments are extremely variable, and in many states, DSH money is diverted to wholly un-related areas, such as long-term care (Ku and Coughlin, 1995; IOM, 2003). It is of note that hospitals that serve a large proportion of Medicaid patients but few uninsured will fare better than hospitals that serve few Medicaid patients but a large proportion of uninsured (Fagnani and Toblert, 1999; IOM, 2003). Current legislative proposals would fold DSH payments into block grants, further diluting their contribution to the funding of safety net emergency and trauma care. According to AHA, 73 percent of hospitals lose money providing emergency care to Medicaid patients, while 58 percent lose money on care provided to Medicare patients (AHA, 2002).

Medicare

Medicare enrollees represent 16.3 percent of ED utilization and visit the ED at a rate in between that of Medicaid and uninsured patients—52.4 per 100 enrollees in 2003 (McCaig and Burt, 2005). Medicare reimburses hospitals through a prospective payment system that pays a set amount for a given type of care. Over 80 percent of ED care falls under the five emergency care Current Procedural Terminology (CPT) codes that are based on the intensity of the service—from Code 99281 for a self-limited or minor problem through Code 99285 for an ED visit of high severity that requires urgent evaluation and poses an immediate and significant threat to the patient's life or physiological function (AMA, 2003). When ED patients are admitted to the hospital, however, the emergency care payment is subsumed by the hospital diagnosis-related group (DRG) payment instead of the CPT-based payment being used. Medicare considers all emergency care provided within 72 hours prior to a hospital inpatient admission as related to that admission. From the perspective of the hospital's accounting ledger, the ED may appear to be less profitable because the hospital can readily tabulate the costs of operating the ED, but revenue for admissions that enter the hospital through the ED is credited to its inpatient units (MedPAC, 2003).

Medicare DSH payments are a percentage addition to the basic DRG payments and are applied to hospitals that provide a certain level of un-compensated care. The calculation of DSH payments is based on a complex formula (CMS, 2004).

Private Health Insurance

Privately insured individuals represent the largest single group making visits to the ED but have the lowest rate of use (21.5 per 100) (McCaig and Burt, 2005). Private insurance companies use a wide variety of reimbursement methods, and payment rates generally are not known to the public. In some cases, services are not reimbursed because of denial of payment by the insurer. According to guidelines established in the Medicare Modernization Act, payment is to be based on Medicare's "reasonable and necessary" requirement on the basis of signs and symptoms at the time of treatment, not retrospective evaluation of the primary diagnosis (ACEP, 2003b). Nonetheless, a recent study of two health maintenance organizations (HMOs) in California found that one of the most frequent categories of denial was emergency care (between 16 and 17 percent of coverage requests were denied) (Kapur et al., 2003). The reason cited for almost every denial was that the visit was not deemed an emergency according to the "prudent layperson standard."[1] But a follow-up study found that patients prevailed in over 90 percent of appeals involving ED care (Gresenz and Studdert, 2004).

Payment for services may be denied for a number of reasons. Insurers may have some incentive to delay physician credentialing because doing so may offer a legally valid reason to deny payment if patients have not seen a "participating provider." There may also be some instances in which payment is denied if a patient's primary care provider was not contacted, although the more stringent forms of gatekeeping of the 1990s have diminished.

Undocumented Immigrants

Undocumented immigrants, many of whom are uninsured and have no means of paying for medical expenses, represent a significant burden for hospitals and other providers throughout the United States, particularly in states that border Mexico. The estimated annual cost of emergency care for just the 28 counties along the border in Texas, New Mexico, Arizona, and California is $232 million (MGT of America, 2002). A recent change in Medicare provides a special funding mechanism to assist providers serving large numbers of undocumented immigrants. Section 1011 of the Medicare Modernization Act provides $250 million per year for fiscal years 2005–2008 in payments to hospitals, certain physicians, and ambulances for unreimbursed emergency health services provided to undocumented and other specified immigrants (CMS, 2006).

---

[1]According to this standard, health insurers must cover emergency services obtained by patients if a reasonable layperson would have interpreted the symptoms as requiring emergency care, regardless of whether the patient sought prior authorization from the insurer. This standard has been adopted by 47 states (Sloan and Hall, 2002).

Trends in Reimbursement

According to data from the Medical Expenditure Panel Survey (MEPS),[2] there is a growing gap between charges and payments for emergency services. The average combined charge for physician and hospital/facility services in the MEPS 2001 sample was $943, a 49 percent increase since 1996. The average payment was $492, a 29 percent increase since 1996. Thus, payments have increased but have not kept pace with charges, with average reimbursement rates declining from approximately 60 percent in 1996 to 52 percent in 1998.[3]

Financial Impact on Emergency and Trauma Care

In most hospitals, if reimbursements fail to cover ED and trauma costs, these operations are cross-subsidized by the admissions that originate in the ED. But uncompensated care is an extreme burden at many large urban safety net hospitals that have large numbers of uninsured patients (Burt and Arispe, 2004). These hospitals often bear an increasing burden as surrounding community hospitals go on diversion to preserve the relative calm of their EDs. Further, surrounding hospitals tend to transfer complex, high-risk patients to the large safety net hospitals for specialized care (Reilly et al., 2005). In many cases, the condition of these patients has deteriorated considerably since their arrival at the first hospital (Byrne and Bagan, 2004). The spate of hospital, ED, and trauma center closures in California and elsewhere (see Chapter 1) is indicative of the severity of the problem (Lambe et al., 2002; Vogt, 2004; Melnick et al., 2004; Kellermann, 2004; Fields, 2004; Dauner, 2004).

Public hospitals, which provide a substantial amount of safety net care, are especially hard hit. A survey conducted by the National Association of Public Hospitals (NAPH) found that while NAPH members represent only 2 percent of all U.S. hospitals, they provide almost a quarter (24 percent) of all uncompensated hospital care nationwide (Huang et al., 2005); 21 percent of NAPH hospitals' costs were uncompensated, versus 5.5 percent for all hospitals. For 56 percent of those hospitals, Medicaid payments did not cover costs, and for 90 percent of NAPH hospitals, Medicare payments did not cover costs—in the aggregate, Medicare covered only 80 percent of costs. A

---

[2]MEPS data given here are based on Tsai and colleagues (2003) and calculations by McConnell and Lindrooth, as reported in their commissioned paper for this study, "The Financing of Hospital-Based Emergency Department Services and Emergency Medical Services" (available upon request).

[3]It should be noted that neither the charge nor the payment represents the true cost of care, which is very difficult to determine. The concern with the growing gap is based on an assumption that the increase in charges reflects the increase in true costs.

significant portion of the losses of public hospitals was associated with the provision of emergency and trauma care; on average, these hospitals had three times more emergency visits than all U.S. acute care hospitals.

While these problems are national in scope, certain localities have experienced particular problems. For example, Los Angeles has seen nine hospital EDs close since 2003 (Robes, 2005), bringing its total ED closures to over 60 in the last decade (California Medical Association, 2003). That figure includes the recent closure of the East Los Angeles hospital, in operation for 90 years and serving primarily the Latino population. It lost more than $800,000 in ED operations in 2001–2002 (Coalition to Preserve Emergency Care, 2004). In addition, Los Angeles has lost 10 trauma centers since the 1980s (Chong, 2004). These closures reflect a statewide trend in ED financial losses: California EDs lost $460 million statewide in fiscal year 2001–2002, an increase of 18 percent over the year before and 58 percent since fiscal year 1998–1999 (California Medical Association, 2004).

Trauma services represent a particular financial drain on safety net hospitals. In Houston, for example, the two level I and five level III trauma centers had $32 million in unreimbursed costs in fiscal year 2001, resulting in losses of $19 million (Bishop+Associates, 2002a). Statewide, the state's 21 trauma centers had total losses of $181 million in direct trauma costs, not including standby/readiness costs (Bishop+Associates, 2002b).

A separate study examined trauma costs in five public and five private/nonprofit trauma centers in Texas in fiscal year 2001. Public trauma centers had a median operating loss of $18.6 million, a 54 percent increase over the previous year. Private/nonprofit trauma centers had a median operating loss for trauma care of $5.5 million. These losses were attributed to the increasing number of uninsured in Texas, which leads the nation with 24 percent of its population uninsured, and a decline in DSH payments of $26 million relative to the previous year (Clifton, 2002).

In Florida, an analysis of 18 of the state's 21 trauma centers in 2003–2004 found that these centers had an aggregate loss of $92 million in combined uncompensated direct care and standby/readiness costs (e.g., the costs of maintaining standby ICU facilities, staff, and on-call specialists for trauma services around the clock) (The University of South Florida, 2005). One study measured three components of the cost of maintaining readiness for trauma care—around-the-clock specialist coverage, verification, and outreach and prevention. The median annual costs were $2.7 million, with the majority of this figure consisting of stipends for specialist coverage (median = $2.1 million) (Taheri et al., 2004).

Consistent with all of these findings was a study of a single medical center in 1999 that found the mean reimbursement for trauma care to be only 36 percent of charges. No reimbursement was obtained for 26 percent of patients, and reimbursement did not cover costs for 56 percent of patients.

Reimbursement was significantly lower for transfers than for other trauma cases, indicating the potential dumping of patients from community hospitals (Lanzarotti et al., 2003). In contrast to these findings for safety net hospitals, one study found that trauma services contributed substantially to the profitability of a hospital with a favorable payer mix—43 percent of trauma patients in this study had private insurance (Breedlove et al., 2005).

The evidence suggests that the burden of providing uncompensated services is placing communities at risk by failing to ensure the continued financial viability of a critical public safety asset—the 24-hour availability of critical lifesaving emergency and trauma care services. Consequently, the committee believes that the emergency care system requires a special funding source, separate from the regular DSH formula, to compensate hospitals and physicians adequately for the burden of providing services to uninsured and underinsured populations. To ensure the continued viability of a critical public safety function, the committee recommends that **Congress establish dedicated funding, separate from Disproportionate Share Hospital payments, to reimburse hospitals that provide significant amounts of uncompensated emergency and trauma care for the financial losses incurred by providing those services (2.1).**[4]

The committee believes that accurate determination of the optimal amount of funding to allocate for this purpose, which could run in the hundreds of millions of dollars, is beyond its expertise, but that the government must begin to address this issue immediately. The committee therefore recommends that **Congress initially appropriate $50 million for the purpose, to be administered by the Centers for Medicare and Medicaid Services (2.1a). The Centers for Medicare and Medicaid Services should establish a working group to determine the allocation of these funds, which should be targeted to providers and localities at greatest risk; the working group should then determine funding needs for subsequent years (2.1b).** Implementation of this recommendation would help staunch the loss of ED capacity in many communities, protect nearby hospitals from a domino effect of spikes in demand, and help ensure the continued viability of the nation's vital emergency and trauma system. The new funding, however, should be targeted only to hospitals that provide a substantial amount of unreimbursed care to uninsured or underinsured patients in their EDs. Also, this new funding should be tied to hospital performance reporting, participation in coordinated regional systems, improvements in efficiency, reduced boarding and diversion, and improved quality of emergency and trauma care.

---

[4]The committee's recommendations are numbered according to the chapter of the main report in which they appear. Thus, for example, recommendation 2.1 is the first recommendation in Chapter 2.

State Funding for Emergency and Trauma Care Capacity

EMS and emergency and trauma care are often supported through local and state taxes, but only a handful of states have established dedicated funding sources to support emergency care. A summary of funding sources used by the states is shown in Table 2-1. Maryland, for example, imposes a surcharge on motor vehicle registration fees to fund its statewide trauma care and EMS system (National Conference of State Legislatures, 2005). Pennsylvania uses fees from the accreditation process to support a state agency charged with verifying and accrediting all trauma centers on a 3-year basis. In addition, this agency must meet or exceed the standards for trauma centers, programs, providers, data reporting, and performance improvement of the American College of Surgeons. The results of the process are public and reported to the state department of health. Pennsylvania guaranteed support to its trauma care system by modifying its insurance statutes to ensure that accredited trauma centers would receive hospital and professional reimbursement at the charges level, rather than the more common and lower Medicare level, for all motor vehicle crash–related care and workmen's compensation patients.

Other states rely on a wide range of funding mechanisms. California collects funds from traffic fines, but in the last election, voters declined to impose an additional 3 percent surcharge on telephone bills to support EMS. Ohio uses penalties from failure to wear a seat belt, license reinstatement fines, and forfeited bails. Wisconsin has considered adding $1 to the vehicle registration or driver's license renewal fee. Surcharges for 9-1-1 phone service have also been used to generate funds to subsidize trauma care. Firearms registration and fines for illegal discharge of firearms are two other potential sources of subsidies that are directly related to the incidence of trauma. It is extraordinary that more states do not support EMS and trauma and emergency care in this manner. The situation may relate to the wide gap between public perception and the reality of the emergency care system. A recent survey found that the public has extremely high expectations of the system but a limited appreciation of the problems that exist (Harris Interactive, 2004).

CHALLENGES OF CARE FOR MENTAL HEALTH CONDITIONS AND SUBSTANCE ABUSE

Patients with mental health conditions and substance-abuse problems represent a small proportion of ED utilization, but they place an inordinate burden on the emergency care system. There is also evidence that the psychiatric and substance-abuse care received in EDs is sometimes less than optimal. On the other hand, it fills a critical need, as the broader health system often fails to provide adequate access to this care.

TABLE 2-1 Revenue Sources to Fund Trauma Care, Organized by Topic

Source	AZ	CO	FL	IL	KS	MD	MI	NE	OH	OK	PA	TX	UT	VA	WA
911 System Surcharges												X			
Controlled Substances Act Violations													X		
Court Fees, Fines, and Penalties					X								X		
Intoxication Offenses—Not Limited to Motor Vehicles								X				X		X	X
Motor Vehicle Fees, Fines, and Penalties		X	X	X		X	X	X		X	X	X		X	X
• Motor vehicle registration		X				X		X		X		X			
• Tax on motor vehicle license			X												
• Driving under the influence (DUI)-related				X								X		X	
• Fee for distinctive license tags							X								
• Violations of child restraint laws									X			X			
• Seat belt violations									X			X			
• Open container violations										X					
• Driver's license fee										X					
• Fee for reinstating revoked license								X		X					
• Driving with revoked or suspended license										X					
• Fine on specific traffic violation											X	X		X	
• Non–motor vehicle intoxication												X			
• Sale or lease of new vehicle															X
Sales Surtax			X												
Tobacco Tax	X														
Trauma Facility Penalty		X													
Tribal Gaming	X														
Weapons Violations				X											

SOURCE: HRSA, 2004.

Care for Mental Health Conditions

Patients with mental illness represent a considerable and growing number of all ED visits. Between 1992 and 2001, the proportion of all ED visits related to mental health problems grew from 6.5 to 8.1 percent; however, fewer than half of those patients (3.3 percent) had a primary diagnosis of mental illness (Larkin et al., 2004). It is estimated that more than 200,000 children present to the ED with mental health problems each year (Melese-d'Hospital et al., 2002). The prevalence of impaired mental status among elderly patients is also high; studies indicate that 26 to 27 percent of patients aged 70 or older present to the ED with an impaired mental state (Hustey et al., 2001, 2003), and 10 percent suffer from delirium (Hustey and Meldon, 2002; Hustey et al., 2003). In a recent national survey, 70 percent of ED physicians reported an increase in patients with mental illness boarding in the ED. Most attribute this trend to cutbacks in state health care budgets and a decrease in the number of psychiatric beds (ACEP, 2004).

Some evidence suggests that the quality of care provided to these patients is substandard. Evidence indicates that mental illness often goes unrecognized and untreated in hospital EDs (Horowitz et al., 2001). One study reported a failure to document mental status for 56 percent of psychiatric patients admitted to one community hospital (Tintinalli et al., 1994). The authors suggested that the lack of documentation may be due to a tendency among ED staff to attribute psychiatric symptoms to physical problems. The inability or refusal of psychiatric patients to respond to a list of questions may also result in an incomplete evaluation (Tintinalli et al., 1994). A study of elderly ED patients with mental illness found that documentation of any mental impairment by the emergency physician was uncommon and that many elderly mentally impaired patients (including those with delirium) were discharged home without plans for addressing the impairment. The authors suggested that the lack of documentation and referrals indicates a lack of recognition of mental illness by emergency physicians (Hustey and Meldon, 2002). A third study found that emergency physicians failed to detect depression in most geriatric patients identified as depressed through a validated self-rated depression scale. As a result, few of those patients received a mental health or psychiatric referral (Meldon et al., 1997).

Studies have also pointed to shortcomings in the care of children with mental illness in the ED. A mid-1990s survey of hospitals revealed that formal mental health services for children are unavailable in most EDs (U.S. Consumer Product Safety Commission, 1997). In a study of pediatric ED records from 10 hospitals, evaluation of pediatric patients with mental health problems appeared to be inconsistent with presenting classifications (Melese-d'Hospital et al., 2002). Three-fourths of emotionally disturbed children received an evaluation by a mental health professional at the ED, compared with 69 percent who had attempted suicide (Melese-d'Hospital et al., 2002). Studies also indicate that proper management of adolescent suicide attempts in the ED is lacking. While the importance of follow-up psychiatric treatment has been demonstrated, psychotherapy is recommended for fewer than half of adolescent suicidal patients evaluated in the ED (Piacentini et al., 1995). Additionally, adolescents with somatic complaints are infrequently screened for depression (Porter et al., 1997).

Training and Capacity

ED providers often lack the training, skills, and resources to deal effectively with mentally ill patients. Standardized psychiatric training is not required of residents in emergency medicine and pediatric emergency medicine. Fewer than one-quarter of emergency medicine residency programs provide formal psychiatric training for residents (Santucci et al., 2003). Moreover, surveys of nurses—even those working in designated pediatric EDs—show that they are uncomfortable with pediatric psychiatric emergencies (Fredrickson et al., 1994). ED physicians also may not have the time to perform a thorough mental health evaluation, and many rely on psychiatrists, psychologists, or social workers to perform such an evaluation. When that assistance is not available, patients may not receive an evaluation at all. The ED setting also makes it difficult to care for a mentally ill patient. The lack of privacy and the noisy, high-stimulus environment may make it uncomfortable for patients to participate in a mental health evaluation (Hoyle and White, 2003).

Impact on the ED

Patients with mental illness have an important impact on EDs. They tend to require resource-intensive care, and their admission rates are high—22 percent in one study (Larkin et al., 2004). These patients are also more likely to arrive by ambulance and to be classified as "urgent" than are ED patients who present without mental health problems (Larkin et al., 2004). Because hospital EDs often do not have specialized psychiatric facilities or psychiatric specialists available and find it difficult to place such patients—many of whom are indigent or uninsured—in outside facilities, ED staff spend more than twice as long seeking beds for these patients than for those without psychiatric problems. Psychiatric patients board in hospital EDs more than twice as long as other patients (ACEP, 2004).

According to the administrator of the Division of Mental Health and Developmental Services for the State of Nevada, the single overarching challenge facing the agency is the number of mentally ill patients who are crowding EDs in the southern part of the state. In 2004, the state had an average of 42 patients waiting 61 hours in EDs for an inpatient mental health bed. More recently, the average was 62 patients waiting an average of 93 hours for an inpatient bed (Ryan, 2005). In a recent national survey, 6 in 10 emergency physicians said the increase in psychiatric patients seeking care at EDs is negatively affecting access to emergency care for all patients by generating longer waiting times and limiting the availability of ED staff and ED beds for other patients (ACEP, 2004).

Care for Substance Abuse

Data from the 2004 National Survey on Drug Use and Health indicate that 50 percent of the U.S. population aged 12 or older were current drinkers of alcohol in 2004; 23 percent were binge drinkers, meaning they had consumed five or more drinks on at least one occasion in the 30 days prior to the survey; and 7 percent were heavy drinkers, defined as binge drinking on 5 or more days in the past month. The survey data also indicate that 8 percent of the U.S. population over age 12 were illicit drug users in 2004 (SAMHSA, 2005).

Alcohol and other drug-related dependence is a pervasive problem in patients presenting to the ED. Between 1992 and 2000, approximately 8 percent of all ED visits each year were attributable to alcohol, and the total number of alcohol-related visits increased by 18 percent during that time (McDonald et al., 2004). Despite this statistic, a much higher percentage of patients would test positive for alcohol use if screened. One study found that one-third of adolescent patients tested as a part of routine care were alcohol-positive, but were not necessarily given an alcohol-related diagnosis (Barnett et al., 1998).

Estimates from the Drug Abuse Warning Network, a surveillance system operated by the Substance Abuse and Mental Health Services Administration (SAMHSA) that collects data on drug-related ED visits (including those involving alcohol) across the country, indicate that there were approximately 628,000 drug-related ED visits in the United States in the second half of 2003. Of those visits, 33 percent were for an adverse reaction, 17 percent for overmedication, 10 percent for detoxification, and 6 percent for drug-related suicide attempts (SAMHSA, 2005). Among drug-related visits in 2002, 80 percent involved only seven categories: alcohol in combination with another drug (31 percent); cocaine (30 percent); marijuana (18 percent); heroin (14 percent); and benzodiazepines, antidepressants, and analgesics, which together accounted for 30 percent of such visits (SAMHSA, 2004).

Again, however, many more patients would likely test positive for drug use if screened. In a study of alcohol and drug use in seven Tennessee general hospital EDs, marijuana was identified in 15 percent of all patients willing and able to participate in a drug screen, benzodiazepines in 11 percent, opioids in 9 percent, and stimulants in 6 percent (Rockett et al., 2003).

Patients often present to the ED with acute or chronic manifestations of alcohol or drug problems. Chronic problems related to alcohol and other drug use include skin infections from drug injections, cirrhosis and its complications, and gastrointestinal disorders. Alcohol and other drug use often occurs in the presence of, or may lead to, physical illness and injury. Among patients that present to the ED with injuries, those that report alcohol or drug use are significantly more likely to report violence associated with the episode (Cunningham et al., 2003). Drug abuse can complicate the evaluation of the injured patient by masking signs and symptoms of injury (Fabbri et al., 2001). Conversely, ED staff may focus on the patient's injury and neglect to screen for drug abuse.

Screening and on-site interventions and referrals for alcohol have been demonstrated in a variety of health care settings, including the ED, to reduce ED and hospital use and decrease the amount that patients drink (Bernstein et al., 1997; Wright et al., 1998; Monti et al., 1999; Helmkamp et al., 2003). In one study of 700 trauma patients admitted for alcohol-related injuries, those that received 30 minutes of counseling at the hospital experienced a 47 percent reduction in serious injuries requiring trauma center admission in the following 3 years and a 48 percent reduction in less serious injuries requiring ED care (Gentilello et al., 1999). A recent meta-analysis of screening and brief intervention identified 39 published studies, 30 of which found a positive effect (D'Onofrio and Degutis, 2002). Additionally, studies have shown that ED patients are often accepting of screening and brief interventions for alcohol problems (Cherpitel et al., 1996; Leikin et al., 2001).

However, research has shown that ED physicians usually fail to identify those at risk for problems with alcohol or to provide such interventions (Gentilello et al., 1999; O'Rourke et al., 2001; Manley et al., 2002). Similar studies have found a high prevalence of undetected substance abuse and an unmet need for treatment among ED patients (Bernstein et al., 1999; Rockett et al., 2003). This situation has been demonstrated by a number of studies even though numerous federal and expert panels have recommended routine screening of injured patients in the ED for substance abuse and the provision of brief interventions for those that test positive (Gentilello, 2003). According to a survey sponsored by the West Virginia Chapter of the American College of Emergency Physicians (ACEP), barriers to screening include provider attitudes of disinterest, avoidance, disdain, and pessimism, as well as inadequate time, insufficient education, and a lack of resources. The survey found that a minority of ED physicians routinely screen and council ED patients on alcohol abuse (Williams et al., 2000).

Reimbursement

Another important barrier to screening of patients for alcohol or drug abuse by ED staff is that the care provided may not be reimbursed if the screen is positive. In some states, laws permit insurance companies to refuse payment for injuries sustained if the patient is found to be under the influence of alcohol or drugs. The intent of these laws is to punish drunk drivers, thereby reducing the cost of insurance for others (Gentilello, 2003). However, physicians may be reluctant to screen patients for alcohol or drugs because of the potential financial impact on patients, the hospital, and themselves.

Impact on the ED

Like mental health patients, those with identified substance-abuse problems tend to be a resource-intensive group. In a statewide study, ED patients with unmet substance-abuse treatment needs generated much higher hospital and ED charges than other patients (Rockett et al., 2005). Yet treatment for addiction requires continuing care, adherence to medications, and behavioral change (D'Onofrio, 2003), none of which are likely to be accomplished during the course of an ED visit. The ED does, however, offer an opportunity to identify, intervene with, and refer patients who have substance-abuse problems (D'Onofrio et al., 1998; Rockett et al., 2003).

Not only do substance-abuse patients require extra time and effort on the part of ED staff, but drug-related ED visits have become a major cause of violence in the ED (Anonymous, 1990). For example, a patient who is primarily seeking drugs may turn violent if not able to obtain them (van Steenburgh, 2002). The types of patient presentations most associated with violence are intoxicant use, states of withdrawal from drugs, delirium, head injury, psychiatric problems, and social factors (Lavoie et al., 1988).

RURAL EMERGENCY CARE

According to the U.S. Census Bureau (2000), more than 59 million people, or 21 percent of the total U.S. population, reside in rural areas. Rural EDs face a number of problems that differ from those of urban hospitals, including limited availability of hospitals and equipment, an inadequate supply of qualified staff, an unfavorable payer mix, and long distances and emergency response times. A recent IOM study, *Quality through Collaboration: The Future of Rural Health*, documented the difficulties faced by rural communities in providing high-quality medical services, particularly emergency care (IOM, 2004).

Availability of Hospitals and Equipment

There are nearly 2,200 rural community hospitals in the United States, representing 44 percent of all community hospitals (AHA, 2005a). Between 1980 and 2002, more than 400 rural hospitals closed. Rural hospitals are smaller than their urban counterparts, with a median of 58 beds compared with 186 for urban hospitals (The Lewin Group, 2002). Smaller hospitals tend to have lower margins than larger ones; more than 50 percent of hospitals with fewer than 25 beds have negative margins, versus only 13 percent of those with 200 or more (The Lewin Group and AHA, 2000). The modest size of rural hospitals and their correspondingly small capital and financial assets make them less able to survive significant changes in financial performance; when the financial survival of a hospital is at stake, investments in the latest technologies and recruitment of highly qualified personnel are assigned low priority.

Given the high cost of maintaining trauma centers and the difficulty of maintaining them even in busy urban areas (Taheri et al., 2004), it is unrealistic to expect that each rural ED will have the full spectrum of trauma resources available. When caring for a traumatized patient, the rural emergency physician's focus is primarily on rapid patient assessment, stabilization, and transfer. Rural EDs also lack many of the newer diagnostic modalities. Such shortages impair the establishment of definitive diagnoses, as well as the application of the latest potential improvements in emergency practice. For example, acute stroke treatment with tissue plasminogen activator (TPA) requires immediate access to a computed tomography (CT) scanner and a fast accurate reading, neither of which may be available at most rural EDs (Drummond, 1998).

Payer Mix

The population served by rural hospitals tends to be poorer, to be uninsured, and to make greater use of various forms of public health insurance. While 72 percent of urban residents had private insurance coverage in 1998, this was the case for only 60 percent of those living in remote rural areas. Rural workers tend to be self-employed, to work for smaller companies, and to earn lower wages. These factors compromise access to private health insurance. The impingement of private health insurance and managed care, public and private, is a major factor determining the financial environment in which rural hospitals are situated (Kaiser Commission on Medicaid and the Uninsured, 2003).

In 2001, over 7 million people living in rural areas were uninsured, including 24 percent of those living in remote rural areas, defined as rural counties nonadjacent to a county with an urban center. This high level of uninsured is compounded by the fact that the rural uninsured tend to lack insurance for longer periods of time than their urban counterparts. They are also older, and their self-reported health is poorer. One-quarter of rural uninsured are aged 45–64, and 42 percent of rural uninsured residents report less than very good health, compared with 38 percent of urban uninsured residents (Kaiser Commission on Medicaid and the Uninsured, 2003). The large numbers of uninsured in rural areas can have spillover effects on the community, reducing access to emergency services, trauma care, specialists, and hospital-based services (Kellermann and Snyder, 2004). Unreimbursed care for emergency physicians and hospitals can result in cutbacks, closure, or relocation of services (Irvin et al., 2003a).

The low levels of private insurance and low incomes in rural America contribute to the important role played by Medicaid and other forms of public insurance in these areas. Public programs insure 16 percent of those in rural areas, compared with 10 percent in urban settings. Therefore, rural hospitals are much more dependent on these programs for their existence. The Balanced Budget Act (BBA) of 1997 and the Balanced Budget Refinement Act (BBRA) of 1999 have had a significant impact on the access to emergency care in rural environments. The BBA mandated that Medicare outpatient payments become prospective, saving $110 billion from 1998 to 2004. Medicare payment reductions to rural hospitals were projected to have a cumulative impact of $16.7 billion over this time frame (IOM, 2000). The BBRA preferentially reinstated cost-based reimbursement to rural hospitals for some services and included higher payments to Medicare-dependent hospitals. The restoration of these payments is expected to reduce the cumulative impact of the BBA by $1.8 billion to approximately $15 billion overall. Yet the impact on rural hospitals remains tremendous, as these acts have projected Medicare margins in rural hospitals to decrease by 3.3–8.4 percent by 2004. Particularly hard hit are outpatient services, expected to decrease by 20–28 percent (IOM, 2000). Given the marginal financial existence of many rural hospitals, these reductions may have detrimental effects on hospitals' survival and provision of services, including outpatient ED services, and may even precipitate closure.

To increase the access of rural residents to urgent and emergency services, Congress established the Critical Access Hospital (CAH) program as part of the BBA. A CAH is exempt from the prospective payment system for both inpatient and outpatient care. Instead, hospitals that receive this designation bill Medicare on a fee-for-service basis. Medicare reimburses at a rate of 100–101 percent of reasonable and customary charges. CAHs are specially designated under the Medicare Rural Hospital Flexibility Grant Program. These rural, low-volume hospitals must meet distinct criteria regarding location, number of available beds, and average length of stay, or may be state certified as a "necessary provider." Emergency services must also be available 24 hours daily. A hospital can be designated as a CAH if it is located in a rural area, provides 24-hour emergency services, has an average length of stay of 96 hours or less, is more than 35 miles from a neighboring hospital or 15 miles in areas with mountainous terrain, or is certified as a necessary provider (prior to 2006), and has fewer than 25 acute care beds (as of January 2004). It is still too early to assess whether the CAH program has been successful in increasing access to emergency care. More research is needed to determine whether new capacity is being built, or hospitals are changing to qualify for the CAH program. For example, a hospital may have to reduce its number of acute care beds to be designated as a CAH. Others hospitals may add 24-hour care, which in turn increases the existing ED capacity.

Workforce Supply

The limited supply of medical workers in rural areas affects many aspects of medicine, not just emergency care. The most difficult aspect of rural emergency care is finding qualified emergency physicians, specialists to provide on-call services, and ancillary staff. Many rural EDs have only part-time physicians on staff and are often not available 24 hours a day. Although 21 percent of Americans live in rural areas, only slightly more than 12 percent of emergency physicians, regardless of training or certification status, practice in these settings (Moorhead et al., 2002). This maldistribution has worsened since 1997, when 15 percent of emergency physicians practiced in rural areas (Moorhead et al., 1998; Williams et al., 2001). The proportion of physicians who are board certified in emergency medicine is also very low in rural areas—67 percent of rural emergency medicine physicians are neither emergency medicine residency trained nor board certified. Rural EDs have lower levels of staffing, and when they are staffed by physicians, it is much more likely for these physicians to be trained in family practice or other primary care specialties than in emergency medicine. In one study, rural EDs were shown to have only 44 percent of the average specialists and referral sources of an urban academic center, with the subspecialties in shortest supply being neurosurgery, gastroenterology, neurology, and cardiology (Sklar et al., 2002).

Even when the resources for appropriate treatment are available, however, the medical care provided in rural EDs may fall short of established guidelines. In one study of acute stroke care in nonurban EDs, treatment was found to be inconsistent with AHA recommendations. For example, hypertension was often treated too aggressively, and inappropriate medications were sometimes used. Additionally, it was suggested that nonmotor symptoms were less likely to be recognized or apt to be treated with less urgency than motor symptoms (Burgin et al., 2001). Although these data are far from conclusive, the results of such studies may explain in part the lower levels of competence attributed to rural emergency physicians (Leap, 2000). Yet the reality is that rural emergency physicians are often called upon to care single-handedly for critically ill and injured patients in a challenging setting typically lacking in manpower, equipment, and access to consultants. The fact that the patient census in a rural ED may be very low likely contributes to the difficulty experienced by physicians and midlevel providers in maintaining a high level of proficiency in emergency medicine.

Distance and Time Factors

Long distances and times involved in the transportation of acutely ill and traumatized patients in rural regions likely affect health outcomes adversely. The negative correlation between prolonged response times and ultimate outcomes inherent in many rural EMS systems has been a focal point of some studies (Bachman et al., 1986; Eitel et al., 1988). In one study of 566 patients with primary cardiac arrest in Wisconsin, the average response time for survivors was 3.7 minutes, while that for nonsurvivors was 7.3 minutes. There were no survivors when the response time was greater than 8 minutes (Olson et al., 1989).

Other studies have demonstrated that poor survival rates in rural patient populations are not related exclusively to prolonged response times. In one study of EMS with advanced coronary life support (ACLS), response time was not predictive of survival from refractory prehospital cardiac arrest. Although rural patients in the study had the lowest survival rate and longest average response time (9 percent and 10.6 minutes, compared with 23 percent and 8.7 minutes for urban sites), the survival rate in suburban locales was only 14 percent, even though these areas had the fastest average response time of 6.9 minutes (Vukmir and Sodium Bicarbonate Study Group, 2004). Adverse outcomes are likely related to multiple factors in rural emergency care systems. These include the absence of a 9-1-1 system, low rates of bystander performance of cardiopulmonary resuscitation (CPR), lack of full-time emergency medical technicians (EMTs) and paramedics, and less well equipped emergency facilities (Vukov et al., 1988; Gallehr and Vukov, 1993; Richless et al., 1993).

Training

Rural emergency care practice involves unique challenges with respect to professional training. Access to university-based centers is usually limited, making it more difficult for rural providers to maintain and upgrade knowledge and skills. Special training is needed in a number of areas, including care and treatment given limited staff and resources, use of telemedicine, the making of appropriate transfer decisions, and how to address patient needs with respect to decisions about local versus regional delivery sites. Current approaches to these training needs include encouraging joint training programs with rural hospitals and funding rural training programs.

Quality of Care

Disparities in the quality of care between rural and nonrural areas and the resulting potential for adverse events and suboptimal outcomes have repeatedly been demonstrated (Bachman et al., 1986; Vukov et al., 1988; Eitel et al., 1988; Olson et al., 1989; Gallehr and Vukov, 1993; Richless et al., 1993). Low population density has been strongly associated with increased trauma-related death rates (Rutledge et al., 1994), and preventable death rates in rural areas have been demonstrated to be twice those in urban areas (Esposito et al., 1995). In some studies, death rates from trauma among rural children have been reported to be nearly double those among urban children (Svenson et al., 1996). Likewise, geriatric trauma patients in rural areas have higher complication rates and in-hospital mortality (Rogers et al., 2001). Killien and colleagues (1996) pointed out that with respect to out-of-hospital cardiac arrest, rates of survival to discharge were reported to be as high as 32 percent in urban studies, compared with less than 10 percent in most rural studies.

SUMMARY OF RECOMMENDATIONS

2.1: Congress should establish dedicated funding, separate from Disproportionate Share Hospital payments, to reimburse hospitals that provide significant amounts of uncompensated emergency and trauma care for the financial losses incurred by providing those services.

2.1a: Congress should initially appropriate $50 million for the purpose, to be administered by the Centers for Medicare and Medicaid Services.

2.1b: The Centers for Medicare and Medicaid Services should establish a working group to determine the allocation of these funds, which should be targeted to providers and localities at greatest risk; the working group should then determine funding needs for subsequent years.

REFERENCES

ACEP (American College of Emergency Physicians). 2003a. *Study Confirms Emergency De-partment "Boarding" Major Cause of Crowding.* [Online]. Available: http://www.acep. org/webportal/Newsroom/PressReleases/AnnalsOfEmergencyMedicinePressReleases/ Arvchive2003/StudyConfirmsEmergencyDepartmentBoardingMajorCauseofCrowding. htm [accessed June 7, 2005].

ACEP. 2003b. *New Medicare Legislation Includes Significant Changes.* [Online]. Available: http://www.acep.org/1,33226,0.html [accessed January 26, 2005].

ACEP. 2004. *Emergency Departments See Dramatic Increase in People with Mental Illness— Emergency Physicians Cite State Health Care Budget Cuts at Root of Problem.* [Online]. Available: http://www.acep.org/1,33706,0.html [accessed July 20, 2004].

Aday LA, Andersen R. 1974. A framework for the study of access to medical care. *Health Services Research* 9(3):208–220.

AHA (American Hospital Association). 2002. *Hospitals Face a Challenging Operating En-vironment: Statement of the American Hospital Association Before the Federal Trade Commission Health Care Competition Law and Policy Workshop.* Chicago, IL: AHA.

AHA. 2005a. *Fast Facts on U.S. Hospitals from AHA Hospital Statistics.* [Online]. Available: http://www.aha.org/aha/resource_center/fastfacts/fast_facts_US_hospitals.html [accessed August 10, 2005].

AHA. 2005b. *TrendWatch Chartbook 2005.* [Online]. Available: http://www.ahapolicyforum. org/ahapolicyforum/trendwatch/chartbook2005.html [accessed May 22, 2006].

AMA (American Medical Association). 2003. *Current Procedural Terminology 2004: Profes-sional Edition.* Chicago, IL: AMA Press.

Andren KG, Rosenqvist U. 1985. Heavy users of an emergency department: Psycho-social and medical characteristics, other health care contacts and the effect of a hospital social worker intervention. *Social Science & Medicine* 21(7):761–770.

Andrulis DP, Kellermann A, Hintz EA, Hackman BB, Weslowski VB. 1991. Emergency depart-ments and crowding in United States teaching hospitals. *Annals of Emergency Medicine* 20(9):980–986.

Anonymous. 1990. Emergency room violence: An update. *Hospital Security & Safety Manage-ment* 11(8):5–8.

Asplin BR, Magid DJ, Rhodes KV, Solberg LI, Lurie N, Camargo CA Jr. 2003. A con-ceptual model of emergency department crowding. *Annals of Emergency Medicine* 42(2):173–180.

Asplin BR, Rhodes KV, Levy H, Lurie N, Crain AL, Carlin BP, Kellermann AL. 2005. Insur-ance status and access to urgent ambulatory care follow-up appointments. *Journal of the American Medical Association* 294(10):1248–1254.

Bachman JW, McDonald GS, O'Brien PC. 1986. A study of out-of-hospital cardiac arrests in northeastern Minnesota. *Journal of the American Medical Association* 256(4):477–483.

Baker DW, Stevens CD, Brook RH. 1991. Patients who leave a public hospital emergency department without being seen by a physician. Causes and consequences. *Journal of the American Medical Association* 266(8):1085–1090.

Baker LC, Baker LS. 1994. Excess cost of emergency department visits for nonurgent care. *Health Affairs* 13(5):164–171.

Bamezai A, Melnick G, Nawathe A. 2005. The cost of an emergency department visit and its relationship to emergency department volume. *Annals of Emergency Medicine* 45(5):483–490.

Barnett NP, Spirito A, Colby SM, Vallee JA, Woolard R, Lewander W, Monti PM. 1998. Detection of alcohol use in adolescent patients in the emergency department. *Academic Emergency Medicine* 5(6):607–612.

Bazzoli GJ, Brewster LR, Liu G, Kuo S. 2003. Does U.S. hospital capacity need to be expanded? *Health Affairs* 22(6):40–54.

Begley CE, Chang YWRC, Weltge A. 2004. Emergency department diversion and trauma mortality: Evidence from Houston, Texas. *The Journal of Trauma Injury, Infection, and Critical Care* 57(6):1260–1265.

Berenson RA, Kuo S, May JH. 2003. Medical malpractice liability crisis meets markets: Stress in unexpected places. *Issue Brief (Center for Studying Health System Change)* (68):1–7.

Bernstein E, Bernstein J, Levenson S. 1997. Project assert: An ED-based intervention to increase access to primary care, preventive services, and the substance abuse treatment system. *Annals of Emergency Medicine* 30(2):181–189.

Bernstein E, Bernstein J, D'Onofrio G. 1999. Patients who abuse alcohol and other drugs: Emergency department identification, intervention, and referral. In: Tintinalli J, Kelen G, Stapczynski J, eds. *Emergency Medicine: A Comprehensive Study Guide*. Princeton, NJ: McGraw Hill.

Bindman A, Grumbach K, Keane D, Rauch L, Luce J. 1991. Consequences of queuing for care at a public hospital emergency department. *Journal of the American Medical Association* 266(8):1091–1096.

Bishop+Associates. 2002a. *Houston Trauma Economic Assessment and System Survey*. Prepared for Save Our ERs. St. Charles, IL: Bishop+Associates.

Bishop+Associates. 2002b. *Texas Trauma Economic Assessment and System Survey*. Prepared for Save Our ERs. St. Charles, IL: Bishop+Associates.

Bradley VM. 2005. Placing emergency department crowding on the decision agenda. *Journal of Emergency Nursing* 31(3):247–258.

Breedlove LL, Fallon WF Jr, Cullado M, Dalton A, Donthi R, Donovan DL. 2005. Dollars and sense: Attributing value to a level I trauma center in economic terms. *Journal of Trauma-Injury Infection & Critical Care* 58(4):668–673; discussion 673–674.

Brown EM, Goel V. 1994. Factors related to emergency department use: Results from the Ontario health survey 1990. *Annals of Emergency Medicine* 24(6):1083–1091.

Burgin WS, Staub L, Chan W, Wein TH, Felberg RA, Grotta JC, Demchuk AM, Hickenbottom SL, Morgenstern LB. 2001. Acute stroke care in non-urban emergency departments. *Neurology* 57(11):2006–2012.

Burt CW, Arispe IE. 2004. Characteristics of emergency departments serving high volumes of safety-net patients: United States, 2000. *Vital Health Statistics* 13(155):1–16.

Burt CW, McCaig LF, Valverde RH. 2006. *Analysis of Ambulance Transports and Diversions among U.S. Emergency Departments*. Hyattsville, MD: National Center for Health Statistics.

Byrne RW, Bagan B. 2004. Academic center ERs bear brunt of Chicago-area transfers. *American Association of Neurological Surgeons Bulletin* 13(4):14–15.

California Medical Association. 2003. *A System in Crisis: More ERs Shut; Losses Grow*. San Francisco, CA: California Medical Association.

California Medical Association. 2004. *A System in Continued Crisis: CMA's Annual ER Losses Report*. Sacramento, CA: California Medical Association.

Cherpitel CJ, Soghikian K, Hurley LB. 1996. Alcohol-related health services use and identification of patients in the emergency department. *Annals of Emergency Medicine* 28(4):418–423.

Chong J-R. 2004, November 28. L.A. to get downtown trauma center. *Los Angeles Times*. *CAL/AAEM News Service*.

Clifton GL. 2002. Cost of treating uninsured jeopardizing trauma centers. *The Internet Journal of Emergency and Intensive Care Medicine* 6(1).

CMS (Centers for Medicare and Medicaid Services). 2004. *Acute Inpatient Prospective Payment System: Disproportionate Share Hospital (DSH)*. [Online]. Available: http://www.cms.hhs.gov/providers/hipps/dsh.asp [accessed September 29, 2004].

CMS. 2006. *Service Furnished to Undocumented Aliens*. [Online]. Available: http://www.cms.hhs.gov/UndocAliens [accessed September 25, 2006].

Coalition to Preserve Emergency Care. 2004. *Hospital ER Closure Points to Need for Proposition 67: Emergency department diversions increasing statewide.* [Online]. Available: http://www.lacmanet.org/news/CPEC_elastar_closes.pdf [accessed September 5, 2005].

Conn AK. 1993. Critical care in the emergency department: Stress within the system. *Critical Care Medicine* 21(7):952–953.

Cunningham P, Hadley J. 2004. Expanding care versus expanding coverage: How to improve access to care. *Health Affairs (Millwood, VA)* 23(4):234–244.

Cunningham P, May J. 2003. Insured Americans drive surge in emergency department visits. *Issue Brief (Center for Studying Health System Change)* (70):1–6.

Cunningham PJ, Clancy CM, Cohen JW, Wilets M. 1995. The use of hospital emergency departments for nonurgent health problems: A national perspective. *Medical Care Research and Review* 52(4):453–474.

Cunningham R, Walton MA, Maio RF, Blow FC, Weber JE, Mirel L. 2003. Violence and substance use among an injured emergency department population. *Academic Emergency Medicine* 10(7):764–775.

D'Onofrio G. 2003. Treatment for alcohol and other drug problems: Closing the gap. *Annals of Emergency Medicine* 41(6):814–817.

D'Onofrio G, Degutis LC. 2002. Preventive care in the emergency department: Screening and brief intervention for alcohol problems in the emergency department. A systematic review. *Academic Emergency Medicine* 9(6):627–638.

D'Onofrio G, Bernstein E, Bernstein J, Woolard RH, Brewer PA, Craig SA, Zink BJ. 1998. Patients with alcohol problems in the emergency department, part 2: Intervention and referral. SAEM Substance Abuse Task Force. Society for Academic Emergency Medicine. *Academic Emergency Medicine* 5(12):1210–1217.

Dauner CD. 2004. Emergency capacity in California: A look at more recent trends. *Health Affairs Web Exclusive* W4-152–154.

Delays in treatment. 2002. *Sentinel Event Alert* (26):1–3.

DeNavas-Walt C, Proctor BD, Hill Lee C. 2005. *Income, Poverty, and Health Insurance Coverage in the United States: 2004*. Washington, DC: U.S. Government Printing Office.

Derlet R, Richards J. 2000. Overcrowding in the nation's emergency departments: Complex causes and disturbing effects. *Annals of Emergency Medicine* 35(1):63–68.

Derlet R, Richards J, Kravitz R. 2001. Frequent overcrowding in U.S. emergency departments. *Academic Emergency Medicine* 8(2):151–155.

Drummond A. 1998. Physician services in small and rural emergency departments: A critique of the Scott Report. *Journal of Emergency Medicine* 16(2):241–244.

Eitel DR, Walton SL, Guerci AD, Hess DR, Sabulsky NK. 1988. Out-of-hospital cardiac arrest: A six-year experience in a suburban-rural system. *Annals of Emergency Medicine* 17(8):808–812.

Esposito TJ, Sanddal ND, Hansen JD, Reynolds S. 1995. Analysis of preventable trauma deaths and inappropriate trauma care in a rural state. *The Journal of Trauma* 39(5):955–962.

Fabbri A, Marchesini G, Morselli-Labate AM, Rossi F, Cicognani A, Dente M, Iervese T, Ruggeri S, Mengozzi U, Vandelli A. 2001. Blood alcohol concentration and management of road trauma patients in the emergency department. *Journal of Trauma Injury Infection & Critical Care* 50(3):521–528.

Fagnani L, Toblert J. 1999. *The Dependence of Safety Net Hospitals and Health Systems on the Medicare and Medicaid Disproportionate Share Hospital Payment Programs*. New York: The Commonwealth Fund.

Fernandes CM, Daya MR, Barry S, Palmer N. 1994. Emergency department patients who leave without seeing a physician: The Toronto hospital experience. *Annals of Emergency Medicine* 24(6):1092–1096.

Fernandes CMB, Price A, Christenson JM. 1997. Does reduced length of stay decrease the number of emergency department patients who leave without seeing a physician? *Journal of Emergency Medicine* 15(3):397–399.

Fields WW. 2004. Emergency care in California: Robust capacity or busted access? *Health Affairs Web Exclusive* W4–143–145.

Fleming NS, Jones HC. 1983. The impact of outpatient department and emergency room use on costs in the Texas Medicaid Program. *Medical Care* 21(9):892–910.

Fredrickson JM, Bauer W, Arellano D, Davidson M. 1994. Emergency nurses' perceived knowledge and comfort levels regarding pediatric patients. *Journal of Emergency Nursing* 20(1):13–17.

Gallehr JE, Vukov LF. 1993. Defining the benefits of rural emergency medical technician-defibrillation. *Annals of Emergency Medicine* 22(1):108–112.

GAO (U.S. Government Accountability Office). 2003. *Hospital Emergency Departments: Crowded Conditions Vary among Hospitals and Communities*. Washington, DC: GAO.

Gentilello L. 2003. *Effectiveness and Influence of Insurance Statutes and Policies on Reimbursement for Emergency Care*. Presentation at Crossing Barriers in the Emergency Care of the Alcohol-Impaired Patient meeting, Washington, DC.

Gentilello LM, Villaveces A, Ries RR, Nason KS, Daranciang E, Donovan DM, Copass M, Jurkovich GJ, Rivara FP. 1999. Detection of acute alcohol intoxication and chronic alcohol dependence by trauma center staff. *Journal of Trauma Injury Infection & Critical Care* 47(6):1131–1135.

Gill JM, Riley AW. 1996. Nonurgent use of hospital emergency departments: Urgency from the patient's perspective. *Journal of Family Practice* 42(5):491–496.

Gresenz CR, Studdert DM. 2004. Disputes over coverage of emergency department services: A study of two health maintenance organizations. *Annals of Emergency Medicine* 43(2):155–162.

Guttman N, Zimmerman DR, Nelson MS. 2003. The many faces of access: Reasons for medically nonurgent emergency department visits. *Journal of Health Politics, Policy & Law* 28(6):1089–1120.

Harris Interactive. 2004. *Trauma Care: Public's Knowledge and Perception of Importance*. New York: Harris Interactive.

Helmkamp JC, Hungerford DW, Williams JM, Manley WG, Furbee PM, Horn KA, Pollock DA. 2003. Screening and brief intervention for alcohol problems among college students treated in a university hospital emergency department. *Journal of American College Health* 52(1):7–16.

Hobbs D, Kunzman SC, Tandberg D, Sklar D. 2000. Hospital factors associated with emergency center patients leaving without being seen. *American Journal of Emergency Medicine* 18(7):767–772.

Horowitz L, Kassam-Adams N, Bergstein J. 2001. Mental health aspects of emergency medical services for children: Summary of a consensus conference. *Academic Emergency Medicine* 8(12):1187–1196.

Hoyle J, White L. 2003. Treatment of pediatric and adolescent mental health emergencies in the United States: Current practices, models, barriers, and potential solutions. *Prehospital Emergency Care* 7(1):66–73.

HRSA (Health Resources and Services Administration). 2004. *State Trauma Care Systems: Revenue Statutes Organized by Topics*. Trauma-EMS Systems Program.

HRSA Bureau of Primary Health Care. 2006. *President's Health Centers Initiative*. [Online]. Available: http://bphc.hrsa.gov/chc/pi.htm [accessed February 19, 2006].

Huang J, Silbert J, Regenstein M. 2005. *America's Public Hospitals and Health Systems, 2003: Results of the Annual NAPH Hospital Characteristics Survey*. Washington, DC: National Association of Public Hospitals and Health Systems.

Hustey FM, Meldon SW. 2002. The prevalence and documentation of impaired mental status in elderly emergency department patients. *Annals of Emergency Medicine* 39(3):248–253.

Hustey FM, Meldon SW, Palmer RM, Parikh N. 2001. Prevalence and documentation of impaired mental status in elder emergency department (ED) patients. *Academic Emergency Medicine* 8(5):451-b, 452.

Hustey FM, Meldon SW, Smith MD, Lex CK. 2003. The effect of mental status screening on the care of elderly emergency department patients. *Annals of Emergency Medicine* 41(5):678–684.

IOM (Institute of Medicine). 1996. *Primary Care: America's Health in a New Era*. Washington, DC: National Academy Press.

IOM. 2000. *America's Health Care Safety Net: Intact but Endangered*. Washington, DC: National Academy Press.

IOM. 2003. *A Shared Destiny: Community Effects of Uninsurance*. Washington, DC: The National Academies Press.

IOM. 2004. *Quality Through Collaboration: The Future of Rural Health*. Washington, DC: The National Academies Press.

Irvin CB, Fox JM, Pothoven K. 2003a. Financial impact on emergency physicians for nonreimbursed care for the uninsured. *Annals of Emergency Medicine* 42(4):571–576.

Irvin CB, Fox JM, Smude B. 2003b. Are there disparities in emergency care for uninsured, Medicaid, and privately insured patients? *Academic Emergency Medicine* 10(11):1271–1277.

Kaiser Commission on Medicaid and the Uninsured. 2003. *Medicaid Benefits*. [Online]. Available: http://www.kff.org/medicaid/benefits/index.cfm [accessed August 20, 2004].

Kapur K, Gresenz CR, Studdert DM. 2003. Managing care: Utilization review in action at two capitated medical groups. *Health Affairs (Millwood, VA)* W3–275–282.

Kellermann AL. 1991. Too sick to wait. *Journal of the American Medical Association* 266(8):1123–1125.

Kellermann AL. 2004. Emergency care in California: No emergency? *Health Affairs Web Exclusive* W4–149–151.

Kellermann AL, Snyder LP. 2004. A shared destiny: Community effects of uninsurance. *Annals of Emergency Medicine* 43(2):178–180.

Killien SY, Geyman JP, Gossom JB, Gimlett D. 1996. Out-of-hospital cardiac arrest in a rural area: A 16-year experience with lessons learned and national comparisons. *Annals of Emergency Medicine* 28(3):294–300.

Ku L, Coughlin TA. 1995. Medicaid disproportionate share and other special financing programs. *Health Care Financial Review* 16(3):27–54.

Kusserow RP. 1992. *Use of Emergency Rooms by Medicaid Recipients*. Washington, DC: U.S. Department of Health and Human Services.

Lambe S, Washington DL, Fink A, Herbst K, Liu H, Fosse JS, Asch SM. 2002. Trends in the use and capacity of California's emergency departments, 1990–1999. *Annals of Emergency Medicine* 39(4):389–396.

Lanzarotti S, Cook CS, Porter JM, Judkins DG, Williams MD. 2003. The cost of trauma. *The American Surgeon* 69(9):766–770.

Larkin GL, Claassen CA, Emond JA, Camargo CA Jr. 2004. Trends in U.S. emergency department visits for mental health, 1992–2001. *Academic Emergency Medicine* 11(5):486-a.

Lavoie F, Carter G, Danzl D, Berg R. 1988. Emergency department violence in United States teaching hospitals [Abstract]. *Annals of Emergency Medicine* 17(11):1127–1133.

Leap E. 2000. The stigma of being a rural EP. *EM News*. P. 12.

Leikin JB, Morris RW, Warren M, Erickson T. 2001. Trends in a decade of drug abuse presentation to an inner city ED. *American Journal of Emergency Medicine* 19(1):37–39.

The Lewin Group. 2002. *Emergency Department Overload: A Growing Crisis. The Results of the AHA Survey of Emergency Department (ED) and Hospital Capacity*. Washington, DC: American Hospital Association.

The Lewin Group, AHA (The Lewin Group, American Hospital Association). 2000. Redefining hospital capacity. *TrendWatch* 2(3).

Litvak E, Long MC, Cooper AB, McManus ML. 2001. Emergency department diversion: Causes and solutions. *Academic Emergency Medicine* 8(11):1108–1110.

Liu T, Sayre MR, Carleton SC. 1999. Emergency medical care: Types, trends, and factors related to nonurgent visits. *Academic Emergency Medicine* 6(11):1147–1152.

Lowe RA, Bindman AB. 1997. Judging who needs emergency department care: A prerequisite for policy-making. *American Journal of Emergency Medicine* 15(2):133–136.

Lowe RA, Localio JR, Schwarz D, Williams SV, Tuton L, Maroney S, Nicklin D, Goldfarb N, Vojta DD, Feldman HI. 2003. Characteristics of primary care practices affect patients' emergency department use [Abstract]. *Academic Emergency Medicine* 10(5):512.

Manley WG, Williams JM, Furbee PM, Hungerford DW, Helmkamp JC, Horn K. 2002. Do emergency department staff identify patients at risk for alcohol problems? *Academic Emergency Medicine* 9(5):465-a.

Massachusetts Department of Public Health. 2001. *The DPH Ambulance Diversion Survey.* Boston, MA: Massachusetts Department of Public Health.

McCaig LF, Burt CW. 2004. *National Hospital Ambulatory Medical Care Survey: 2002 Emergency Department Summary.* Hyattsville, MD: National Center for Health Statistics.

McCaig LF, Burt CW. 2005. *National Hospital Ambulatory Medical Care Survey: 2003 Emergency Department Summary.* Hyattsville, MD: National Center for Health Statistics.

McDonald A, Wang N, Camago C. 2004. U.S. emergency department visits for alcohol-related diseases and injuries between 1992 and 2000. *Archives of Internal Medicine* 164:531–537.

The Medicaid Access Study Group. 1994. Access of Medicaid recipients to outpatient care. *New England Journal of Medicine* 330(20):1426–1430.

MedPAC (Medicare Payment Advisory Committee). 2003, March. *Appendix A: How Medicare Pays for Services: An Overview.* Report to Congress: Medicare Payment Policy. Washington, DC: MedPAC.

Meldon SW, Emerman CL, Schubert DS. 1997. Recognition of depression in geriatric ED patients by emergency physicians. *Annals of Emergency Medicine* 30(4):442–447.

Melese-d'Hospital IA, Olson LM, Cook L, Skokan EG, Dean JM. 2002. Children presenting to emergency departments with mental health problems. *Academic Emergency Medicine* 9(5):528-a.

Melnick G, Nawathe A, Bamezai A, Green L. 2004. Emergency department capacity and access in California, 1990–2001: An economic analysis. *Health Affairs Web Exclusive.* W4-136–142.

Merrill CT, Elixhauser A. 2005. *Hospitalization in the United States, 2002.* HCUP Fact Book No. 6, AHRQ Publication No. 05-0056. Rockville, MD: Agency for Healthcare Research and Quality.

MGT of America. 2002. *Medical Emergency: Costs of Uncompensated Care in Southwest Border Counties.* Washington, DC: U.S./Mexico Border Counties Coalition.

Monti PM, Colby SM, Barnett NP, Spirito A, Rohsenow DJ, Myers M, Woolard R, and Lewander, W. 1999. Brief intervention for harm reduction with alcohol-positive older adolescents in a hospital emergency department. *Journal of Consulting & Clinical Psychology* 67(6):989–994.

Moorhead JC, Gallery ME, Mannle T, Chaney WC, Conrad LC, Dalsey WC, Herman S, Hockberger RS, McDonald SC, Packard DC, Rapp MT, Rorrie CC Jr, Schafermeyer RW, Schulman R, Whitehead DC, Hirschkorn C, Hogan P. 1998. A study of the workforce in emergency medicine. *Annals of Emergency Medicine* 31(5):595–607.

Moorhead JC, Gallery ME, Hirshkorn C, Barnaby DP, Barsan WG, Conrad LC, Dalsey WC, Fried M, Herman SH, Hogan P, Mannle TE, Packard DC, Perina DG, Pollack CV Jr, Rapp MT, Rorrie CC Jr, Schafermeyer RW. 2002. A study of the workforce in emergency medicine: 1999. *Annals of Emergency Medicine* 40(1):3–15.

Moroney S. 2002. *Emergency and Acute Care System Background Research.* Minneapolis, MN: National Institute of Health Policy. [Online]. Available: http://www.nihp.org/Reports/EACS-Research1.htm [accessed May 15, 2006].

Murphy AW, Bury G, Plunkett PK, Gibney D, Smith M, Mullan E, Johnson Z. 1996. Randomised controlled trial of general practitioner versus usual medical care in an urban accident and emergency department: Process, outcome, and comparative cost. *British Medical Journal* 312(7039):1135–1142.

National Conference of State Legislatures. 2005. *State Funding for Emergency Medical Services and Trauma Care.* [Online]. Available: http://www.ncsl.org/programs/health/traumafund. htm [accessed November 7, 2005].

Needleman J, Buerhaus P, Mattke S, Stewart M, Zelevinsky K. 2002. Nurse-staffing levels and the quality of care in hospitals. *New England Journal of Medicine* 346(22):1715–1722.

NHAAP (National Heart Attack Alert Program) Coordinating Committee. 2004. *Use of Emergency Medical Services (EMS) by Patients with Acute Coronary Syndrome Symptoms: Summary of the Evidence and Future Directions.* Bethesda, MD: National Institutes of Health.

O'Brien GM, Stein MD, Fagan MJ, Shapiro MJ, Nasta A. 1999. Enhanced emergency department referral improves primary care access. *American Journal of Managed Care* 5(10):1265–1269.

O'Rourke M, Pillai S, Richardson LD. 2001. ED patients and alcohol use: Are emergency physicians missing an opportunity to help? *Academic Emergency Medicine* 8(5):462-b, 463.

Olson DW, LaRochelle J, Fark D, Aprahamian C, Aufderheide TP, Mateer JR, Hargarten KM, Stueven HA. 1989. EMT-defibrillation: The Wisconsin experience. *Annals of Emergency Medicine* 18(8):806–811.

Oster A, Bindman AB. 2003. Emergency department visits for ambulatory care sensitive conditions: Insights into preventable hospitalizations. *Medical Care* 41(2):198–207.

Petersen LA, Burstin HR, O'Neil AC, Orav EJ, Brennan TA. 1998. Nonurgent emergency department visits: The effect of having a regular doctor. *Medical Care* 36(8):1249–1255.

Piacentini J, Rotheram-Borus MJ, Gillis JR, Graae F, Trautman P, Cantwell C, Garcia-Leeds C, Shaffer D. 1995. Demographic predictors of treatment attendance among adolescent suicide attempters. *Journal of Consulting & Clinical Psychology* 63(3):469–473.

Porter SC, Fein JA, Ginsburg KR. 1997. Depression screening in adolescents with somatic complaints presenting to the emergency department. *Annals of Emergency Medicine* 29(1):141–145.

Quinn JV, Polevoi SK, Kramer NR, Callaham ML. 2003. Factors associated with patients who leave without being seen. *Academic Emergency Medicine* 10(5):523-b, 524.

Reilly PM, Schwab CW, Kauder DR, Dabrowski GP, Gracias V, Gupta R, Pryor JP, Braslow BM, Kim P, Wiebe DJ. 2005. The invisible trauma patient: Emergency department discharges. *Journal of Trauma-Injury Infection & Critical Care* 58(4):675–683; discussion 683–685.

Richardson LD, Asplin BR, Lowe RA. 2002. Emergency department crowding as a health policy issue: Past development, future directions. *Annals of Emergency Medicine* 40(4): 388–393.

Richless LK, Schrading WA, Polana J, Hess DR, Ogden CS. 1993. Early defibrillation program: Problems encountered in a rural/suburban EMS system. *Journal of Emergency Medicine* 11(2):127–134.

Robes K. 2005, August 4. Medical center may close ER: Rising cost of uninsured patient care part of the problem. *Long Beach Press Telegram.* P. A3.

Rockett IR, Putnam SL, Jia H, Smith G. 2003. Assessing substance abuse treatment need: A statewide hospital emergency department study. *Annals of Emergency Medicine* 41(6):802–813.

Rockett IR, Putnam SL, Jia H, Chang CF, Smith GS. 2005. Unmet substance abuse treatment need, health services utilization, and cost: A population-based emergency department study. *Annals of Emergency Medicine* 45(2):118–127.

Rogers FB, Osler TM, Shackford SR, Morrow PL, Sartorelli KH, Camp L, Healey MA, Martin F. 2001. A population-based study of geriatric trauma in a rural state. *Journal of Trauma-Injury Infection & Critical Care* 50(4):604–609; discussion 609–611.

Rosen P. 1995. *History of Emergency Medicine.* New York: Josiah Macy, Jr. Foundation. Pp. 59–79.

Roth JA. 1971. Utilization of the hospital emergency department. *Journal of Health & Social Behavior* 12(4):312–320.

Rutledge R, Fakhry SM, Baker CC, Weaver N, Ramenofsky M, Sheldon GF, Meyer AA. 1994. A population-based study of the association of medical manpower with county trauma death rates in the United States. *Annals of Surgery* 219(5):547–563; discussion 563–567.

Ryan C. 2005, January 12. Report to legislature shows rising mental illness. *Las Vegas Sun.*

SAMHSA (Substance Abuse and Mental Health Services Administration). 2004. *2003 National Survey on Drug Use and Health.* Rockville, MD: Office of Applied Studies.

SAMHSA. 2005. *2004 National Survey on Drug Use and Health.* Rockville, MD: Office of Applied Studies.

Santucci KA, Sather J, Baker MD. 2003. Emergency medicine training programs' educational requirements in the management of psychiatric emergencies: Current perspective. *Pediatric Emergency Care* 19(3):154–156.

Sarver JH, Cydulka RK, Baker DW. 2002. Usual source of care and nonurgent emergency department use. *Academic Emergency Medicine* 9(9):916–923.

Schappert SM, Burt CW. 2006. *Ambulatory Care Visits to Physician Offices, Hospital Outpatient Departments, and Emergency Departments: United States, 2001–02.* Hyattsville, MD: National Center for Health Statistics.

Schull MJ, Lazier K, Vermeulen M, Mawhinney S, Morrison LJ. 2003. Emergency department contributors to ambulance diversion: A quantitative analysis. *Annals of Emergency Medicine* 41(4):467–476.

Schull MJ, Vermeulen M, Slaughter G, Morrison L, Daly P. 2004. Emergency department crowding and thrombolysis delays in acute myocardial infarction. *Annals of Emergency Medicine* 44(6):577–585.

Simmons HE, Goldberg MA. 2003. *Charting the Cost of Inaction.* Washington, DC: National Coalition on Health Care.

Sklar D, Spencer D, Alcock J, Cameron S, Saiz M. 2002. Demographic analysis and needs assessment of rural emergency departments in New Mexico (DANARED–NM). *Annals of Emergency Medicine* 39(4):456–457.

Sloan FA, Hall MA. 2002. Market failures and the evolution of state regulation of managed care. *Law & Contemporary Problems* 65(4):169–206.

Smith RD, McNamara JJ. 1988. Why not your pediatrician's office? A study of weekday pediatric emergency department use for minor illness in a community hospital. *Pediatric Emergency Care* 4(2):107–111.

St. Luke's Health Initiative. 2004. *Fact and Fiction: Emergency Department Use and the Health Safety Net in Maricopa County.* Phoenix, AZ: St. Luke's Health Initiatives.

Stratmann WC, Ullman R. 1975. A study of consumer attitudes about health care: The role of the emergency room. *Medical Care* 13(12):1033–1043.

Studdert DM, Mello MM, Sage WM, DesRoches CM, Peugh J, Zapert K, Brennan TA. 2005. Defensive medicine among high-risk specialist physicians in a volatile malpractice environment. *Journal of the American Medical Association* 293(21):2609–2617.

Svenson JE, Spurlock C, Nypaver M. 1996. Factors associated with the higher traumatic death rate among rural children. *Annals of Emergency Medicine* 27(5):625–632.

Taheri PA, Butz DA, Lottenberg L, Clawson A, Flint LM. 2004. The cost of trauma center readiness. *American Journal of Surgery* 187(1):7–13.

Tintinalli JE, Peacock FW 4th, Wright MA. 1994. Emergency medical evaluation of psychiatric patients. *Annals of Emergency Medicine* 23(4):859–862.

Tsai AC, Tamayo-Sarver JH, Cydulka RK, Baker DW. 2003. Characterizing payments for emergency department visits: Do the uninsured pay their way? *Academic Emergency Medicine* 10(5):523-a.

University of Michigan. 2003. *The Emergence of Emergency Medicine.* [Online]. Available: http://www.medicineatmichigan.org/magazine/2003/summer/classnotes/wiegenstein.asp [accessed August 15, 2005].

The University of South Florida. 2005. *A Comprehensive Assessment of the Florida Trauma System.* Tampa, FL: The University of South Florida.

U.S. Census Bureau. 2000. *Statistical Abstract of the United States, 2000: The National Data Book.* Washington, DC: Commerce Department.

U.S. Consumer Product Safety Commission. 1997. *Hospital-Based Pediatric Emergency Resources Survey.* Bethesda, MD: Division of Hazard and Injury Data Systems.

van Steenburgh J. 2002. Strategies to help you cope with violent patients. *ACP-ASIM Observer.*

Vogt K. 2004. Backers of a tax initiative say it could ease the burden on hospitals. *American Medical News.*

Vukmir RB, Sodium Bicarbonate Study Group. 2004. The influence of urban, suburban, or rural locale on survival from refractory prehospital cardiac arrest. *American Journal of Emergency Medicine* 22(2):90–93.

Vukov LF, White RD, Bachman JW, O'Brien PC. 1988. New perspectives on rural EMT defibrillation. *Annals of Emergency Medicine* 17(4):318–321.

Walker AF. 2002. The legal duty of physicians and hospitals to provide emergency care. *Canadian Medical Association Journal* 166(4):465–469.

Weiss SJ, Derlet R, Arndahl J, Ernst AA, Richards J, Fernandez-Frackelton M, Schwab R, Stair TO, Vicellio P, Levy D, Brautigan M, Johnson A, Nick TG, Fernandez-Frankelton M. 2004. Estimating the degree of emergency department overcrowding in academic medical centers: Results of the national ED overcrowding study (NEDOCS). *Academic Emergency Medicine* 11(1):38–50.

White-Means SI, Thornton MC. 1995. What cost savings could be realized by shifting patterns of use from hospital emergency rooms to primary care sites? *The American Economic Review* 85(2):138–142.

Williams JM, Chinnis AC, Gutman D. 2000. Health promotion practices of emergency physicians. *American Journal of Emergency Medicine* 18(1):17–21.

Williams JM, Ehrlich PF, Prescott JE. 2001. Emergency medical care in rural America. *Annals of Emergency Medicine* 38(3):323–327.

Williams RM. 1996. The costs of visits to emergency departments. *New England Journal of Medicine* 334(10):642–646.

Wright S, Moran L, Meyrick M, O'Connor R, Touquet R. 1998. Intervention by an alcohol health worker in an accident and emergency department. *Alcohol & Alcoholism* 33(6):651–656.

Young GP, Wagner MB, Kellermann AL, Ellis J, Bouley D. 1996. Ambulatory visits to hospital emergency departments. Patterns and reasons for use. 24 Hours in the ED Study Group. *Journal of the American Medical Association* 276(6):460–465.

3

Building a 21st-Century
Emergency Care System

Hospitals are part of a continuum of emergency care services that includes 9-1-1 and ambulance dispatch, prehospital emergency medical services (EMS) care and transport, hospital-based emergency and trauma care, and inpatient services. While today's emergency care system offers significantly more medical capability than was available in years past, it continues to suffer from severe fragmentation, an absence of systemwide coordination, and a lack of accountability. These shortcomings diminish the care provided to emergency patients and often result in worsened medical outcomes. To address these challenges and chart a new direction for emergency care, the committee envisions a system in which all communities will be served by well-planned and highly coordinated emergency care services that are accountable for performance and serve the needs of patients of all ages within the system.

In this new system, 9-1-1 dispatchers, EMS personnel, medical providers, public safety officers, and public health officials will be fully interconnected and united in an effort to ensure that each patient receives the most appropriate care, at the optimal location, with the minimum delay. From the patient's point of view, delivery of services for every type of emergency will be seamless. All service delivery will also be evidence based, and innovations will be rapidly adopted and adapted to each community's needs. Hospital emergency department (ED) closures and ambulance diversions will never occur, except in the most extreme situations, such as a hospital fire or a communitywide mass casualty event. Standby capacity appropriate to each community based on its disaster risks will be embedded in the system. The performance of the system will be transparent, and the public will be actively engaged in its operation through prevention, bystander training, and monitoring of system performance.

While these objectives will require substantial, systemwide change, they are achievable. Early progress toward the goal of more integrated, coordinated, regionalized emergency care systems became derailed over the last two decades. Efforts stalled because of deeply entrenched interests and cultural attitudes, as well as funding cutbacks and practical impediments to change. These obstacles remain today, and represent the primary challenges to achieving the committee's vision. However, the need for change is clear. The committee calls for concerted, cooperative efforts at multiple levels of government and the private sector to finally achieve the objectives outlined above.

This chapter describes the committee's vision for a 21st-century emergency care system. This vision rests on the broad goals of improved coordination, expanded regionalization, and increased transparency and accountability, each of which is discussed in turn. Next, current approaches of states and local regions that exhibit these features are profiled. The chapter then details the committee's recommendation for a federal demonstration program to support additional state and local efforts aimed at attaining the vision of a more coordinated and effective emergency care system. The chapter ends with a discussion of the need for system integration and a presentation of the committee's recommendation regarding a federal lead agency to meet that need.

THE GOAL OF COORDINATION

The value of integrating and coordinating emergency care has long been recognized. The 1996 National Academy of Sciences/National Research Council (NAS/NRC) report *Accidental Death and Disability* called for better coordination of emergency care through Community Councils on Emergency Medical Services that would bring together physicians, medical facilities, EMS, public health agencies, and others "to procure equipment, construct facilities and ensure optimal emergency care on a day-to-day basis as well as in a disaster or national emergency" (NAS and NRC, 1966, p. 7). The National Highway Traffic Safety Administration's (NHTSA) 1996 report *Emergency Medical Services Agenda for the Future* also emphasized the goal of system integration:

> EMS of the future will be community-based health management that is fully integrated with the overall health care system. It will have the ability to identify and modify illness and injury risks, provide acute illness and injury care and follow-up, and contribute to treatment of chronic conditions and community health monitoring. . . . [P]atients are assured that their care is considered part

of a complete health care program, connected to sources for continuous and/or follow-up care, and linked to potentially beneficial health resources. . . . EMS maintains liaisons, including systems for communication with other community resources, such as other public safety agencies, departments of public health, social service agencies and organizations, health care provider networks, community health educators, and others. . . . EMS is a community resource, able to initiate important follow-up care for patients, whether or not they are transported to a health care facility. (NHTSA, 1996, Pp. 7, 10)

In 1972, the NAS/NRC report *Roles and Responsibilities of Federal Agencies in Support of Comprehensive Emergency Medical Services* promoted an integrated, systems approach to planning at the state, regional, and local levels and called for the Department of Health, Education and Welfare (DHEW) to take an administrative and leadership role in federal EMS activities. The Emergency Medical Services Systems Act of 1973 (P.L. 93-154) created a new grant program in DHEW's Division of EMS to foster the development of regional EMS systems. The Robert Wood Johnson Foundation added support by funding the development of 44 regional EMS systems. Although the drive toward system development waned after the demise of the DHEW program and the subsequent absorption of federal EMS funding into federal block grants in 1981, the goals of system planning and coordination remained paramount within the emergency care community.

Limited Progress

While the concept of a highly integrated emergency care system as articulated in NHTSA's *Emergency Medical Services Agenda for the Future* is not new, progress toward its realization has been slow. Prehospital EMS, hospital-based emergency and trauma care, and public health have traditionally worked in silos (NHTSA, 1996), a situation that largely persists today. For example, public safety and EMS agencies often lack common communications frequencies and protocols for communicating with each other during emergencies. Jurisdictional borders contribute to fragmentation under the current system. For example, one county in Michigan has 18 different EMS systems with a range of different service models and protocols. Coordination of services across state lines is particularly challenging.

Trauma systems provide a valuable model for how such coordination could and should operate. The inclusive trauma system is meant to ensure that each patient is directed to the most appropriate setting, including a level I trauma center, when necessary. To this end, many elements within the regional system—community hospitals, trauma centers, and particularly prehospital EMS—must coordinate the regional flow of patients effectively. Such coordination not only improves patient care, but also is a critical tool in reducing overcrowding in EDs.

Unfortunately, only a handful of systems nationwide coordinate transport effectively throughout the region. Short of formally going on diversion, there is typically little information sharing between hospitals and EMS regarding overloaded emergency and trauma centers and availability of ED beds, operating suites, equipment, trauma surgeons, and critical specialists—information that could be used to balance the load among EDs and trauma centers in the region. Too often hospitals are located such that one is overloaded with emergency and trauma patients, while just several blocks away another works at a comfortable 50 percent of capacity. There is little incentive for ambulances to drive by a hospital to take patients to a facility that is less overloaded.

The benefits to patients of better regional coordination have been demonstrated. Furthermore, the technologies needed to facilitate such approaches exist; police and fire departments are ahead of the emergency care system in this regard. The main impediment appears to be entrenched interests and a lack of sufficient vision to change the current system.

The problem is intensified in some regions by turf wars between firefighters and EMS personnel that were documented in a series of articles for *USA Today* (Davis, 2003). Moreover, air medical services typically operate outside the control of the EMS system and have a poor record of safety and effectiveness in transporting patients. The situation is exacerbated in cities with both private and public EMS agencies that sometimes compete for patients and transport based on hospital ownership of the agency rather than what is best for the patient. Even within EDs, there may be friction between emergency staff trying to admit patients and personnel on inpatient units who have no incentive to speed up the admissions process. Lack of coordination between EMS and hospitals can result in delays that compromise care, and emergency physicians sometimes clash with on-call specialists and admitting physicians over delays in response.

Linkages with Public Health

The ED has a special relationship with the community and state and local public health departments because it serves as a community barometer of both illness and injury trends (Malone, 1995). In her analysis of heavy users of ED services, Malone argued that "emergency departments remain today a 'window' on wider social issues critical to health care reforms" (Malone, 1995, p. 469). A commonly cited example is the use of seat belts. We now know that increased use of seat belts reduces the number of seriously injured car crash victims in the ED—the ED served as a proving ground for documenting the results of seat belt enforcement initiatives. Although prevention activities have been limited in the emergency care setting, that setting represents an important teaching opportunity. To take advantage of that opportunity, emergency care providers would benefit from the resources and experiences of public health agencies and experts in the implementation of injury prevention measures.

Perhaps now more than ever, with the threat of bioterrorism and outbreaks of such diseases as avian influenza and severe acute respiratory syndrome (SARS), it is essential that EMS, EDs, trauma centers, and state and local public health agencies partner to conduct surveillance for disease prevalence and outbreaks and other health risks. Hospital EDs can recognize the diagnostic clues that may indicate an unusual infectious disease outbreak so that public health authorities can respond quickly (GAO, 2003c). However, a solid partnership must first be in place—one that allows for easy communication of information between emergency providers and public health officials.

Linkages with Other Medical Care Providers

As discussed earlier, EDs fill a variety of gaps within the health care network and serve as key safety net providers in many communities (Lewin and Altman, 2000). Studies have shown that a significant number of patients use the ED for nonurgent purposes because of financial barriers, lack of access to clinics after hours, transportation barriers, convenience, and lack of a usual source of care (Grumbach et al., 1993; Young et al., 1996; Peterson et al., 1998; Koziol-McLain et al., 2000; Cunningham and May, 2003) (see Chapter 2). There is also evidence that clinics and physicians are increasingly using EDs as an adjunct to their practice, referring patients to the ED for a variety of reasons, such as their own convenience after regular hours, reluctance to take on a complicated case, the need for diagnostic tests they cannot perform in the office, and liability concerns (Berenson et al., 2003; Studdert et al., 2005). (See the detailed discussion of these issues in Chapter 2.) Unfortunately, in many communities there is little interaction between emergency care services and community safety net providers—this even though they share a common base of patients, and their actions may affect one another substantially. The absence of coordination represents missed opportunities for enhanced access; improved diagnosis, patient follow-up, and adherence to treatment; and enhanced quality of care and patient satisfaction.

Successes Achieved

While progress toward a highly integrated emergency care system has been slow, some important successes in the coordination of emergency care services point the way toward solutions to the fragmentation that dominates the system today. For example, the trauma system in Maryland, described in more detail later in this chapter, provides a comprehensive and coordinated approach to the care of injured children. Children's hospitals have also been successful in accomplishing regional coordination to ensure the transport and appropriate care of children needing specialized services. The pediatric intensive care system is a leading example of regional coordination among hospitals, community physicians, and emergency medical technicians (EMTs) (Gausche-Hill and Wiebe, 2001). These are but a few examples demonstrating the possibilities for enhancing coordination of the system as a whole.

One promising public health surveillance effort is Insight, a computer-based clinical information system at the Washington Hospital Center (WHC) in Washington, D.C., designed to record and track patient data, including geographic and demographic information. The software proved useful during the 2001 anthrax attacks, when it enabled WHC to transmit complete, real-time data to the Centers for Disease Control and Prevention (CDC) while other hospitals were sending limited information with a lag time of one or more days. The success of Insight attracted considerable grant funding for the system's expansion; WHC earmarked $7 million for the system to link it to federal and regional agencies and to integrate it with other hospital systems (Kanter and Heskett, 2002).

Many communities have established primary care networks that integrate hospital EDs into their planning and coordination efforts. A rapidly growing number of communities, such as San Francisco and Boston, have developed regional health information organizations that coordinate the development of information systems to facilitate patient referrals and track the sharing of medical information between providers to optimize a patient's care across settings. The San Francisco Community Clinic Consortium brings together primary and specialty care providers and EDs in a planning and communications network that closely coordinates the care of safety net patients throughout the city.

The Importance of Communications

Communications are a critical factor in establishing systemwide coordination. An effective communications system is the glue that can hold together effective, integrated emergency care services. It provides the key link between 9-1-1/dispatch and EMS responders and is necessary to ensure that on-line medical direction is available when needed. It enables ambulance dispatchers to tell callers what to do until help arrives and to track a patient's progress following the arrival of EMS responders. An effective communications system also enables ambulance dispatchers to assist EMS personnel in directing patients to the most appropriate facility based on the nature of their illness or injury and the capacity of receiving facilities. It links the emergency medical system with other public safety providers—such as police and fire departments, emergency management services, and public health agencies—and facilitates coordination between the medical response system and incident command in both routine and disaster situations. It helps hospitals communicate with each other to organize interfacility transfers and arrange for mutual aid. And it facilitates medical and operational oversight and quality control within the system.

THE GOAL OF REGIONALIZATION

The objective of regionalization is to improve patient outcomes by directing patients to facilities with optimal capabilities for any given type of illness or injury. Substantial evidence demonstrates that doing so improves outcomes and reduces costs across a range of high-risk conditions and procedures, including cardiac arrest and stroke (Grumbach et al., 1995; Imperato et al., 1996; Nallamothu et al., 2001; Chang and Klitzner, 2002; Bardach et al., 2004). The literature also supports the benefits of regionalization for severely injured patients in improving patient outcomes and lowering costs (Jurkovich and Mock, 1999; Mann et al., 1999; Mullins and Mann, 1999; Chiara and Cimbanassi, 2003; Bravata et al., 2004; MacKenzie et al., 2006), although the evidence in this regard is not uniformly positive (Glance et al., 2004). MacKenzie and colleagues (2006) have provided the strongest evidence to date for the benefits of such regionalized trauma systems. In their study, mortality among patients receiving trauma center and comparable non–trauma center care in 14 states was compared after adjustment for differences in case mix. Mortality among patients with serious injuries was significantly lower at trauma centers. Other studies have likewise documented the value of regionalized trauma systems in improving outcomes and reducing mortality from traumatic injury (Jurkovich and Mock, 1999; MacKenzie, 1999; Mullins, 1999; Nathens et al., 2000). Organized trauma systems have also been shown to add value in facilitating performance measurement and promoting research. Formal protocols within a region for prehospital and hospital care contribute to improved patient outcomes as well (Bravata et al., 2004).

While regionalization to distribute trauma services to high-volume centers is optimal when feasible in terms of transport, Nathens and Maier (2001) argued for an inclusive trauma system in which smaller facilities have been verified and designated as lower-level trauma centers. They suggested that care may be substantially better in such facilities than in those outside the system, and comparable to national norms (Nathens and Maier, 2001). An inclusive trauma system addresses the needs of all injured patients across the entire continuum of care and utilizes the resources of all committed and qualified personnel and facilities, with the goal of ensuring that every injured patient is triaged expeditiously to a level of care commensurate with his or her injuries.

Research has demonstrated a number of additional benefits of regionalization. Regionalizing inventories (pooling supplies at regional warehouses) has been shown to reduce inventories, improve the capacity to serve the target population, and save money. Regionalization may also be a cost-effective strategy for developing and training teams of response personnel. Regionalization benefits outbreak investigations, security management, and emergency management as well. Both the Health Resources and Services Administration (HRSA) and CDC have made regional planning a condition for preparedness funding (GAO, 2003a).

Concerns About Regionalization

Not all aspects of regionalization are positive. If not properly implemented, regionalizing key clinical services may adversely impact their overall availability in a community. For example, regional allocation of patients with suspected acute myocardial infarction could result in the closure of a cardiac unit or even an entire hospital, particularly in rural areas. The survival of small rural facilities may require identification and treatment of those illnesses and injuries that do not require the capacities and capabilities of larger facilities, as well as repatriation to the local facility for long-term care and follow-up after stabilization at the tertiary center. A systems approach to regionalization considers the full effects of regionalizing services on a community. Determining the appropriate metrics for this type of analysis and defining the process for applying them within each region are significant research and practical issues. Nonetheless, in the absence of rigorous evidence to guide the process, planning authorities should take these factors into account in developing regionalized systems of emergency care.

The committee believes communities will best be served by emergency care systems in which services are organized so as to provide the optimal care based on the patient's location and condition. To the extent that the movement toward specialty hospitals impacts the configuration of services and therefore the ability of the system to optimize emergency services, it is an appropriate subject for the committee to address. While the committee does not advocate for or against the further development of specialty hospitals, it does believe that their development would potentially impact emergency care and that this impact, which in some cases could be adverse, should be considered in the regionalization of emergency care. Specialty hospitals that do not provide emergency care can drain financial resources from those that do (GAO, 2003b; Dummit, 2005). Also, specialty hospitals present an attractive option for some specialists, potentially luring them away from the medical staffs of general hospitals. In such cases, general hospitals may be forced to subsidize specialists, or recruit new ones, to remain compliant with the Emergency Medical Treatment and Active Labor Act (EMTALA) (Asplin and Knopp, 2001; Iglehart, 2005; Johnson et al., 2001). Specialty hospitals may also siphon commercially insured patients away from general hospitals while retaining the option of sending their sickest patients to the nearest general hospital ED.

Despite these problems, the movement toward specialty hospitals is gathering strength. The number of ambulatory surgery centers increased by about 6 percent per year between 1997 and 2003, to a total of 3,735 recorded nationally in 2003; the number of specialty hospitals increased by approximately 20 percent per year between 1997 and 2003, to a total of 113 in 2003 (Iglehart, 2005). In December 2003, Congress declared an 18-month moratorium on the development of new specialty hospitals partly owned by physicians who refer their patients to those facilities. Federal agencies were directed to study these facilities and recommend an extension of the moratorium or a new policy. The moratorium expired in 2005, but the Centers for Medicare and Medicaid Services (CMS) is studying how to revise its payment rates and procedures for approving specialty hospitals.

Configuration of Services

The design of the emergency care system envisioned by the committee bears similarities to the inclusive trauma system concept originally conceived and first proposed and developed by CDC, and adapted and disseminated by the American College of Surgeons. Under this approach, every hospital in the community can play a role in the trauma system by undergoing verification and designation as a level I to level IV/V trauma center, based on its capabilities. Trauma care is optimized in the region through protocols and transfer agreements that are designed to direct trauma patients to the most appropriate level of care available given the type of injury and relative travel times to each center.

The committee's vision expands this concept beyond trauma care to include all serious illnesses and injuries, and extends beyond hospitals to include the entire continuum of emergency care—including 9-1-1 and dispatch and prehospital EMS, as well as clinics and urgent care providers. In this model, every provider organization can potentially play a role in providing emergency care services according to its capabilities. Provider organizations undergo a process by which their capabilities are identified and categorized in a manner not unlike trauma verification and designation, which results in a complete inventory of emergency care provider organizations within a community. Initially, this categorization may simply be based on the existence of a service—for example, capacity to achieve cardiac reperfusion or perform emergency neurosurgery. Over time, the categorization process may evolve to include more detailed information, such as the times specific emergency procedures are available; the arrangements for on-call specialty care; service-specific outcomes; or general emergency service indicators, such as time to treatment, frequency of diversion, and ED boarding. Prehospital EMS services are similarly categorized according to ambulance capacity; availability; credentials of EMS providers; advanced life support (ALS) and pediatric advanced life support (PALS); treat and release and search and rescue capabilities; disaster readiness (e.g., extrication capability and personal protective equipment); and outcomes for sentinel indicators, such as out-of-hospital cardiac arrest.

A standard national approach to the categorization of emergency care providers is needed. Categories should reflect meaningful differences in the types of emergency care available, yet be simple enough to be understood easily by emergency care organizations and the public at large. The use of national definitions would ensure that the categories would be understood by providers and by the public across states or regions of the country, and would also promote benchmarking of performance.

The committee concludes that a standard national approach to the categorization of emergency care, defined in the broadest possible sense, is essential for the optimal allocation of resources and provision of critical information to an informed public. Therefore the committee recommends that **the Department of Health and Human Services and the National Highway Traffic Safety Administration, in partnership with professional organizations, convene a panel of individuals with multidisciplinary expertise to develop evidence-based categorization systems for emergency medical services, emergency departments, and trauma centers based on adult and pediatric service capabilities (3.1).** The results of this process would be a complete inventory of emergency care assets for each community, which should be updated regularly to reflect the rapid changes in delivery systems nationwide. The development of the initial categorization system should be completed within 18 months of the release of this report.

Treatment, Triage, and Transport

Once the basic classification system proposed above is understood, it can be used to determine the optimal destination for patients based on their condition and location. However, more research and discussion are needed to determine the circumstances under which patients should be brought to the closest hospital for stabilization and transfer as opposed to being transported directly to the facility offering the highest level of care, even if that facility is farther away. A debate remains over whether EMS providers should perform ALS procedures in the field, or rapid transport to definitive care is best (Wright and Klein, 2001). It is likely that this answer depends, at least in part, on the type of emergency condition. It is evident, for example, that whether a patient will survive out-of-hospital cardiac arrest depends almost entirely on actions taken at the scene, including rapid defibrillation, provision of cardiopulmonary resuscitation (CPR), and perhaps other ALS interventions. Delaying these actions until the unit reaches a hospital results in dismal rates of survival and poor neurological outcomes. Conversely, there is little that prehospital personnel can do to stop internal bleeding from major trauma. In this instance, rapid transport to definitive care in an operating room offers the victim the best odds of survival. For example, a recent study showed that bypassing a level II trauma center in favor of a more distant level I trauma center may be optimal for head trauma patients (McConnell et al., 2005).

EMS responders who provide stabilization before the patient arrives at a critical care unit are sometimes subject to criticism because of a strongly held bias among many physicians that out-of-hospital stabilization only delays definitive treatment without adding value; however, there is little evidence that the prevailing "scoop and run" paradigm of EMS is always optimal (Orr et al., 2006). For example, in cases of out-of-hospital cardiac arrest, properly trained and equipped EMS personnel can provide all needed interventions at the scene. In fact, research has shown that failure to reestablish a pulse on the scene virtually ensures that the patient will not survive, regardless of what is done at the hospital (Kellermann et al., 1993). On the other hand, a scoop and run approach makes sense when a critical intervention needed by the patient can be provided only at the hospital (for example, surgery to control internal bleeding).

Decisions regarding the appropriate steps to take should be resolved using the best available evidence. The committee concludes that there should be a national approach to the development of prehospital protocols. It therefore recommends that **the National Highway Traffic Safety Administration, in partnership with professional organizations, convene a panel of individuals with multidisciplinary expertise to develop evidence-based model prehospital care protocols for the treatment, triage, and transport of patients (3.2).** The transport protocols should also reflect the state of readiness of given facilities within a region at a particular point in time. Real-time, concurrent information on the availability of hospital resources and specialists should be made available to EMS providers to support transport decisions. Development of an initial set of model protocols should be completed within 18 months of the release of this report. Treatments may require modification to reflect local resources, capabilities, and transport times; however, the basic pathophysiology of human illness is the same in all areas of the country. Once in place, the national protocols could be tailored to local assets and needs. The process for updating the protocols will also be important because it will dictate how rapidly patients receive the current standard of care.

The 1966 report *Accidental Death and Disability* anticipated the need to categorize care facilities and improve transport decisions:

> The patient must be transported to the emergency department best prepared for his particular problem. . . . Hospital emergency departments should be surveyed . . . to determine the numbers and types of emergency facilities necessary to provide optimal emergency treatment for the occupants of each region. . . . Once the required numbers and types of treatment facilities have been determined, it may be necessary to lessen the requirements at some institutions, increase them in others, and even redistribute resources to support space, equipment, and personnel in the major emergency facilities. Until patient, ambulance driver, and hospital staff are in accord as to what the patient might reasonably expect and what the staff of an emergency facility can logically be expected to administer, and until effective transportation and adequate communication are provided to deliver casualties to proper facilities, our present levels of knowledge cannot be applied to optimal care and little reduction in mortality and/or lasting disability can be expected. (NAS and NRC, 1966, P. 20)

This concept was echoed in the 1993 Institute of Medicine (IOM) report *Emergency Medical Services for Children*, which stated that "categorization and regionalization are essential for full and effective operation of systems" (IOM, 1993, p. 171).

Once the decision has been made to transport a patient, the responding ambulance unit should be instructed—either by written protocol or by on-line medical direction—which hospital should receive the patient. This instruction should be based on developed transport protocols to ensure that the patient is taken to the optimal facility given the severity and nature of the illness or injury, the status of the various care facilities, and the travel times involved. Ideally, this decision will take into account a number of complex and fluctuating factors, such as hospital ED closures and diversions and traffic congestion that hinders transport times for the EMS unit (The SAFECOM Project, 2004). Some potential transport options in a coordinated, regionalized system are depicted in Figure 3-1.

In addition to the use of ambulance units and the EMS system to direct patients to the optimum location for emergency care, hospital emergency care designations should be posted prominently to improve patients' self-triage decisions. Such postings can educate the public about the types of emergency services available in their community and enable patients who are not using EMS to direct themselves to the optimal facility.

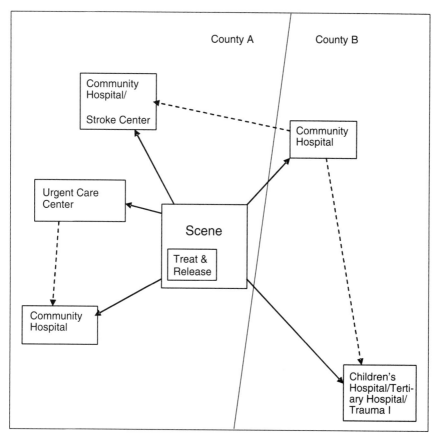

FIGURE 3-1 Potential transport options within a coordinated, regionalized system. The basic structure of current EMS systems is not altered, but protocols are refined to ensure that patients go to the optimal facility given the type of illness or injury, the travel time involved, and facility status (e.g., ED and intensive care unit [ICU] bed availability). For example, instead of taking a stroke victim to the closest general community hospital or to a tertiary medical center that is farther away, there may be a third option—transport to a community hospital with a stroke center. Over time, based on evidence on the effectiveness of alternative delivery models, some patients may be transported to a nearby urgent care center for stabilization or treated on the street and released. Whichever pathway the patient follows, communications are enhanced, data are collected, and the performance of the system is evaluated and reported so that future improvements can be made.

THE GOAL OF ACCOUNTABILITY

Accountability is perhaps the most important of the three goals of the emergency care system envisioned by the committee because it is necessary to achieving the other two. Lack of accountability has contributed to the failure of the emergency care system to adopt needed changes in the past. Without accountability, participants in the system need not accept responsibility for failure and can avoid making changes necessary to avoid the same outcomes in the future.

Accountability is difficult to establish in emergency care because responsibility is dispersed across many different components of the system; thus it is difficult for policy makers to determine when and where breakdowns occur and how they can be prevented in the future. Ambulance diversion is a good example. Because diversion statistics are rarely published or announced, the problem is likely to remain outside the public eye. When a city finally recognizes it has an unacceptably high frequency of diversion, whom should it hold accountable? EMS can blame the hospitals for crowded conditions and excessively long offload times; hospitals can blame the on-call specialists or the discharge sites that are unwilling to take additional referrals; and everyone can blame the public health department for inadequate funding of community-based clinics.

The unpredictable and infrequent nature of emergency care contributes to the lack of accountability. Most people have limited exposure to the emergency care system—for most Americans, an ambulance call or a visit to the ED is a relatively rare event. Further, public awareness is hindered by the lack of nationally defined indicators of system performance. Few localities can answer basic questions about their emergency care services, such as "What is the overall performance of the emergency care system?"; "How well do 9-1-1, ambulance services, hospital emergency and trauma care, and other components of the system perform?"; and "How does performance compare with that in other parts of the state and the country?" Consequently, few understand the crisis presently facing the system. By and large, the public assumes that the system functions better than it does (Harris Interactive, 2004).

The committee believes several steps are required to bring accountability to the emergency care system. These include the development of national performance indicators, implementation of performance measurement, and public dissemination of performance information.

Development of National Performance Indicators

There is currently no shortage of performance measurement and standards-setting projects. For example, ED performance measures have been developed by Qualis Health and Lindsay (Lindsay et al., 2002). In addition, the Data Elements for Emergency Department Systems (DEEDS) project and Health Level Seven (HL7) are working to develop uniform specifications for ED performance data (Pollock et al., 1998; Centers for Disease Control and Prevention and National Center for Injury Control and Prevention, 2001).

The EMS Performance Measures Project is working to develop consensus measures of EMS system performance that will assist in demonstrating the system's value and defining an adequate level of EMS service and preparedness for a given community (measureEMS.org, 2005). The consensus process of the project has sought to unify disparate efforts to measure performance previously undertaken nationwide that have lacked consistency in definitions, indicators, and data sources. In 2004, the project developed 138 indicators of EMS performance, which were pared down to 25 indicators in 2005. The list included system measures, such as "What are the time intervals in a call?" and "What percentage of transports is conducted with red lights and sirens?", and clinical measures, such as "How well was my pain relieved?" The questions were defined using data elements from the National EMS Information System (NEMSIS) dataset so that results could be compared with validity across EMS systems. The EMS Performance Measures Project is coordinated by the National Association of State EMS Officials in partnership with the National Association of EMS Physicians and is supported by NHTSA and HRSA. CDC, the Association of American Medical Colleges, and Emory University are currently developing a simple cardiac arrest registry that will allow communities across the United States to determine their rate of successful resuscitations and identify opportunities for improvement.

In addition, statewide trauma systems and EMS systems have been evaluated by the American College of Surgeons' Committee on Trauma; NHTSA's Office of EMS; and, until it was recently defunded, HRSA's Division of Trauma and EMS Systems. There are also various components of the system with independent accrediting bodies. Hospitals, for example, are accredited by the Joint Commission on Accreditation of Healthcare Organizations (JCAHO); ambulance services are accredited by the Commission on Accreditation of Ambulance Services; and air medical services are voluntarily accredited by the Commission on Accreditation of Medical Transport Systems. Each of these organizations collects performance information.

What is missing is a standard set of measures that can be used to assess the performance of the full emergency care system within each community, as well as the ability to benchmark that performance against statewide and national performance metrics. A credible entity to develop such measures would not be strongly tied to any one component of the emergency care continuum.

One approach would be to form a collaborative entity that would include representation from all of the system components, including hospitals, trauma centers, EMS agencies, physicians, nurses, and others. Another approach would be to work with an existing organization, such as the National Quality Forum (NQF), to develop a set of emergency care–specific measures. NQF grew out of the President's Advisory Commission on Consumer Protection and Quality in the Health Care Industry in 1998. It operates as a not-for-profit membership organization made up of national, state, regional, and local groups representing consumers, public and private purchasers, employers, health care professionals, provider organizations, health plans, accrediting bodies, labor unions, supporting industries, and organizations involved in health care research or quality improvement. NQF has reviewed and endorsed measure sets applicable to several health care settings and clinical areas and services, including hospital care, home health care, nursing-sensitive care, nursing home care, cardiac surgery, and diabetes care (NQF, 2002, 2003, 2004, 2005).

The committee concludes that a standard national approach to the development of performance indictors is essential, and therefore recommends that **the Department of Health and Human Services convene a panel of individuals with emergency and trauma care expertise to develop evidence-based indicators of emergency and trauma care system performance (3.3).** This should be an independent, national process with the broad participation of every component of emergency care, and with the federal government playing a lead role in its promotion and funding. The development of the initial set of performance indicators should be completed within 18 months of the release of this report.

The measures developed should include structure and process measures, but evolve toward outcome measures over time. They should be nationally standardized so that comparisons can be made across regions and states. Measures should evaluate the performance of individual providers within the system, as well as that of the system as a whole. Measures should also be sensitive to the interdependence among the components of the system; for example, EMS response times may be adversely affected by ED diversions.

Furthermore, because an episode of emergency care can span multiple settings, each of which can have a significant impact on the final outcome, it is important that patient-level data from each setting be captured and combined. Currently it is difficult to piece together a complete picture of an episode of emergency care. To address this need, states should develop guidelines for the sharing of patient-level data from dispatch through post–hospital release. The federal government should support such efforts by sponsoring the development of model procedures that can be adopted by states to minimize their administrative costs and liability exposure as a result of sharing these data.

Measurement of Performance

Performance data should be collected on a regular basis from all of the emergency care providers in a community. Over time, emerging technologies may support more simplified and streamlined data collection methods, such as wireless transmission of clinical data and direct links to patient electronic health records. However, these types of technical upgrades would likely require federal financial support, and EMS personnel would have to be persuaded to transition from paper-based run records, which are less amenable to efficient performance measurement. The data collected should be tabulated in ways that can be used to measure, report on, and benchmark system performance, generating information useful for ongoing feedback and process improvement. Using their regulatory authority over health care services, states should play a lead role in collecting and analyzing these performance data.

While a full-blown data collection and performance measurement and reporting system is the desired ultimate outcome, the committee believes a handful of key indicators of regional system performance should be collected and promulgated as soon as possible. These could include, for example, indicators of 9-1-1 call processing times, EMS response times for critical calls, and ambulance diversions. In addition, consensus measurement of EMS outcomes could be applied to two to three sentinel conditions. For example, emergency care systems across the country might be tasked with providing data on such conditions as cardiac arrest (see Box 3-1), pediatric respiratory arrest, and major blunt trauma with shock. Data from the different system components would allow researchers to measure how well the system performs at each level of care (9-1-1, first response, EMS, and ED). In addition, registries could provide a rich source of data for use in research and identification of trends.

Public Dissemination of Information on System Performance

Public dissemination of performance data is crucial to drive the needed changes in the delivery of emergency care services. Dissemination could take various forms, including public report cards, annual reports, and state public health reports, which could be viewed either in hard copy format or on line. A key to success would be ensuring that important information regarding the performance of the community's emergency care system could be retrieved by the public with a minimum of effort in a format that was highly organized and visually compelling.

Public dissemination of health care information is still in a state of development, despite the proliferation of such initiatives over the past two decades. Problems include the costs associated with data collection, the sensitivity of individual provider information, concerns about interpretation

---

BOX 3-1
Cardiac Arrest Registry to Enhance Survival

A new 18-month initiative funded by the Centers for Disease Control and Prevention (CDC) is under way in Fulton County, Georgia. Cardiac Arrest Registry to Enhance Survival (CARES) is intended to develop a prototype national registry to help local EMS administrators and medical directors identify when and where cardiac arrest occurs, which elements of their EMS system are functioning properly in dealing with these cases, and what changes can be made to improve outcomes. The initiative is engaging Atlanta-area 9-1-1, EMS and first responder services, and EDs in systematically collecting minimum data essential to improving survival in cases of cardiac arrest and submitting these data to the registry. Area hospitals log on to a simple, Health Insurance Portability and Accountability Act (HIPAA)-compliant website to report each patient's outcome. Data compilation and analysis are conducted by researchers at Emory University. Using information gathered from the CARES registry, a community consortium organized by the American Heart Association (AHA) will orchestrate various community interventions to reduce disparities and improve outcomes among victims of cardiac arrest. CARES is designed to enable cities across the country to collect similar data quickly and easily, and use these data to improve cardiac arrest treatment and outcomes.

Sudden cardiac arrest results from an abrupt loss of heart function and is the leading cause of death among adults in the United States. Its onset is unexpected, and death occurs minutes after symptoms develop (AHA, 2005). Survival rates in the event of sudden cardiac arrest are low, but vary as much as 10-fold across communities. Victims' chances of survival increase with early activation of 9-1-1 and prompt handling of the call, early provision of bystander cardiopulmonary resuscitation (CPR), rapid defibrillation, and early access to definitive care. CARES is designed to allow communities to measure each link in their "chain of survival" quickly and easily and use this information to save more lives.

---

of data by the public, and lack of public interest. There are many examples from which to learn—the Health Plan Employer Data and Information Set (HEDIS), which reports on managed care plans to purchasers and consumers; CMS's reports on home health and nursing home care—the *Home Health Compare* and *Nursing Home Compare* websites, respectively (CMS, 2005a); and *Hospital Compare* from the Hospital Quality Alliance, which reports comparative quality data on hospitals (CMS, 2005b). A number of states and regional business coalitions have also developed report cards on managed care plans and hospitals (State of California Office of the Patient Advocate, 2005). Because of the unique status of the emergency care system as an essential public service and the public's limited awareness of the significant problems facing the system, the public is likely to take an active interest in this information. The committee believes dissemination of these data would have an important impact on public awareness and the development of integrated regional systems.

Public reporting can be at a detailed or aggregate level. Because of the potential sensitivity of performance data, they should initially be reported in the aggregate at the national, state, and regional levels rather than at the level of the individual provider. Prematurely reporting provider performance data could inhibit participation and divert providers' resources to public relations rather than corrective efforts. At the same time, however, individual providers should have full access to their own data so they can understand and improve their individual performance, as well as their contribution to the overall system. Over time, information on individual provider organizations should become an important part of the public information on the system. Eventually, the data may be used to drive performance-based payment for emergency care.

Approaches for Reducing Barriers to Implementation

Institutional barriers to the adoption of integrated, regionalized care exist. These include payment systems and the legal framework that defines much of the structure of emergency care delivery.

Aligning Payments with Incentives

No major change in health care can take place without strong financial incentives. The way emergency care services are reimbursed reinforces certain modes of delivery that are inefficient and stand in the way of achieving the committee's vision of emergency care. For example, under Medicare and Medicaid, prehospital providers do not receive payment unless they transport a patient to the hospital. This payment system makes it difficult for regional systems to implement treat and release or other innovative nontransport approaches that could result in better care for patients and more efficient system design. CMS and all other payers should eliminate this requirement and develop a payment system for prehospital care that reflects the costs of providing those services.

Similarly, many hospitals do not have a strong economic motivation to address the problems of ED crowding, boarding, and ambulance diversion. In fact, these practices may even benefit them financially. Several payment approaches could eliminate incentives that degrade emergency care. One is to eliminate the discrepancies in reimbursement between scheduled and ED admissions that relate to differences in both payer mix and severity of illness. CMS should evaluate the effect of existing Diagnosis-Related Group (DRG) payments for elective admissions as opposed to patients admitted from the ED. For example, DRG payments could be adjusted to reflect the average costs of scheduled surgical admissions versus ED medical admissions at safety net hospitals. Care would have to be exercised to ensure that this did not result in physicians simply admitting their elective patients through the ED. Another method is to assess direct financial rewards or penalties for hospitals based on their management of patient throughput. Through its purchaser and regulatory power, CMS has the ability to drive hospitals to address and manage patient flow and ensure timely access to quality care for its clients. All payers, including Medicare, Medicaid, and private insurers, could also develop contracts that would penalize hospitals for chronic delays in treatment, ED crowding, and EMS diversions. One strategy would be to refuse to pay for inpatient care unless it was provided in a designated inpatient unit. CMS and JCAHO should lead the way in the development of innovative payment approaches that can accomplish these objectives. All payers should be encouraged to do the same. States with strong certificate of need (CON) laws could include boarding and diversion as criteria in CON decisions.

Adapting the Legal and Regulatory Framework

The way hospitals and EMS agencies deliver emergency care is shaped largely by federal and state laws—in particular, EMTALA, the Health Insurance Portability and Accountability Act (HIPAA), and medical malpractice laws. The application of these laws to the actual provision of care is guided by regulatory rules and advisories, enforcement decisions, and court decisions, as well as by providers' understanding of these. EMTALA and HIPAA are discussed below, and medical malpractice in Chapter 6.

EMTALA was passed in 1986 to prevent hospitals from refusing to serve uninsured patients and "dumping" them on other hospitals. EMTALA established a mandate for hospitals and physicians who provide emergency and trauma care to provide a medical screening exam to all patients and appropriately stabilize patients or transfer them to an appropriate facility if an emergency medical condition exists (GAO, 2001). This requirement applies regardless of patients' ability to pay. This aspect of EMTALA and its impact on the availability of EDs, trauma centers, and on-call specialists are described in Chapter 2.

EMTALA also has implications for the regional coordination of care. The act was written to provide individual patient protections—it focuses on the obligations of an individual hospital to an individual patient (Rosenbaum and Kamoie, 2003). The statute is not clearly adaptable to a highly integrated regional emergency care system in which the optimal care of patients may diverge from conventional patterns of emergency treatment and transport.

Until recently, EMTALA appeared to hinder the regional coordination of services in several specific ways—for example, requiring a hospital-owned ambulance to transport a patient to the parent hospital even if it is not the optimal destination for that patient; requiring a hospital to interrupt the transfer to administer a medical screening exam for a patient being transferred from ground transport to helicopter and using the hospital's helipad; and limiting the ability of hospitals to direct nonemergent patients who enter the ED to an appropriate and readily available ambulatory care setting. Interim guidance published by CMS in 2003, however, appeared to mitigate these problems (DHHS, 2003). This guidance established, for example, that a patient visiting an off-campus hospital site that does not normally provide emergency care does not create an EMTALA obligation, that a hospital-owned ambulance need not return the patient to the parent hospital if it is operating under the authority of a communitywide EMS protocol, and that hospitals are not obligated to provide treatment for clearly nonemergency situations as determined by qualified medical personnel. Further, hospitals involved in disasters need not adhere strictly to EMTALA if operating under a community disaster plan. Despite these changes, however, uncertainty surrounding the interpretation and enforcement of EMTALA remains a damper on the development of coordinated, integrated emergency care systems.

In 2005, CMS convened a technical advisory group to study EMTALA and address additional needed changes (CMS 2005a,b,c). To date, the advisory group has focused on incremental modifications to the act.

While the recent CMS guidance and deliberations of the EMTALA advisory group are positive steps, the committee envisions a more fundamental rethinking of the act that would support and facilitate the development of regionalized emergency systems rather than simply addressing each obstacle on a piecemeal basis. The new EMTALA would continue to protect patients from discrimination in treatment while enabling and encouraging communities to test innovations in the design of emergency care systems, such as direct transport of patients to non–acute care facilities—dialysis centers and ambulatory care clinics, for example—when appropriate.

HIPAA was enacted to facilitate electronic transmission of data between providers and payers while protecting the privacy of patient health information. In protecting patient confidentiality, HIPAA can present certain challenges for providers, such as making it more complicated for a physician to send information about a patient to another physician for a consultation.

Regional coordination is based on the seamless delivery of care across multiple provider settings. Patient-specific information must flow freely between these settings—from dispatch to emergency response to hospital care—to ensure that appropriate information will be available for clinical decision making and coordination of services in emergency situations. Current interpretations of HIPAA would make it difficult to achieve the required degree of information fluidity.

Both EMTALA and HIPAA protect patients from potential abuses and serve invaluable purposes. As written and frequently interpreted, however, they can impede the exchange of lifesaving information and hinder the development of regional systems. The committee believes appropriate modifications could be made to both acts that would preserve their original purpose while reducing their adverse impact on the development of regional systems. The committee recommends that **the Department of Health and Human Services adopt regulatory changes to the Emergency Medical Treatment and Active Labor Act and the Health Insurance Portability and Accountability Act so that the original goals of the laws will be preserved, but integrated systems can be further developed (3.4).**

CURRENT APPROACHES

A number of current efforts to establish emergency care systems achieve some or all of the committee's goals of coordination, regionalization, and accountability. Some are purely voluntary, while others have the force of state regulation. Some are local and regional in scope, while others are statewide or national. This section highlights several such efforts that provide insights for future initiatives.

The Maryland EMS and Trauma System

Maryland has a unique statewide system that coordinates all EMS and trauma activity throughout the state. The Maryland Institute for EMS Systems (MIEMSS) is an independent state agency governed by an 11-member board that is appointed by the governor. The system provides training and certification, has established statewide EMS protocols, coordinates care through a central communications center, and operates the air medical system in coordination with the Maryland State Police. The system is funded in part through a surcharge on state driver's license fees.

Coordination

The key to coordination in Maryland is the statewide communications center, which coordinates all communications between EMS and other components of the system. The center links ambulances, helicopters, and hospitals and enables direct communications between components at any time. For example, a paramedic in western Maryland can talk directly with a local ED physician or obtain on-line consultation with a specialty hospital in Baltimore. While the local 9-1-1 centers initiate dispatch, they are usually too busy to follow patients through the continuum of care. The statewide communications center provides support by maintaining communications links, providing medical direction, and maintaining continuity of care. The center has direct links to incident command to facilitate management of EMS resources as an event unfolds.

The state also is developing a new wireless digital capability that will connect EMS with other public safety entities (police, fire, emergency management, public health) throughout the state. In addition, the state has developed a County Hospital Alert Tracking System (CHATS) to monitor the status of hospitals and EMS assets so ambulances can be directed to less crowded facilities. This capability can also be applied to individual services—for example, patients with acute coronary syndrome can be directed to facilities based on the current availability of reperfusion suites. The Facility Resource Emergency Database system was designed to gather detailed information electronically from hospitals on bed availability, staffing, medications, and other critical capacity issues during disasters, but is also used to monitor and report on system capacity issues on a regular basis.

The state ensures coordination and compliance with protocols through its statewide training, provider designation, and licensure functions. In addition to providing EMS training and certification, the system offers statewide disaster preparedness training for members of the National Disaster Medical System.

Regionalization

While EMS and 9-1-1 are operated locally, they utilize statewide protocols that promote regionalization of services to designated centers. In addition to multiple trauma levels, these centers are designated for stroke, burn, eye, pediatric, perinatal, and hand referrals. A relatively new stroke protocol, for example, designates regional stroke care centers according to three levels: level I provides comprehensive stroke care; level II initial emergency management, including fibrinolytic therapy; and level 3 screening and immediate transport to a level I or II center. There is also a designated center for the injury of hands, a common form of trauma that requires specialized expertise, within a non–trauma center. The control of air medical services by the state facilitates the regionalization of care through the active operation of dispatch.

Accountability

The state monitors performance at the provider and system levels through a provider review panel that regularly evaluates the operation of the system. As a state agency, the system reports on its performance goals and improvements. Also, CHATS enables participating hospitals and the public to view the status of hospitals at all times through its website, including data on availability of cardiac monitor beds, ED beds, and trauma beds. Paper ambulance run sheets are being replaced with an electronic system so that data can be collected and analyzed quickly to facilitate real-time performance improvement.

Conclusion

While Maryland is relatively advanced in achieving the goals of coordination, regionalization, and accountability, it is not clear how easily its system could be replicated in other states. The system has benefited from strong and stable leadership in the state office, adequate funding, a high concentration of resources, and limited geography—features that many states do not currently enjoy.

Austin/Travis County, Texas

Austin/Travis County and four surrounding counties agreed to form a single EMS and trauma system to provide seamless care to emergency and trauma patients throughout the region. The initiative, 10 years in the making, started with a fragmented delivery system consisting of the Austin EMS system, 13 separate fire departments, and a 9-1-1 service run through the sheriff's office that lacked any unified protocols. These different entities agreed to come together to form a unified system that would coordinate all emergency care within the region. The system operates through a Combined Clinical Council that includes representatives of the different agencies and providers within the geographic area, including fire departments, 9-1-1, EMS, air medical services, and corporate employers. This is a "third service" system—it is separate from fire and other public safety entities. The system is supported financially by the individual entities.

Coordination

Coordination of care is achieved through several means. A unified set of clinical guidelines was developed and is maintained by the system in accordance with current clinical evidence. These guidelines provide a common framework for the care and transport of patients throughout the system. Any changes to the guidelines must be evaluated and approved by the Combined Clinical Council.

All providers in the region have a common set of credentials and are given badges that identify them as certified providers within the system, substantially reducing the multijurisdictional fragmentation that is common across metropolitan areas. In addition, there is no distinction within the system between volunteer and career providers. The integrated structure facilitates both incident command and disaster planning.

Regionalization

The unified system supports the regional emergency and trauma care system through clinical operating guidelines that determine the care and transport of all emergency and trauma patients. But the system is focused more on coordination and medical direction of EMS than on regionalization of care.

Accountability

A Healthcare Quality Committee is charged with reviewing the performance of the system and recommending specific actions to improve quality.

Palm Beach County, Florida

An initiative currently under way in Palm Beach County, Florida, is more limited in scope than the Maryland and Austin/Travis County systems. The goal of the initiative is to find regional solutions to the limited availability of physician specialists who provide on-call emergency care services. In spring 2004, physician leaders, hospital executives, and public health officials formed the Emergency Department Management Group to address this problem. The initiative is in the early stages of development, and approaches are evolving. One approach is to attack the rising cost of malpractice insurance for emergency care providers, which discourages specialists from serving on on-call panels. The organization is developing a group captive insurance company to offer liability coverage for physicians providing care in county EDs.

Coordination

The group is developing a web-based, electronic ED call schedule so the EMS system can track which specialists are available at all hospitals throughout the county. This will enable the system to direct transport to the most appropriate facility based on a patient's type of injury or illness.

Regionalization

The group is exploring the regionalization of certain high-demand specialties, such as hand surgery and neurosurgery, so that the high costs of maintaining full on-call coverage can be concentrated in a few high-volume hospitals, where the number of cases makes it feasible to maintain such coverage. Hospitals throughout the county would pay a "subscription fee" to support the cost of on-call coverage at designated hospitals. The fee would be set at a level below what it would cost to have hospitals manage their on-call coverage problems individually.

Accountability

The initiative includes the development of a countywide quality assurance program under which all hospitals would submit certain data elements for assessment. It is unclear at this time how far this system would go toward public disclosure of system performance.

San Diego County, California

San Diego County has a regionalized trauma system that is characterized by a strong public–private partnership between the county and its five adult and one children's trauma centers. Public health, assessment, policy development, and quality assurance are core components of the system, which operates under the auspices of the state EMS Authority.

Coordination

A countywide electronic system (QA Net) provides the real-time status of every trauma center and ED in the county, including the reason for diversion status, ICU bed availability, and trauma resuscitation capacity. The system has been in place for over 10 years and is a critical part of the coordination of emergency and trauma care in the county.

A regional communications system serves as the backbone of the EMS and emergency and trauma care systems for both day-to-day operations and disasters. It includes an enhanced 9-1-1 system and a countywide network that allows all ambulance providers and hospitals to communicate. The network is used to coordinate decisions on EMS destinations and bypass information, and allows each hospital and EMS provider to know the status of every other hospital and provider on a real-time basis. Because the system's authority comes from the state to the local level, all prehospital and emergency hospital services are coordinated through one lead agency. This arrangement provides continuity of services, standardized triage, treatment and transport protocols, and an opportunity to improve the system as issues are identified.

Regionalization

The county is divided into five service areas, each of which has at least a level II trauma center. Adult trauma patients are triaged and transported to the appropriate trauma center, while the children's trauma center provides care to all seriously injured children below the age of 14. Serious burn cases are taken to the University of California-San Diego Burn Center. The county is considering regionalization for other conditions, such as stroke and heart attack, based on the trauma model. The system includes the designation of regional trauma centers, designation of base hospitals to provide medical direction to EMS personnel, establishment of regional medical policies and procedures, and licensure of EMS services.

Accountability

Accountability is driven by a quality improvement program in which a medical audit committee meets monthly to review systemwide patient deaths and complications. The committee includes trauma directors; trauma nurse managers; the county medical examiner; the chief of EMS; and representatives of key specialty organizations, including orthopedic surgeons and neurosurgeons, as well as a representative for nondesignated facilities. A separate prehospital audit committee that includes ED physicians and prehospital providers also meets monthly and discusses any relevant prehospital issues.

A PROPOSAL FOR FEDERAL, STATE, AND LOCAL COLLABORATION THROUGH DEMONSTRATION PROJECTS

States and regions face a variety of situations, and no one approach to building EMS systems will achieve the goals discussed in this chapter. There is, for example, substantial variation across states and regions in the level of development of trauma systems; the effectiveness of state EMS offices and regional EMS councils; and the degree of coordination and integration among fire departments, EMS, hospitals, trauma centers, and emergency management. The baseline conditions and needs also vary. For example, rural areas face very different problems from those of urban areas, and an approach that works for one may be counterproductive for the other.

In addition to these varying needs and conditions, the problems involved are too complex for the committee to prescribe an a priori solution. A number of different avenues should be explored and evaluated to determine what does and does not work. Over time and over a number of controlled initiatives, such a process should yield important insights about what works and under what conditions. These insights could provide best-practice models that could be widely adopted to advance the nation toward the committee's vision.

The process described here is one that could be supported effectively through federal demonstration projects. Such an approach could provide funding critical to project success; guidance for design and implementation; waivers from federal laws that might otherwise impede the process; and standardized, independent evaluations of projects and overall national assessment of the program. At the same time, the demonstration approach would allow for significant variations according to state and regional needs and conditions within a set of clearly defined parameters. The IOM report *Fostering Rapid Advances in Health Care: Learning from System Demonstrations* articulated the benefits of the demonstration approach: "There is no accepted blueprint for redesigning the health care sector, although there is widespread recognition that fundamental changes are needed. . . . For many important issues, we have little experience with alternatives to the status quo . . . the committee sees the launching of a carefully crafted set of demonstrations as a way to initiate a 'building block' approach" (IOM, 2002, p. 3).

The committee therefore recommends that **Congress establish a demonstration program, administered by the Health Resources and Services Administration, to promote coordinated, regionalized, and accountable emergency care systems throughout the country, and appropriate $88 million over 5 years to this program (3.5).** The essential features of the proposed program are described below.

Recipients

Grants would be targeted at states, which could define projects at the state, regional, or local level; cross-state collaborative proposals would be encouraged. Projects would be selected so as to ensure that each of the three goals discussed in this chapter would be well represented in the final set of projects. Grantees would be selected through a competitive process based on the quality of proposals, assessment of the likelihood of success in achieving the stated goal(s), and the potential sustainability of the approach after the end of the grant period. Proposals should explicitly address the implications of the proposed project for both pediatric and adult patients.

Purpose of the Grants

Grantees could propose approaches addressing one, two, or all three of the goals of coordination, regionalization, and accountability. Proposals would not have to address more than one goal, but doing so would not be discouraged.

Initiatives could be statewide, regional, or local and could include collaborations between adjacent states. Each proposal would be required to describe the proposed approach in detail, explain how it would achieve the stated goal(s), identify who would carry out the responsibilities associated with the initiative, identify the costs associated with its implementation, and describe how success would be measured. Proposals should describe the state's current stage of development and sophistication with regard to the stated goal(s) and explain how the grant would be used to enhance system performance in that regard.

Grants could be used in a number of different ways. Grant funds could be used to enhance communications so as to improve coordination of services; of particular interest would be the development of centralized communications centers at the regional or state level. Grants could be used to establish convening and planning functions, such as the creation of a regional or state advisory group of stakeholders for the purposes of building collaboration and designing and executing plans to improve coordination. Grant funds could be used to hire consultants and staff to manage the planning and coordination functions, as well as to pay for data collection, analysis, and public reporting. In very limited circumstances, they could also be used to implement information systems for the purpose of improving coordination of services. Grant funds should not, however, be used for routine functions that would be performed in the absence of the demonstration project, such as the hiring or training of EMS providers or the purchase of EMS equipment. Funds could also be used to enhance linkages between rural and urban emergency services within broadly defined regions so as to improve rural emergency care through communications, telemedicine, training, and coordination activities.

Funding Levels

The committee proposes a two-phase program. In phase I, the program would fund up to 10 projects at up to $6 million over 3 years. Funding 10 projects would likely result in considerable variation in the types of projects proposed and the range of lessons learned. Based on successful results that appeared to be reproducible in other states, the program would launch phase II, in which smaller, 2-year demonstration grants—up to $2 million each—would be made available to up to 10 additional states. This phase

of the program would also include a technical assistance program designed
to disseminate results and practical guidance to all states. Program administration would include evaluation of the program throughout its 5 years,
including reports and public comments at 2.5 and 5 years after program
initiation. The committee estimates funding for the program as follows:

- Phase I grants: $60 million (over 3 years)
- Phase II grants: $20 million (over 2 years)
- Phase II technical assistance: $4 million (over 2 years)
- Overall program administration: $4 million (over 5 years)
- Total program funding: $88 million (over 5 years)

Granting Agency

No single federal agency has responsibility for the various components
of the nation's emergency care system. As noted earlier, this responsibility
is currently shared among multiple agencies—principally NHTSA, HRSA,
CDC, and the Department of Homeland Security (DHS). If, as recommended below, a lead agency is established to consolidate funding and
provide leadership for these multiple activities, it would be the appropriate
agency to lead this proposed effort. Until that consolidation occurs, however, the committee believes this demonstration program should be placed
within HRSA. HRSA currently directs a successful, related demonstration
program—Emergency Medical Services for Children (EMSC)—and sponsors the Trauma-EMS Systems Program, both of which share many of the
broad goals of the proposed demonstration program. HRSA has already
demonstrated a willingness and ability to collaborate effectively with other
relevant federal agencies, including NHTSA, CDC, and, increasingly, DHS,
and should be encouraged to consider them as partners in this enterprise.

NEED FOR SYSTEM INTEGRATION AND
A FEDERAL LEAD AGENCY

If the process of redesigning the emergency and trauma care system to
achieve the goals outlined by the committee is to be successful, it must be
supported. As stated in *Fostering Rapid Advances*, ". . . we must both plant
the seeds of innovation and create an environment that will allow success to
proliferate. Steps must be taken to remove barriers to innovation and to put
in place incentives that will encourage redesign and sustain improvements"
(IOM, 2002, p. 3). The process used to redesign the system must include
payment policies that reward successful strategies. It must recognize the
interdependencies within emergency care and address systemic problems.

It must balance the interests of many different stakeholders. And it must involve leadership at many levels taking responsibility for creating change.

Underlying the committee's vision of a coordinated, regionalized, and accountable emergency care system is the recognition that the system is complex, with many interdependent components. If the system is to function effectively, these components must be highly integrated. Operationally, this means that all of the key players in a given region—hospital EDs, EMS dispatchers, state public health officials, trauma surgeons, EMS agencies, ED nurses, hospital administrators, firefighters, police, community safety net providers, and others—must work together to make decisions, deploy resources, and monitor and adjust system operations based on performance feedback.

As documented throughout this report, however, fragmentation, silos, and entrenched interests prevail throughout emergency care. The organization of federal government programs that support and regulate emergency services largely reflects the fragmentation of emergency services at the state and local levels. Prehospital EMS, hospital-based emergency care, trauma care, injury prevention and control, and medical disaster preparedness are scattered across numerous agencies within the Department of Health and Human Services (DHHS), the U.S. Department of Transportation (DOT), and DHS. This situation reflects the history and inherent nature of emergency and trauma care—essential public services that operate at the intersection of medical care, public health, and public safety (police and fire departments and emergency management agencies).

In the 1960s, the mounting toll of highway deaths led NHTSA to become the first government home for EMS, where it has remained. Thus although EMS is primarily a medical discipline, federal responsibility for EMS rests with DOT. This responsibility was recently reinforced by the elevation of NHTSA's EMS program to the status of an Office of EMS within the agency. Today, NHTSA sponsors a number of workforce and research initiatives and the development of NEMSIS, and it recently received funding for a major nationwide initiative to promote the development of next-generation 9-1-1 service.

DHHS has played an important supporting role in the development of EMS and has taken the lead role with respect to hospital-based emergency and trauma care. It housed the Division of Emergency Medical Services and the Division of Trauma and EMS for many years, and most recently the Trauma/EMS Systems program. All of these programs have been eliminated; the latter was recently zeroed out of the federal budget for fiscal year 2006. DHHS continues to support CDC's National Center for Injury Prevention and Control (NCIPC), the EMSC program, and the National Bioterrorism Hospital Preparedness Program. These programs have made important contributions to emergency and trauma care, despite inconsistent funding and the frequent threat of elimination. The Agency for Healthcare Research and Quality (AHRQ), another DHHS agency, has historically been the principal federal agency funding research in emergency care delivery, including much of the early research on management of out-of-hospital cardiac arrest. Recently, AHRQ has funded important studies of ED crowding, operations management, and patient safety issues. It is active as well in funding research on preparedness, bioterrorism planning, and response.

DHS also plays an important role in emergency and trauma care. The Federal Emergency Management Agency (FEMA), once an independent cabinet-level agency now housed in DHS, provides limited amounts of grant funding to local EMS agencies through the U.S. Fire Administration. DHS also houses the Metropolitan Medical Response System (MMRS), a grant program designed to enhance emergency and trauma preparedness in major population centers. This program was migrated from DHHS to DHS in 2003. In addition, DHS houses the Disaster Medical Assistance Team (DMAT) program, through which health professionals volunteer and train as locally organized units so they can be deployed rapidly, under federal direction, in response to disasters nationwide.

While most of these agencies attempt to develop programs within a systemwide framework, the divisions among them make it difficult to plan and to allocate federal dollars in the most effective manner. For example, continuing to fund EMS grants through the U.S. Fire Administration has led to limited overall EMS funding and neglect of EMS representation in both day-to-day planning and disaster preparedness. There is also substantial overlap in the responsibilities of these agencies. For example, almost every agency is involved in disaster preparedness, and some of those efforts overlap considerably. Programs addressing hospital surge capacity, for instance, are currently taking place in AHRQ, CDC's NCIPC, HRSA's Office of Domestic Preparedness, and DHS.

Efforts have been made to improve interagency collaboration at the federal level, especially in recent years. Over the last decade, federal agencies have worked collaboratively to provide leadership in the emergency and trauma care field, to minimize gaps and overlaps across programs, and to pool resources to fund promising research and demonstration programs. For example, NHTSA and HRSA jointly supported the development of the *Emergency Medical Services Agenda for the Future*, which was published in 1996. This degree of collaboration has not been universal, however, and has been evident in some agencies more than others. Furthermore, collaborative efforts are limited by the constraints of agency authorization and funding. At some point, agencies must pursue their own programmatic goals at the expense of joint initiatives. Furthermore, to the degree that successful collaboration has occurred, it has generally depended on the good will of key individuals in positions of leadership, limiting the sustainability of these efforts when personnel changes occur.

In an effort to enhance the sustainability of collaborative initiatives, a number of agencies have participated in informal planning groups. For example, the Interagency Committee on EMSC Research (ICER), which is sponsored by HRSA, brings together representatives from a number of federal programs for the purposes of sharing information and improving research in emergency and trauma care for children.

A broader initiative is the Federal Interagency Committee on EMS (FICEMS), a planning group designed to coordinate the efforts of the various federal agencies involved in emergency and trauma care. FICEMS was established in the late 1970s. After a subsequent period of dormancy, it was reconstituted in the mid-1980s. The organization had no statutory authority until 2005, when it was given formal status by the Safe, Accountable, Flexible, Efficient Transportation Equity Act: A Legacy for Users (SAFETEA-LU), DOT's reauthorization legislation (P.L. 109-59). While the focus of FICEMS is EMS, the group has in practice reached beyond the strict boundaries of prehospital care to facilitate coordination and collaboration with agencies involved in other aspects of hospital-based emergency and trauma care (see Box 3-2). NHTSA is charged with providing administrative support for FICEMS, which must submit a report to Congress annually. The central aims of the group are as follows:

• To ensure coordination among the federal agencies involved with state, local, and regional EMS and 9-1-1 systems.
• To identify state, local, and regional needs in EMS and 9-1-1 services.
• To recommend new or expanded programs, including grant programs, for improving state, local, and regional EMS and implementing improved EMS communications technologies, including wireless 9-1-1.
• To identify ways of streamlining the process through which federal agencies support state, local, and regional EMS.
• To assist state, local, and regional EMS agencies in setting priorities based on identified needs.
• To advise, consult, and make recommendations on matters relating to the implementation of coordinated state EMS programs.

Problems with the Current Structure

Despite recent efforts at improved federal collaboration, there is widespread agreement that the various components of emergency care (EMS for adults and children, trauma, care, hospital-based care) individually have not received sufficient attention, stature, and funding within the federal

BOX 3-2
FICEMS Membership

The Safe, Accountable, Flexible, Efficient Transportation Equity Act: A Legacy for Users (SAFETEA-LU) designated the following agencies as members of FICEMS. Each year, members elect a representative from one of these member organizations as the FICEMS chairperson:

- National Highway Traffic Safety Administration (DOT)
- Preparedness Division, Directorate of Emergency Preparedness and Response (DHS)
- Health Resources and Services Administration (DHHS)
- Centers for Disease Control and Prevention (DHHS)
- U.S. Fire Administration, Directorate of Emergency Preparedness and Response (DHS)
- Centers for Medicare and Medicaid Services (DHHS)
- Under Secretary of Defense for Personnel and Readiness (Department of Defense [DoD])
- Indian Health Service (DHHS)
- Wireless Telecommunications Bureau, Federal Communications Commission
- A representative of any other federal agency appointed by the Secretary of Transportation or the Secretary of Homeland Security through the Under Secretary for Emergency Preparedness and Response, in consultation with the Secretary of Health and Human Services, having a significant role in relation to the purposes of the interagency committee

government. The scattered nature of federal responsibility for emergency care limits the visibility necessary to secure and maintain funding within the federal government. The result has been marked fluctuations in budgetary support and the constant risk that key programs will be dramatically downsized or eliminated. The lack of a clear point of contact for the public and for stakeholders makes it difficult to build a unified constituent base that can advocate effectively for funding and provide feedback to the government on system performance. The lack of a unified budget has created overlaps, gaps, and idiosyncratic funding of various programs. Finally, lack of unified accountability disperses responsibility for system failures and perpetuates divisions between public safety– and medical-based emergency and trauma care professionals. The degree to which the scattered responsibility for emergency and trauma care at the federal level has contributed to this disappointing performance is unclear. Regardless, the committee believes a new approach is warranted.

Alternative Approaches

Strong federal leadership for emergency and trauma care is at the heart of the committee's vision for the future, and continued fragmentation of responsibility at the federal level is unacceptable. The committee considered two options for remedying the situation: (1) maintain the status quo, giving the FICEMS approach time to strengthen and mature, or (2) designate or create a new lead agency within the federal government for emergency and trauma care. Some of the key differences between these two approaches are summarized in Table 3-1.

Option 1: Maintain the Status Quo, Allowing FICEMS to Gain Strength

The committee considered the ramifications of maintaining the status quo. The problems associated with fragmented federal leadership of emergency care, documented above, include variable funding, periodic program cuts, programmatic duplication, and critical program gaps. With the recent enactment of a statutory framework for FICEMS, however, the committee considered the possibility that the need for a federal lead agency has diminished. The committee carefully examined the rationale for delaying the move toward a federal lead agency and allowing FICEMS time to gain strength. The central argument in support of this strategy is that there have been a number of recent improvements in collaboration at the federal level, and these efforts should be given a chance to work before an unproven and politically risky approach is pursued. A number of recent developments support this view: the enactment of a statutory framework for FICEMS; the increasing level of collaboration among some federal agencies; the substantial new NHTSA funding for a next-generation 9-1-1 initiative; and the elevation of the NHTSA EMS program to the Office of EMS, which has the potential to improve visibility and funding for EMS, and perhaps other aspects of emergency and trauma care, within the federal government.

While the committee applauds these positive developments, setbacks have occurred as well. As noted above, DHHS's Division of Emergency Medical Services, its Division of Trauma and EMS, and most recently its Trauma/EMS Systems program were recently zeroed out of the federal budget. Federal funding for AHRQ, nonbioterrorism programs at CDC, and other federal programs related to emergency and trauma care at the federal level has been cut. These developments suggest that a fragmented organizational structure at the federal level will significantly hinder the creation of a coordinated, regionalized, accountable emergency and trauma care system.

TABLE 3-1 Comparison of the Current FICEMS Approach and the
Committee's Lead Agency Proposal

	Maintain the Status Quo, Allowing FICEMS to Gain Strength	Designate or Create a New Federal Lead Agency
Description	• Current agencies retain autonomy, but the FICEMS process fosters collaboration in planning.	• Combines emergency care functions from several agencies into a new lead agency.
Authority	• FICEMS has the authority to convene meetings, but no authority to enforce planning, evaluation, and coordination of programs and funding.	• Lead agency would have planning and budgetary authority over the majority of emergency care activities at the federal level.
Funding	• No guarantee of coordinated program funding. • Distributed responsibility for federal functions means that if programs are cut, others remain, reducing the risk of losing all federal support for emergency and trauma care.	• Consolidates visibility and political representation of emergency care, enhancing federal funding opportunities. • Emergency care funding is fully coordinated. • Risk of losing significant funding for emergency care in a hostile budget environment.
Collaboration	• Brings together the key emergency and trauma care agencies. • FICEMS cannot enforce coordination or collaboration.	• Unified agency would drive collaboration among all components of emergency and trauma care to achieve systemwide performance goals.
Public Identity	• Still lacks a unified point of authority from the public's perspective. • FICEMS facilitates response to the public.	• Provides for a unified federal emergency care presence for interaction with the public and stakeholder groups.
Professional Identity	• Fragmented federal representation makes it difficult to break down silos in the field.	• Provides a home for emergency and trauma care, which can project and enhance the professional identity of emergency and trauma care providers over time. • Lead agency could consolidate constituencies and engender stronger political representation.

continued

TABLE 3-1 Continued

	Maintain the Status Quo, Allowing FICEMS to Gain Strength	Designate or Create a New Federal Lead Agency
Efficiency	• May reduce redundancy through enhanced collaboration. • Very low administrative overhead costs.	• Eliminates redundant administrative structure, reducing administrative overhead costs. • Consolidated funding would allow for better allocation of federal dollars across the various emergency care needs (e.g., would eliminate overlapping programs).
Transition	• FICEMS is established in law, and implementation is under way. • Given FICEMS' limited powers, risks to individual programs and constituencies are minimal.	• Substantial startup costs associated with the transition to a single agency. • Potential for changes in program and funding emphasis during the transition, which could create winners and losers. • Potential dissension among emergency care agencies and constituencies could impact the organization's effectiveness.

FICEMS can be a valuable body, but it is a poor substitute for formal agency consolidation. FICEMS is expressly focused on EMS, and ultimately has limited power over even this sphere. It is not a federal agency and therefore cannot regulate, or allocate or withhold funding. It cannot even hold its own member agencies accountable for their actions—or lack of action.

Option 2: Designate or Create a New Federal Lead Agency

The possibility of a lead agency for emergency and trauma care has been discussed for years and was highlighted in the 1996 report *Emergency Medical Services Agenda for the Future*. While the concept of a lead agency promoted in that report was focused on prehospital EMS, the committee believes a lead agency should encompass all components involved in the provision of emergency and trauma care. This lead federal agency would unify federal policy development related to emergency and trauma care, provide a central point of contact for the various constituencies in the field, serve as a federal advocate for emergency and trauma care within the government, and coordinate grants so that federal dollars would be allocated efficiently and effectively.

A lead federal agency could better move the emergency and trauma care system toward improved integration; unify funding and other decisions; and represent all emergency and trauma care patients, providers, and settings, including prehospital EMS (both ground and air), hospital-based emergency and trauma care, pediatric emergency and trauma care, rural emergency and trauma care, and medical disaster preparedness. Specifically, a federal lead agency could:

• Provide consistent federal leadership on policy issues that cut cross agency boundaries.
• Create unified accountability for the performance of the emergency and trauma care system.
• Rationalize funding across the various aspects of emergency and trauma care to optimize the allocation of resources in achieving system outcomes.
• Coordinate programs to eliminate overlaps and gaps in current and future funding.
• Create a large combined federal presence, increasing the visibility of emergency and trauma care within the government and among the public.
• Provide a recognizable entity that would serve as a single point of contact for stakeholders and the public, resulting in consolidated and efficient data collection and dissemination and coordinated program information.
• Enhance the professional identity and stature of emergency and trauma care practitioners.
• Bring together multiple professional groups and cultures, creating cross-cultural and interdisciplinary interaction and collaboration that would model and reinforce the integration of services envisioned by the committee.

Although creating a lead agency could yield many benefits, such a move would also involve significant challenges. Numerous questions would have to be addressed regarding the location of such an agency in the federal government, its structure and functions, and the possible risk of weakening or losing current programs. HRSA's rural EMS and EMS/Trauma Systems programs have already been defunded, and the EMS-C program is under the constant threat of elimination. There is real concern that proposing an expensive and uncertain agency consolidation could jeopardize programs already at risk, such as EMS-C, as well as cripple new programs that are just getting started, such as NHTSA's enhanced 9-1-1 program. This is particularly likely if there is resistance to the consolidation from within the current agency homes for these programs.

A related concern is that the priority currently given to certain programs could shift, resulting in less support for existing programs. EMS advocates have expressed concern that hospital-based emergency and trauma care issues would dominate the agenda of a new unified agency. The pediatric community is worried about getting lost in a new agency, and has fought hard to establish and maintain strong categorical programs supported by historically steady funding streams. There is concern that under the proposed new structure, the current focus of the EMS-C program could get lost or diminished, or simply lose visibility in the multitude of programs addressed by the new agency.

There is also the potential for administrative and funding disruptions. Combining similar agencies, particularly those that reside within the same department, may be straightforward. But combining agencies with different missions across departments with different cultures could prove highly difficult. The problems that were experienced during the consolidation of programs in DHS increase anxiety about this proposal.

Another concern is that removing medical-related functions from DHS and DOT could exacerbate rather than reduce fragmentation. Operationally, nearly half of EMS services are fire department–based. Thus, there is concern that separating EMS and fire responsibilities at the federal level could splinter rather than strengthen relationships.

The Committee's Recommendation

Despite the concerns outlined above, the committee believes the potential benefits of consolidation outweigh the potential risks. A lead federal agency is required to fully realize the committee's vision of a coordinated, regionalized, and accountable emergency and trauma care system. The committee recognizes that a number of challenges are associated with the establishment of a new lead agency, though it believes these concerns can be mitigated through appropriate planning. The committee therefore recommends that **Congress establish a lead agency for emergency and trauma care within 2 years of this report. The lead agency should be housed in the Department of Health and Human Services, and should have primary programmatic responsibility for the full continuum of emergency medical services and emergency and trauma care for adults and children, including medical 9-1-1 and emergency medical dispatch, prehospital emergency medical services (both ground and air), hospital-based emergency and trauma care, and medical-related disaster preparedness. Congress should establish a working group to make recommendations regarding the structure, funding, and responsibilities of the new agency, and develop and monitor the transition. The working group should have representation from federal and state agencies and professional disciplines involved in emergency and trauma care (3.6).**

Objectives of the Lead Agency

The lead agency's mission would be to enhance the performance of the emergency and trauma care system as a whole, as well as to improve the performance of the various components of the system, such as prehospital EMS, hospital-based emergency care, trauma systems, pediatric emergency and trauma care, prevention, rural emergency and trauma care, and disaster preparedness. The lead agency would set the overall direction for emergency and trauma care planning and funding; would be the primary collector and repository of data in the field; and would be the key source of information about emergency and trauma care for the public, the federal government, and practitioners themselves. It would be responsible for allocating federal resources across all of emergency and trauma care to achieve systemwide goals, and should be held accountable for the performance of the system and its components.

Location of the Lead Agency

The lead agency would be housed within DHHS. The committee considered many factors in selecting DHHS over DOT and DHS. The factor that drove this decision above all others was the need to unify emergency and trauma care within a public health/medical care framework. Emergency and trauma care is by its very nature involved in multiple arenas—medical care, public safety, public health, and emergency management. The multiple identities that result from this multifaceted involvement reinforce the fragmentation that is endemic to the emergency and trauma care system. For too long, the gulf between EMS and hospital care has hindered efforts at communication, continuity of care, patient safety and quality of care, data collection and sharing, collaborative research, performance measurement, and accountability. It will be difficult for emergency and trauma care to achieve seamless and high-quality performance across the system until the entire system is organized within a medical/public health framework while also retaining its operational linkages with public safety and emergency management.

Only DHHS, as the department responsible for medical care and public health in the United States, can encompass all of these functions effectively. Although DOT has played an important role in both EMS and acute trauma care and has collaborated effectively with other agencies, its EMS and highway safety focus is too narrow to represent all of emergency and trauma care. DHS houses the Fire Service, which is closely allied with EMS, particularly at the field operations level. But the focus of DHS on disaster preparedness and bioterrorism is also too narrow to encompass the broad scope of emergency and trauma care.

Because emergency and trauma care functions would be consolidated in a department oriented toward public health and medical care, there is a risk that public safety and emergency management components could receive less attention, stature, or funding. Therefore, the committee considers it imperative that the mission of the new agency be understood and clearly established by statute so that the public safety and emergency management aspects of emergency and trauma care will not be neglected.

Programs Included Under the Lead Agency

The committee envisions that the lead agency would have primary programmatic responsibility for the full continuum of EMS; emergency and trauma care for adults and children, including medical 9-1-1 and emergency medical dispatch; prehospital EMS (both ground and air); hospital-based emergency and trauma care; and medical-related disaster preparedness. The agency's focus would be on program development and strategic funding to improve the delivery of emergency and trauma care nationwide. It would not be primarily a research funding agency, with the exception of existing grant programs mentioned above. Funding for basic, clinical, and health services research in emergency and trauma care would remain the primary responsibility of existing research agencies, including the National Institutes of Health (NIH), AHRQ, and CDC. Because of the limited research focus of the lead agency, it would be important for existing research agencies, NIH in particular, to work closely with the new agency and strengthen their commitment to emergency and trauma care research. On the other hand, it may be appropriate to keep certain clinical and health services research initiatives with the programs in which they are housed, and therefore bring them into the new agency. For example, the Pediatric Emergency Care Applied Research Network could be moved into the new agency along with the rest of the EMS-C program.

In addition to existing functions, the lead agency would become the home for future programs related to emergency and trauma care, including new programs that would be dedicated to the development of inclusive systems of emergency and trauma care.

Working Group

While the committee envisions consolidation of most of the emergency care–related functions currently residing in other agencies and departments, it recognizes that many complex issues are involved in determining which programs should be combined and which left in their current agency homes. A deliberate process would be established to determine the exact composition of the new agency and to coordinate an effective transition.

For these reasons, the committee is recommending the establishment of an independent working group to make recommendations regarding the structure, funding, and responsibilities of the new agency and to coordinate and monitor the transition process. The working group would include representatives from federal and state agencies and professional disciplines involved in emergency care. The committee considered whether FICEMS would be an appropriate entity to assume this advisory and oversight role and concluded that, as currently constituted, it lacks the scope and independence to carry out this role effectively.

Role of FICEMS

FICEMS is a highly promising entity that is complementary to the proposed new lead agency. FICEMS would play a vital role during the proposed interim 2-year period by continuing to enhance coordination and collaboration among agencies and providing a forum for public input. In addition, it could play an important advisory role to the independent working group. Once the lead agency had been established, FICEMS would continue to coordinate work between the lead agency and other agencies, such as NIH, CMS, and DoD, that would remain closely involved in various emergency and trauma care issues.

Structure of the Lead Agency

While the principle of integration across the multiple components of emergency and trauma care should drive the structure, operation, and funding of the new lead agency, the committee envisions distinct program offices to provide focused attention and programmatic funding for key areas, such as the following:

- Prehospital EMS, including 9-1-1, dispatch, and both ground and air medical services
- Hospital-based emergency and trauma care
- Trauma systems
- Pediatric emergency and trauma care
- Rural emergency and trauma care
- Disaster preparedness

To ensure that current programs would not lose visibility and stature within the new agency, each program office should have equal status and reporting relationships within the agency's organizational structure. The committee envisions a national dialogue over the coming year—coordinated by the proposed independent working group, aided by input from FICEMS, and with the involvement of the Office of Management and Budget and congressional committees with jurisdiction—to specify the organizational structure in further detail and implement the committee's recommendation.

Funding for the Lead Agency

Existing programs transferring to the new agency would bring with them their full current and projected funding, although this may not be possible for some funds, such as the Highway Trust Funds, which contribute to the operational funding for the Office of EMS. Congress should also establish additional funding to cover the costs of the transition to the lead agency and associated administrative overhead. In addition, Congress should add new funding for the offices of hospital-based emergency and trauma care, rural emergency and trauma care, and trauma systems. In light of the pressing challenges confronting emergency care providers and the American public, this would be money well spent. While the committee is unable to estimate the costs associated with establishing a unified lead agency, it recognizes that those costs would be substantial. At the same time, however, the committee believes that countervailing cost savings would result from reduced duplication and lower overhead. Consequently, new funding that flowed into the agency would result in new programming, rather than an increase in existing overhead.

Mitigation of Concerns Regarding the Establishment of a Lead Federal Agency

The committee recognizes that transitioning to a single lead agency would be a difficult challenge under any circumstances, but would be especially difficult for an emergency and trauma care system that is already under duress from funding cutbacks, elimination of programs, growing public demand on the system, and pressure to enhance disaster preparedness. During this critical period, it is important that support for emergency and trauma care programs already in place in the various federal agencies be sustained. In particular, the Office of EMS within NHTSA has ongoing programs that are critical to the EMS system. Similarly, existing emergency care–related federal programs, such as those in HRSA's EMS-C program and Office of Rural Health Policy and at CDC, should be supported during the transition period. If the committee's proposal is to be successful, the constituencies associated with established programs must not perceive that they are being politically weakened during the transition.

The committee believes the proposed consolidation of agencies would enhance support for emergency and trauma care across the board, benefiting all current programs. But it also believes avoiding disruptions that could adversely affect established programs is critically important. Therefore, the committee believes legislation creating the new agency should protect current levels of funding and visibility for existing programs. The new agency should balance its funding priorities by adding to existing funding levels, not by diverting funds away from existing programs.

The committee acknowledges the concern that removing medical-related emergency and trauma functions from DHS and DOT would create additional fragmentation. The committee believes the public safety aspects of emergency and trauma care must continue to be addressed as a core element of the emergency and trauma care system. But the primary focus of the system should be medical care and public health if the recognition, stature, and outcomes that are critical to the system's success are to be achieved.

SUMMARY OF RECOMMENDATIONS

3.1: The Department of Health and Human Services and the National Highway Traffic Safety Administration, in partnership with professional organizations, should convene a panel of individuals with multidisciplinary expertise to develop evidence-based categorization systems for emergency medical services, emergency departments, and trauma centers based on adult and pediatric service capabilities.

3.2: The National Highway Traffic Safety Administration, in partnership with professional organizations, should convene a panel of individuals with multidisciplinary expertise to develop evidence-based model prehospital care protocols for the treatment, triage, and transport of patients.

3.3: The Department of Health and Human Services should convene a panel of individuals with emergency and trauma care expertise to develop evidence-based indicators of emergency and trauma care system performance.

3.4: The Department of Health and Human Services should adopt regulatory changes to the Emergency Medical Treatment and Active Labor Act and the Health Insurance Portability and Accountability Act so that the original goals of the laws will be preserved, but integrated systems can be further developed.

3.5: Congress should establish a demonstration program, administered by the Health Resources and Services Administration, to promote coordinated, regionalized, and accountable emergency care systems throughout the country, and appropriate $88 million over 5 years to this program.

3.6: Congress should establish a lead agency for emergency and trauma care within 2 years of this report. The lead agency should be housed in the Department of Health and Human Services, and should have primary programmatic responsibility for the full continuum of emergency medical services and emergency and trauma care for adults and children, including medical 9-1-1 and emergency medical dispatch, prehospital emergency medical services (both ground and air), hospital-based emergency and trauma care, and medical-related disaster preparedness. Congress should establish a working group to make recommendations regarding the structure, funding, and responsibilities of the new agency, and develop and monitor the transition. The working group should have representation from federal and state agencies and professional disciplines involved in emergency and trauma care.

REFERENCES

AHA (American Heart Association). 2005. *Sudden Cardiac Death: AHA Scientific Position.* [Online]. Available: http://www.americanheart.org/presenter.jhtml?identifier=4741 [accessed February 15, 2006].

Asplin BR, Knopp RK. 2001. A room with a view: On-call specialist panels and other health policy challenges in the emergency department. *Annals of Emergency Medicine* 37(5):500–503.

Bardach NS, Olson SJ, Elkins JS, Smith WS, Lawton MT, Johnston SC. 2004. Regionalization of treatment for subarachnoid hemorrhage: A cost-utility analysis. *Circulation* 109(18):2207–2212.

Berenson RA, Kuo S, May JH. 2003. Medical malpractice liability crisis meets markets: Stress in unexpected places. *Issue Brief (Center for Studying Health System Change)* (68):1–7.

Bravata DM, McDonald K, Owens DK. 2004. *Regionalization of Bioterrorism Preparedness and Response.* Rockville, MD: Agency for Healthcare Research and Quality.

CDC (Centers for Disease Control and Prevention) National Center for Injury Control and Prevention. 2001. *Web-based Injury Statistics Query and Reporting System (WISQARS).* [Online]. Available: http://www.cdc.gov/ncipc/wisqars/ [accessed September 2004].

Chang RK, Klitzner TS. 2002. Can regionalization decrease the number of deaths for children who undergo cardiac surgery? A theoretical analysis. *Pediatrics* 109(2):173–181.

Chiara O, Cimbanassi S. 2003. Organized trauma care: Does volume matter and do trauma centers save lives? *Current Opinion in Critical Care* 9(6):510–514.

CMS (Centers for Medicare and Medicaid Services). 2005a. *Report Number One to the Secretary, U.S. Department of Health and Human Services, from the Inaugural Meeting of the Emergency Medical Treatment and Labor Act Technical Advisory Group.* Washington, DC: CMS.

CMS. 2005b. *Report Number Two to the Secretary, U.S. Department of Health and Human Services, from the Emergency Medical Treatment and Labor Act Technical Advisory Group.* Washington, DC: CMS.

CMS. 2005c. *Report Number Three to the Secretary, U.S. Department of Health and Human Services, from the Emergency Medical Treatment and Labor Act Technical Advisory Group.* Washington, DC: Centers for Medicare and Medicaid Services.

Cunningham P, May J. 2003. Insured Americans drive surge in emergency department visits. *Center for Studying Health System Change Issue Brief* (70):1–6.

Davis R. 2003, July. The method: Measure how many victims leave the hospital alive. *USA Today.* P. A1.

DHHS (U.S. Department of Health and Human Services). 2003. *Emergency Medical Treatment and Labor Act (EMTALA) Interim Guidance.* Baltimore, MD: Centers for Medicare and Medicaid Services.

Dummit LA. 2005. Specialty hospitals: Can general hospitals compete? *National Health Policy Forum Issue Brief* (804):1–12.

GAO (U.S. Government Accountability Office). 2001. *Emergency Care. EMTALA Implementation and Enforcement Issues.* Washington, DC: U.S. Government Printing Office.

GAO. 2003a. *Hospital Preparedness: Most Urban Hospitals Have Emergency Plans but Lack Certain Capacities for Bioterrorism Response.* Washington, DC: U.S. Government Printing Office.

GAO. 2003b. *Specialty Hospitals: Geographic Location, Services Provided, and Financial Performance.* Washington, DC: U.S. Government Printing Office.

GAO. 2003c. *Infectious Diseases: Gaps Remain in Surveillance Capabilities of State and Local Agencies.* Washington, DC: GAO.

Gausche-Hill M, Wiebe R. 2001. Guidelines for preparedness of emergency departments that care for children: A call to action. *Pediatrics* 107(4):773–774.

Glance LG, Osler TM, Dick A, Mukamel D. 2004. The relation between trauma center outcome and volume in the national trauma databank. *Journal of Trauma-Injury Infection & Critical Care* 56(3):682–690.

Grumbach K, Keane D, Bindman A. 1993. Primary care and public emergency department overcrowding. *American Journal of Public Health* 83(3):372–378.

Grumbach K, Anderson GM, Luft HS, Roos LL, Brook R. 1995. Regionalization of cardiac surgery in the United States and Canada: Geographic access, choice, and outcomes. *Journal of the American Medical Association* 274(16):1282–1288.

Harris Interactive. 2004. *Trauma Care: Public's Knowledge and Perception of Importance.* New York: Harris Interactive.

Iglehart JK. 2005. The emergence of physician-owned specialty hospitals. *New England Journal of Medicine* 352(1):78–84.

Imperato PJ, Nenner RP, Starr HA, Will TO, Rosenberg CR, Dearie MB. 1996. The effects of regionalization on clinical outcomes for a high risk surgical procedure: A study of the Whipple procedure in New York state. *American Journal of Medical Quality* 11(4):193–197.

IOM (Institute of Medicine). 1993. *Emergency Medical Services for Children.* Washington, DC: National Academy Press.

IOM. 2002. *Fostering Rapid Advances in Health Care: Learning from System Demonstrations.* Washington, DC: The National Academies Press.

Johnson LA, Taylor TB, Lev R. 2001. The emergency department on-call backup crisis: Finding remedies for a serious public health problem. *Annals of Emergency Medicine* 37:495–499.

Jurkovich GJ, Mock C. 1999. Systematic review of trauma system effectiveness based on registry comparisons. *Journal of Trauma–Injury Infection & Critical Care* 47(Suppl. 3): S46–S55.

Kanter RM, Heskett M. 2002. *Washington Hospital Center (B): The Power of Insight.* Boston, MA: Harvard Business School.

Kellermann AL, Hackman BB, Somes G, Kreth TK, Nail L, Dobyns P. 1993. Impact of first-responder defibrillation in an urban emergency medical services system. *Journal of the American Medical Association* 270(14):1708–1713.
Koziol-McLain J, Price DW, Weiss B, Quinn AA, Honigman B. 2000. Seeking care for nonurgent medical conditions in the emergency department: Through the eyes of the patient. *Journal of Emergency Nursing* 26(6):554–563.
Lewin ME, Altman S. 2000. *America's Health Care Safety Net*. Washington, DC: National Academy Press.
Lindsay P, Schull M, Bronskill S, Anderson G. 2002. The development of indicators to measure the quality of clinical care in emergency departments following a modified-delphi approach. *Academic Emergency Medicine* 9(11):1131–1139.
MacKenzie EJ. 1999. Review of evidence regarding trauma system effectiveness resulting from panel studies. *Journal of Trauma-Injury Infection & Critical Care* 47(Suppl. 3): S34–S41.
MacKenzie EJ, Rivara FP, Jurkovich GJ, Nathens AB, Frey KP, Egleston BL, Salkever DS, Scharfstein DO. 2006. A national evaluation of the effect of trauma-center care on mortality. *New England Journal of Medicine* 354(4):366–378.
Malone RE. 1995. Heavy users of emergency services: Social construction of a policy problem. *Social Science and Medicine* 40(4):469–477.
Mann NC, Mullins RJ, MacKenzie EJ, Jurkovich GJ, Mock CN. 1999. Systematic review of published evidence regarding trauma system effectiveness. *Journal of Trauma-Injury Infection & Critical Care* 47(Suppl. 3):S25–S33.
McConnell KJ, Newgard CD, Mullins RJ, Arthur M, Hedges JR. 2005. Mortality benefit of transfer to level I versus level II trauma centers for head-injured patients. *Health Services Research* 40(2):435–457.
measureEMS.org. 2005. *Performance Measures in EMS*. [Online]. Available: http://www.measureems.org/performancemeasures2.htm [accessed January 5, 2006].
Mullins RJ. 1999. A historical perspective of trauma system development in the United States. *Journal of Trauma-Injury Infection & Critical Care* 47(Suppl. 3):S8–S14.
Mullins RJ, Mann NC. 1999. Population-based research assessing the effectiveness of trauma systems. *Journal of Trauma-Injury Infection & Critical Care* 47(Suppl. 3):S59–S66.
Nallamothu BK, Saint S, Kolias TJ, Eagle KA. 2001. Clinical problem-solving of nicks and time. *New England Journal of Medicine* 345(5):359–363.
Nathens AB, Maier RV. 2001. The relationship between trauma center volume and outcome. *Advances in Surgery* 35:61–75.
Nathens AB, Jurkovich GJ, Rivara FP, Maier RV. 2000. Effectiveness of state trauma systems in reducing injury-related mortality: A national evaluation. *The Journal of Trauma* 48(1):25–30; discussion 30–31.
NAS, NRC (National Academy of Sciences, National Research Council). 1966. *Accidental Death and Disability: The Neglected Disease of Modern Society*. Washington, DC: National Academy of Sciences.
NHTSA (National Highway Traffic Safety Administration). 1996. *Emergency Medical Services Agenda for the Future*. Washington, DC: U.S. Government Printing Office.
NQF (National Quality Forum). 2002. *National Voluntary Consensus Standards for Adult Diabetes Care*. [Online]. Available: http://www.qualityforum.org/txdiabetes-public.pdf [accessed November 23, 2005].
NQF. 2003. *Safe Practices for Better Health Care*. Washington, DC: NQF.
NQF. 2004. *National Voluntary Consensus Standards for Nursing Home Care*. [Online]. Available: http://www.qualityforum.org/txNursingHomesReportFINALPUBLIC.pdf [accessed November 23, 2005].

NQF. 2005. *National Voluntary Consensus Standards for Home Health Care.* [Online]. Available: http://www.qualityforum.org/webHHpublic09–23–05.pdf [accessed November 23, 2005].

Orr RA, Han YY, Roth K. 2006. Pediatric transport: Shifting the paradigm to improve patient outcome. In: Fuhrman B, Zimmerman J, eds. *Pediatric Critical Care* (3rd edition). St. Louis, MO: Mosby, Elsevier Science Health. Pp. 141–150.

Petersen LA, Burstin HR, O'Neil AC, Orav EJ, Brennan TA. 1998. Nonurgent emergency department visits: The effect of having a regular doctor. *Medical Care* 36(8):1249–1255.

Pollock DA, Adams DL, Bernardo LM, Bradley V, Brandt MD, Davis TE, Garrison HG, Iseke RM, Johnson S, Kaufmann CR, Kidd P, Leon-Chisen N, MacLean S, Manton A, McClain PW, Michelson EA, Pickett D, Rosen RA, Schwartz RJ, Smith M, Snyder JA, Wright JL. 1998. Data elements for emergency department systems, release 1.0: A summary report. Deeds Writing Committee. *Journal of Emergency Nursing* 24(1):35–44.

Rosenbaum S, Kamoie B. 2003. Finding a way through the hospital door: The role of EMTALA in public health emergencies. *Journal of Law, Medicine & Ethics* 31(4):590–601.

The SAFECOM Project. 2004. *Statement of Requirements for Public Safety Wireless Communications & Interoperability.* Washington, DC: Department of Homeland Security.

State of California Office of the Patient Advocate. 2005. *2005 HMO Report Card.* [Online]. Available: http://www.opa.ca.gov/report_card/ [accessed January 12, 2006].

Studdert DM, Mello MM, Sage WM, DesRoches CM, Peugh J, Zapert K, Brennan TA. 2005. Defensive medicine among high-risk specialist physicians in a volatile malpractice environment. *Journal of the American Medical Association* 293(21):2609–2617.

Wright JL, Klein BL. 2001. Regionalized pediatric trauma systems. *Clinical Pediatric Emergency Medicine* 2:3–12.

Young GP, Wagner MB, Kellermann AL, Ellis J, Bouley D. 1996. Ambulatory visits to hospital emergency departments. Patterns and reasons for use. 24 Hours in the ED Study Group. *Journal of the American Medical Association* 276(6):460–465.

4

Improving the Efficiency of Hospital-Based Emergency Care

The emergency care system is but one component of the larger health care delivery system and of the even larger social safety net system. As such, it is subject to many forces far beyond its direct control. There is little that emergency care providers and advocates can do to alter such environmental factors as growing use of the emergency department (ED) by the uninsured; the increasing age and number of chronic conditions of patients; staffing shortages in many key areas, especially nurses and on-call specialists; malpractice insurance rates that grew on average more than 50 percent between 2002 and 2003 (AMA, 2003); and declining public and private reimbursements—not to mention disasters, both natural and man-made. There is, however, a great deal that the emergency care system can do to anticipate, prepare for, and manage the effects of these broader trends. This chapter explores strategies for improving the efficiency of hospital-based emergency care within the context of the broader health care delivery system, with a focus on the special issue of patient flow. The chapter also examines approaches to overcoming barriers to improved ED patient flow and operational efficiency. The committee emphasizes the compelling need for regulatory and policy changes to increase accountability and incentivize the efficient management of patient flow throughout the hospital and beyond.

THE ED IN THE CONTEXT OF
THE HEALTH CARE DELIVERY SYSTEM

Medical science in the United States is arguably the most advanced in the world, but the organization and delivery of health care lags well behind many other U.S. industries in terms of innovation, use of information technology, and management practices. Kleinke (1998, p. 6) described medical delivery in the United States as ". . . a miracle of disorganization, held together through the sheer collective will of overworked professionals tasked with managing tens of millions of patients by memory, pen scrawl, Post-It note, and telephone call." It is a system that, to quote Berwick (1996, p. i3), "is perfectly designed to achieve exactly the results it gets." The results, as documented by the Institute of Medicine (IOM) reports *To Err Is Human: Building a Safer Health System* (IOM, 2000) and *Crossing the Quality Chasm: A New Health System for the 21st Century* (IOM, 2001), include an estimated 98,000 deaths and more than 1 million injuries each year as a result of health care process and system failures (Starfield, 2000). According to the joint National Academy of Engineering (NAE) and IOM (2005, p. 1) report *Building a Better Delivery System: A New Engineering/Health Care Partnership*, "an estimated thirty to forty cents of every dollar spent on health care . . . a half trillion dollars a year . . . is spent on costs associated with: overuse, underuse, misuse, duplication, system failures . . . and inefficiency." While confidence in American medicine remains strong, patients understand that the delivery system is failing. In a survey conducted by the Picker Institute (2000), 75 percent of patients described a system that was fragmented; difficult to navigate; and inconsistent in terms of information, evidence, and treatment.

According to the NAE/IOM report, the U.S. health care system retains a "cottage industry" structure, with physicians and other health care providers operating semiautonomously. As a result, hospitals and other provider organizations lack the hierarchical control of the typical business enterprise, making it difficult to introduce efficiency principles to streamline flows in such areas as production, inputs, and inventory as in other industries. In addition, the prevalent payment structures in health care, which focus on individual encounters and practice settings, tend to reinforce silos, reward inefficient practices, and discourage investment in new technologies and process improvements. As a result, innovations that have swept through other sectors of the economy, including banking, airlines, and manufacturing, have failed to take hold in health care delivery—a sector of the economy that now consumes 16 percent of the nation's gross domestic product and is growing at twice the rate of inflation. Health care information technology has advanced considerably in the last decade, but mainly in the administrative and financial arenas, as opposed to the core processes of delivering clinical services (NAE and IOM, 2005).

Other industries have made use of a number of tools derived from engineering and operations research, which can be referred to collectively as operations management tools (see Box 4-1). Manufacturers, airlines, banks, the military, and others have adopted systems that employ a number of these tools. For example, Motorola's Six Sigma process and the Toyota Production System combine statistical and process controls with worker empowerment and cultural change to minimize defect rates and achieve high levels of quality. Some of these approaches have been promoted and implemented by health care organizations, such as the Joint Commission on Accreditation of Healthcare Organizations (JCAHO), the Veterans Health Administration, Kaiser Permanente, the National Association of Public Hospitals and Health Systems (NAPHHS), the Agency for Healthcare Research and Quality (AHRQ), and several private hospital organizations. But adoption of such approaches has yet to become widespread (Gabow et al., 2005; National Association of Public Hospitals and AHRQ, 2005).

A common thread among these tools is the systems concept, in which the dependence of every component on the others is recognized. To achieve the system's maximum performance, each unit must not only achieve high individual performance, but also cooperate with interdependent units to optimize system objectives. The tools of operations management facilitate the understanding of complex systems and make it possible for managers to control and improve overall system performance.

Nowhere is the interdependence among individual components more evident and the need for tools to manage complex systems more crucial than in the hospital ED. Taking care of emergency patients involves many discreet components, such as registration, emergency physicians, nurses, laboratory services, imaging, inpatient departments, and on-call specialists. These components are highly interdependent, such that optimizing the performance of any one without considering the broader objectives of the system is unlikely to improve the overall performance of the delivery of emergency care. For example, optimizing care in an inpatient department may slow admissions from the ED, worsen ED crowding, and create a host of associated problems. Indeed, that is what often happens.

UNDERSTANDING PATIENT FLOW
THROUGH THE HOSPITAL SYSTEM

Crowding in the nation's EDs poses a serious threat to the quality, safety, and timeliness of emergency care. While many of the factors contributing to ED crowding are outside the immediate control of the hospital, many more are the result of operational inefficiencies in the management of hospital patient flow. EDs receive an almost steady stream of patients. If an individual arriving by ambulance cannot be transferred quickly to an ED stretcher, efficiently triaged, and then rapidly evaluated, stabilized, and admitted or discharged, ED crowding will quickly develop, and patient care will be compromised.

BOX 4-1
Operations Management Tools

Many operations management tools could be applied to achieve better management of patient flow:

Quality functional deployment. This iterative process links stakeholder needs to the resources required to meet those needs throughout the organization. Conflicting demands on the organization emerge and are resolved, with all relevant stakeholders examining the trade-offs from a systems perspective. The process has been used in a variety of industrial applications, including integrated circuit and automobile design.

Failure modes and effects analysis (FMEA). FMEA is a formal process for analyzing failures that might occur under varying conditions so they can be avoided through design features. It has been used in manufacturing for more than 30 years and has recently been applied to health care. The Veterans Health Administration encourages its accredited hospitals to use FMEA or hazard analysis tools in a required annual proactive risk assessment of at least one high-risk process each year.

Root-cause analysis is a qualitative, retrospective variation on FMEA that has been widely used to analyze industrial accidents. The Joint Commission on Accreditation of Healthcare Organizations requires accredited hospitals to use the method to evaluate sentinel patient safety events.

Human factors engineering. This set of techniques attempts to integrate human behavior and limitations into process design. Human factors research has been widely used across industries and has had many recent applica-

Hospital administrators and policy makers have at their disposal a number of promising options for identifying and resolving the patient flow problems that contribute to ED crowding and its consequences. But these leaders must first be compelled to take action, something that will occur only when the causes of ED crowding are clearly understood, and administrators realize that the strategies required to address the problem go well beyond the ED itself. More than 15 years ago, Lynn and Kellermann (1991) described approaches to improving management of the ED in an overcrowded hospital. Key to their thesis, then as now, was the idea that crowding is an inpatient problem that manifests itself in the ED. Accordingly, measures to address crowding should begin on inpatient units, rather than with diversion of inbound ambulances. Moreover, administrators, policy makers, and the public must have the knowledge, incentives, and regulatory obligations needed to inspire change.

tions in health care, such as medication administration, diagnosis, handoffs of patients between shifts, and telemedicine.

Queuing theory. Queuing theory is used to determine the capacity of services that are subject to variable demand over time. It has been widely used in a number of service industries, such as banking and public transportation. It has had limited use in health care, but has been applied to optimize scheduling and staffing in primary care, operating rooms, nursing homes, radiology departments, and emergency departments (Huang, 1995; Siddharthan et al., 1996; Reinus et al., 2000; Lucas et al., 2001; Gorunescu et al., 2002; Murray and Berwick, 2003; McManus et al., 2004; Green et al., 2006). (See the detailed discussion in Box 4-2.)

Supply-chain management. This set of techniques helps match resources with demand in highly complex production processes. Companies such as Dell, Toyota, and Procter & Gamble represent enormously complex systems that use supply-chain management tools, such as linear integer programs, to optimize performance. Airlines use these models to assign crews to thousands of flights per day across hundreds of cities. The techniques have revolutionized production in many industries but have had very little impact in the hospital environment despite substantial successes. For example, both Vanderbilt University Medical Center and Deaconess Hospital in Evansville, Indiana, have achieved substantial savings using these techniques. It has been estimated that the health care industry could save $11 billion by using supply-chain management (NAE and IOM, 2005).

Statistical process control. This technique involves plotting the outcomes of a process over time to see whether variations fall within an acceptable range or fall outside that range and require corrective action. It is widely used in manufacturing.

From arrival in the ED to hospital admission or discharge, emergency patients receive treatment at multiple points of the care delivery process. Patient flow, defined as the movement of patients through this system, is an important indicator of the timeliness, safety, and quality of the care received. Efficient patient flow ensures maximum throughput (the number of patients treated and discharged from the ED per day), minimizing delays at each point of the delivery process with no decrement in the quality of care. Impaired patient flow, on the other hand, results in bottlenecks that prolong delays for patients already in the system, as well as those awaiting entry.

The input/throughput/output (I/T/O) model of patient care, based on engineering principles from queuing theory and compartmental models of flow, applies operations management concepts to patient flow within the acute care system (see Figure 4-1). The I/T/O model defines the acute care system as including unscheduled ambulatory care, urgent care, ED care and

134

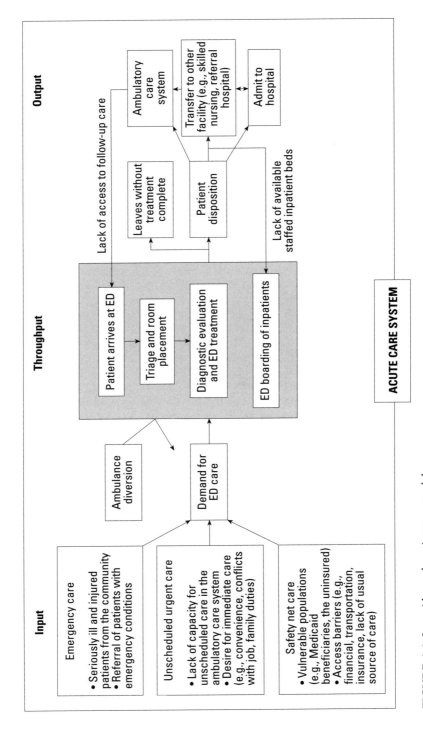

FIGURE 4-1 Input/throughput/output model.
SOURCE: Reprinted from Asplin et al., 2003, with permission from the American College of Emergency Physicians.

its ancillary services, inpatient care for those admitted through the ED, and out-of-hospital emergency medical services (EMS) care. In this way, the I/T/O model allows for the identification of all components of the health care system that contribute to or are affected by ED crowding (Asplin et al., 2003; Solberg et al., 2003).

Under the I/T/O model, ED input, or demand, comprises three distinct categories of care: emergency care (treatment of seriously ill or injured patients), unscheduled urgent care (treatment of patients unable to receive needed care in a timely manner from other components of the acute care system), and safety net care (treatment of patients who experience substantial barriers to accessing unscheduled care from other components of the health care system). Variations in the demand for each of these types of care, both patient- and systems-driven, determine the input fluctuations in the ED. That is, ED input levels depend on both the volume of critically ill and injured patients and the ability of the overall health care system to care for nonemergent and safety net patients (Asplin et al., 2003; Solberg et al., 2003).

The throughput component of the I/T/O model represents a patient's length of stay in the ED and comprises two key phases: (1) triage, room placement, and medical evaluation, and (2) diagnostic testing and ED treatment. ED boarding is also included in the throughput component as it extends ED lengths of stay. The output component of the model represents the disposition of ED patients. It includes hospital admission, transfer to another facility, and patient discharge. It also includes the ability of the ambulatory health care system to provide timely and appropriate postdischarge care (Asplin et al., 2005).

As designed, the structure of the I/T/O model allows hospitals to systematically identify and resolve impediments to patient flow across a spectrum of acute care settings. It also provides direction for researchers, policy makers, and hospital administrators seeking to understand and alleviate ED crowding as a way to improve access to and quality of care (Asplin et al., 2003; Solberg et al., 2003; Wilson et al., 2005).

IMPEDIMENTS TO EFFICIENT PATIENT FLOW IN THE ED

While hospitals are unable to control forces outside the facility that contribute to high levels of demand, they can understand the impact of those forces on operations and structure their organization for optimal response. At the same time, hospitals have direct control over a number of variables that affect operational efficiency, including such factors as inpatient bed capacity, ancillary service delays, the scheduling of surgeries and support staff, and provision of adequate physical space in the ED to permit evaluation and treatment (GAO, 2003). By applying variability methodology, queuing theory, and the I/T/O model, hospitals can identify and eliminate many of the impediments to patient flow caused by operational inefficiencies (Litvak and Long, 2000; Litvak, 2005).

One of the most important factors currently outside the control of most hospitals is the regional flow of patients (see Chapter 3). Short of the need to go on diversion, there is typically little information sharing between hospitals and EMS regarding overloaded EDs and trauma centers and the availability of ED beds, operating suites, equipment, trauma surgeons, and critical specialists. Such information is needed to balance the patient load among EDs and trauma centers in a region, which requires that many elements within the regional system—community hospitals, trauma centers, and particularly prehospital EMS—effectively coordinate the regional flow of patients. In addition to improving patient care, coordinating the regional flow of patients is a critical tool for reducing overcrowding in EDs. Unfortunately, only a handful of systems around the country coordinate transport effectively throughout their region. Some examples were described in Chapter 3.

Inpatient Admissions Bottlenecks

The most commonly cited contributor to ED crowding is the inability to move admitted patients from the ED into inpatient hospital beds, in particular intensive care unit (ICU) beds. This lack of inpatient beds has the immediate effect of forcing ED staff to "board" admitted patients until an inpatient ICU or medical-surgical bed is available (see Chapter 1). Placing ED patients who require hospital admission in hallways or examination spaces temporarily until an inpatient bed becomes available is a poor substitute for inpatient care. EDs are not designed to provide privacy to hallway boarders, and staff are often too busy to meet an admitted patient's needs in a timely manner. Moreover, boarding is the primary cause of ambulance diversion, a practice that delays access to emergency care and can send inbound patients to a hospital where the medical staff does not know them and has no access to their medical records. Ambulance diversion also contributes to reduced EMS capacity as ambulances seeking to offload patients are forced to find an open ED and once there, to wait until the ED staff are able to find an empty stretcher (Gallagher and Lynn, 1990; Thorpe, 1990; Andrulis et al., 1991; Derlet and Richards, 2000; Epstein and Slate, 2001; Derlet et al., 2001; Henry, 2001; Viccellio, 2001; The Lewin Group, 2002; McManus et al., 2003; Asplin et al., 2003; GAO, 2003; Schull et al., 2003; Solberg et al., 2003; Weissert et al., 2003; Eckstein and Chan, 2004; JCAHO, 2004; Kennedy et al., 2004; see also Chapter 1). By failing to manage patient flow effectively, hospitals allow the most time-critical access point in the facility—the ED—to become blocked and ultimately inaccessible.

Financial Incentives

In addition to contributing to an overall shortage of bed space, the current reimbursement structure discourages hospitals from making provision of inpatient beds to ED admissions a management priority. Within the hospital, ED patients compete for beds, staff, and services with patients who have been scheduled for elective admission, particularly elective surgical patients and those being admitted for invasive diagnostic or therapeutic procedures. When beds are scarce, elective admissions generally prevail because they pay better margins and promote loyalty among admitting physicians. ED admissions typically generate less revenue for the hospital, and may even cost the hospital money. Furthermore, since these patients are already in the system, they are unlikely to leave, whereas an elective admission can choose to go to another hospital. Finally, because hospitals benefit financially from increased volume (up to a point), there is a financial disincentive to hold vacant beds open for ED admissions.

Delays in Ancillary Services

Enhanced standards of care and improved medical technology mean that today's ED patients routinely receive a number of complex diagnostic and screening services (McCaig and Burt, 2005). Whether complex or routine, the timely administration of these ancillary services and the prompt availability of test results are imperative for smooth hospital operations and efficient patient flow. Data suggest, however, that delays in diagnostic and screening tests for ED patients are both common and strongly associated with prolonged lengths of stay in the ED. In fact, nearly one-half of all ED service delays were related to wait times for radiology and laboratory results according to one survey conducted by the Emergency Nurses Association (Derlet and Richards, 2000; Weissert et al., 2003; JCAHO, 2004). Housekeeping also is frequently a problem, as most ED admissions occur in the late afternoon to early morning hours, while housekeeping staffs are usually reduced after 5:00 PM.

Overuse of ED Services

Physicians treating patients in the ED have access to a wide range of complex medical screening and evaluation tools, all within the confines of a single physical space—the hospital. This means that ED patients often also have access to the best technology in the community, as hospitals are frequently more able than local providers or smaller health clinics to purchase and operate expensive medical equipment. These factors have resulted in the dual effect of some patients opting to seek care in the ED and some primary or specialty care providers referring their patients to the

ED as a means of streamlining the medical testing process. In short, the ED is assuming, by default, another new role—that of "one-stop shop" for complex medical workups, a phenomenon that improves the efficiency of office-based practitioners, but contributes to ED crowding and hinders the safety and timeliness of true emergency care. Also, because EDs often have limited access to patient records, redundant workups and diagnostic tests are often performed.

Defensive Medicine

The rise in the number and severity of medical malpractice claims, especially in high-risk fields such emergency medicine, has led to an increasingly defensive approach to providing care in the ED. Because emergency physicians have such a range of tests and diagnostic technologies at their fingertips, they are more likely to be blamed if they fail to use them and ultimately miss a diagnosis. For example, missed myocardial infarction has been the leading cause of malpractice claims in emergency medicine, yet definitively excluding the possibility of a myocardial infarction or acute coronary syndrome requires a minimum of 6–12 hours of evaluation and diagnostic tests costing more than a thousand dollars. Fearing potential litigation, ED physicians and on-call specialists may order additional tests or prolong monitoring periods, slowing patient flow and contributing to service delays. ED staff may also hospitalize patients in borderline condition rather than running the risk that a discharged patient will have an adverse outcome. This is even more likely to happen when the physician is concerned that the patient may not be able to secure outpatient follow-up care in a timely manner (Asplin et al., 2005). It should be noted, however, that it is difficult to quantify the increment over and above appropriate evaluation in emergency care that constitutes "defensive medicine."

Staffing Requirements

In contrast to the strict nurse-to-patient ratios on many inpatient units and ICUs, most hospitals have declined to adopt nurse-to-patient ratios for the ED. As a result, an inpatient unit that has vacant beds but has reached its maximum ratio of nurses to patients may block admissions from an ED that may be caring for two or even three times as many patients per nurse. The merits of staffing ratios in general are discussed in Chapter 6.

Inadequate Physical Space

Unlike most high-risk enterprises, health care has been slow to embrace principles of ergonomics or human factors engineering in the design and maintenance of its various workplaces. As a result, ED providers often face limitations on the amount of space available in which to provide care, and they routinely encounter user-unfriendly spatial layouts and equipment placement and design. In many hospitals, for example, computed tomography (CT) scans, operating rooms, or ICUs are located a significant distance from the ED, requiring the staffed transport of patients across multiple hospital divisions or floors. Similarly, desktop-only registration, whiteboard tracking, and land-line phone paging systems routinely pull physicians and other staff away from the bedside, extending patients' lengths of stay and leading to disruptions in the course of care. Fortunately, many of these design failures can be addressed through the adoption of new information technology tools (McKay, 1999; Chisholm et al., 2000; Derlet and Richards, 2000; Wears and Perry, 2002). Additional discussion of these tools is provided in Chapter 6.

STRATEGIES FOR OPTIMIZING EFFICIENCY

A number of initiatives now under way are aimed at improving patient flow in order to reduce ED crowding and its related effects. These include Urgent Matters, a $6.4 million, 10-hospital campaign supported by The Robert Wood Johnson Foundation that aims to eliminate ED crowding and improve public understanding of challenges facing the health care safety net; the IHI IMPACT Network, which, through its Improving Flow Learning and Innovation Community, seeks to increase patient throughput and minimize delays while ensuring that high performance in flow is not achieved at the expense of quality; and the University HealthSystem Consortium (UHC) Patient Flow Benchmarking Project, which targets in-hospital factors that impede or impair efficient patient flow. Recognizing the importance of managing patient flow to addressing ED crowding, JCAHO published a new standard for accredited hospitals: "LD.3.11." "The leaders develop and implement plans to identify and mitigate impediments to efficient patient flow throughout the hospital" (JCAHO, 2004).

Based on the above efforts, a wide range of tools have been developed and tested to address patient flow issues, generally with good success. While controlled studies have yet to be conducted, a growing body of anecdotal evidence suggests that by smoothing the peaks and valleys of patient flow (the movement of patients into and between various hospital areas for care), hospitals can reduce crowding while improving quality and reducing cost (JCAHO, 2004; Wilson and Nguyen, 2004). Boston Medical Center and St. John's Regional Health Center in Springfield, Missouri, for example, reduced crowding by adjusting elective surgery schedules so they did not conflict with predictable peaks in emergency surgeries (Litvak and Long, 2000; Crute, 2005).

Techniques That Address Bottlenecks in Patient Flow

The effective management of patient flow in the ED and between the ED and hospital inpatient units is essential to the quality and safety of patient care (Begley et al., 2004). By smoothing the inherent peaks and valleys of patient flow and eliminating the artificial variabilities that unnecessarily impair that flow, hospitals can minimize the occurrence of queues and improve safety and quality while simultaneously reducing hospital waste and costs (Litvak and Long, 2000). For inherent, patient-driven peaks and valleys, the necessary ED capacity (number of beds, nurses, ancillary services) can be determined by applying queuing theory (see Box 4-2). This approach leads to greater predictability and control and ultimately to improved quality, safety, and timeliness of care (Litvak and Long, 2000; NAE and IOM, 2005).

A number of additional techniques have been tested for improving the

---

BOX 4-2
Queuing Theory

Queuing theory applies analytical expressions to problems involving waiting times, or queues, that develop because of limited resources. Its purpose is to understand and achieve a balance between fixed capacity and the random demands of customer services. Queuing models have long been used in a number of industries, including telecommunications, the Internet, commercial banking, sales, and public transportation. They are increasingly being recognized as a tool that can help identify and manage the variabilities in patient flow that contribute to crowding in the emergency department (ED) (Litvak, 2005; NAE and IOM, 2005).

Many basic queuing models comprise three variables: arrival rate, service time, and number of servers. In the ED setting, the arrival rate is the frequency of patient arrivals, while service time is the average time spent caring for a particular type of patient at a specific point of care in the ED and its related sites. The number of servers can be the number of stations, beds, nurses, or work areas providing similar services to all patients who enter those areas (NAE and IOM, 2005). The problem, however, is that service time frequently has two components: the average time spent caring for patients and boarding time. Since boarding time is frequently a result of artificial variability in hospital patient flow (artificial peaks in inpatient bed census), basic queuing models cannot be applied to determining adequate ED resources. Thus to determine true (versus inflated) resources needed, one must exclude boarding time from the service time (length of stay in the ED).

flow of patients through the hospital, thereby reducing the ED–inpatient bottleneck. Examples are described in Boxes 4-3, 4-4, and 4-5.

Coordinated Surgery Schedule

The two most common routes to hospital admission today are through the ED (e.g., 50 percent) and through scheduled elective surgery in the operating room (OR) (e.g., 35 percent). Variability in admissions is well documented and leads to substantial fluctuations in inpatient capacity. For many hospitals, periods of limited capacity are often followed by periods of excess capacity, and managing this variability has the potential to improve patient flow and ED crowding significantly (DeLia, 2006). While the natural variability associated with emergency care might lead one to assume the ED is responsible for most of the fluctuations in inpatient traffic, data demonstrate that scheduled elective surgery in the OR, when adjusted for patient volume, is in fact the more variable of the two admission routes, thereby creating a significant artificial component of the variability in case volume (Litvak and Long, 2000; Litvak, 2005). Coordinating surgery times for scheduled and unscheduled admissions therefore not only adds organization to the rate and flow of scheduled elective OR admissions, but also allows hospitals to smooth out variabilities in ED and OR patient flow—an effect that serves to alleviate ED crowding (Litvak and Long, 2000; Cedars-Sinai Learns, 2004; Wilson and Nguyen, 2004; Litvak, 2005).

Many of the hospitals participating in the Urgent Matters, IHI, and UHC patient flow initiatives have undertaken systematic reviews and revamping of OR scheduling as a way of improving patient flow; enhancing the quality, safety, and timeliness of emergency care; reducing unnecessary costs; and increasing surgical revenue. Two related tactics are among those employed most frequently by these hospitals: (1) setting aside one OR for unscheduled surgical cases admitted through the ED and (2) smoothing the elective surgery schedule by distributing surgery times more evenly across the entire week (Litvak and Long, 2000). Both techniques have significantly reduced waiting times for surgical cases, especially among ED patients. This in turn has reduced the amount of time ED patients must wait for an inpatient bed, easing ED crowding and its effects. Improved coordination of surgery schedules also has been associated with increased revenue for surgeons, an important compensation for the disruption to the surgeons' schedules (Litvak, 2005; Crute, 2005).

Coordinated Bed Management

One strategy that has been successful in smoothing patient flow and alleviating ED crowding is the creation of "bed czars" or "bed teams" charged

BOX 4-3
Case Study: Boston Medical Center, Boston, Massachusetts

Boston Medical Center (BMC) is a private, nonprofit academic medical center that serves as the primary teaching affiliate for the Boston University School of Medicine. It has nearly 500 licensed beds and is the largest safety net hospital in New England, with an annual operating budget of $1 billion. BMC offers an array of medical services, including a level I trauma center, full-service acute care, pediatric care, and cardiothoracic surgery. Its emergency department (ED), staffed by 26 full-time physicians, treats over 120,000 patients annually.

As recently as 2003, BMC experienced significant ED crowding and ambulance diversion and high rates of patients leaving without being seen. To alleviate these conditions, BMC initiated a comprehensive project to identify and address inefficiencies in hospital operations, particularly those that inhibited patient flow. Before embarking on the initiative, BMC chief executive officer (CEO) Elaine Ullian established a project stakeholders group that included, among others, hospital leadership, the chiefs of surgery and anesthesiology, and key nursing staff. Ullian also convened several issue-focused teams, including an inpatient team, an ED team, and a surgery schedule smoothing team.

BMC employed a rapid cycle change (RCC) model, in which small changes are rapidly implemented and evaluated by staff. The study team first identified a specific aim or goal intended to improve patient flow. It then

with various aspects of bed management. Typically a nurse manager, a bed czar has primary responsibility for accounting for inpatient beds and working with housekeeping to ensure rapid bed turnaround. To fulfill this responsibility, bed czars are given authority to notify staff of impending bed shortages, make decisions regarding inpatient bed transfers, cancel elective procedures, and initiate hospital diversion. Bed teams, on the other hand, usually consist of nurses from multiple units, each of whom has access to real-time hospital census data. Working collaboratively, these teams meet throughout the day to discuss the types of ED patients waiting for inpatient beds and the types of beds expected to become available, making flow changes as necessary (JCAHO, 2004; Wilson and Nguyen, 2004; Wilson et al., 2005).

Among its many advantages, the bed czar or bed team approach offers a consistent, timely mechanism through which hospital staff can be notified about bed status; a centralized patient placement process; and improved ability to anticipate bed needs across multiple settings. Use of coordinated bed management techniques has been associated with significant reductions developed, implemented, and evaluated strategies on a small scale, modifying or rejecting the approach based on the results obtained. For example, one goal of the BMC team was to reduce ED throughput time. In response to suggestions from the nursing staff and nurse manager, the team decided to test a "zone nursing" approach in which nurses were assigned to patients in a particular area of the ED. Historically, ED nurses at BMC had been assigned to patients randomly, meaning that each nurse typically was responsible for a number of patients located throughout the ED. After a week-long, small-scale trial, the zone approach was associated with a 70-minute reduction in ED throughput time. In response to this success, the BMC team subsequently decided to extend the zone approach to the entire ED.

Another BMC project goal was to smooth surgery schedule variations in order to improve operating room (OR) and ED throughput. The team worked with the Cardiothoracic Surgery Department and Vascular Surgery Section to reduce peaks in elective surgical case volume; place a daily cap on the number of elective surgeries; switch surgeons' clinic and surgery days; and dedicate one of the hospital's eight ORs to emergent cases, with the other seven being open for block scheduling. The resulting improvements in patient flow through the ORs were significant; the number of "bumped" surgical cases, for example, fell from 337 between April and September 2003 to 3 between April and September 2004. At the same time, BMC ambulance diversion rates declined by 40 percent and overall ED throughput times by 17 percent.

SOURCE: Wilson et al., 2005.

in bed turnaround times at a number of EDs nationwide. The Regional Medical Center in Memphis, Tennessee, for example, reduced its average bed turnaround time by nearly 70 percent, cutting wait times from 150 to 47 minutes (JCAHO, 2004; Wilson and Nguyen, 2004; Wilson et al., 2005).

Efficiencies can also be achieved by use of a transfer center to coordinate referrals to a tertiary center. Such a center can reduce delays for transfer patients in the ED, ensure the availability of timely resources needed by such patients, and help coordinate transfers between facilities (Southard et al., 2005).

Clinical Decision Units (CDUs), or Observation Units

CDUs, or observation units, are separate areas that allow for the observation of patients to determine whether admission is necessary. Originally, these units were developed to provide a method for monitoring patients with chest pain who had a low to intermediate probability of acute myocardial

---

BOX 4-4
Case Study: Grady Health Systems, Atlanta, Georgia

Grady Health Systems, comprising Grady Memorial Hospital, Hughes Spalding Children's Hospital, and 10 regional health centers, is one of the largest public hospitals in the southeastern United States. Licensed for more than 1,000 beds, Grady Memorial Hospital (Grady) houses the only level I trauma center within a 100-mile radius, the state's only poison control center, and the city of Atlanta's emergency medical services (EMS) ambulance fleet. Grady also serves as the teaching hospital for both Emory and Morehouse schools of medicine. More than 100,000 visits are made to the Grady emergency department (ED) each year.

In 2002, as ED patient satisfaction levels fell to historic lows, Grady found itself experiencing a number of significant ED crowding–related challenges. Average ED throughput times, for example, frequently exceeded 7 hours, with fast-track throughput times reaching 10 hours. Rates of patients leaving the ED without being seen were estimated at 2.4 percent, or 200 patients per month. And by 2003, Grady's ED was operating under diversionary status more than 20 percent of the time.

Attempting to turn the tide on these trends, Grady used the input/throughput/output (I/T/O) model to identify major bottlenecks in patient flow. Under the direction of a project steering committee, led jointly by the hospital chief executive officer and chief operating officer, the Grady team developed and implemented a number of approaches involving a wide range of staff. For example, Grady instituted a new diagnostic test ordering process whereby

---

infarction (AMI) (Zwiche et al., 1982; Fineberg et al., 1984; Talbot-Stern et al., 1986; Vallee et al., 1988; de Leon et al., 1989; Henneman et al., 1989; Mikhail et al., 1997; Rydman et al., 1998; Graff et al., 2000). By observing patients for up to 23 hours, ED staff were able to rule out many patients at risk of AMI while using fewer resources than if these same patients were admitted to the ICU or an inpatient telemetry unit (Graff et al., 1997). Today, observation units are used most frequently for the efficient management of patients with complaints of chest pain, abdominal pain, back pain, dehydration, congestive heart failure, asthma, and shortness of breath (Hostetler et al., 2002; Ross et al., 2003). They are typically overseen full time by a nurse practitioner with assistance from an attending physician and other nursing staff. CDUs have been shown to reduce costs associated with inpatient admissions (Mikhail et al.,1997; Rydman et al., 1998; Graff et al., 2000), although the net impact on hospital costs is unclear (Sinclair and Green, 1998). One recent study found that approximately 30 percent

requests were handled by the unit clerk rather than the charge nurse; under the new process, wait times for test results were reduced by as much as 95 minutes during periods of ED crowding. In addition, Grady improved staff coordination and training in its fast-track unit; these changes were associated with signification reductions in the average time from ED arrival to bed placement (from 219 to 94 minutes) and average ED throughput time (from 340 to 211 minutes) for fast-track patients.

Finally, Grady implemented a care management unit (CMU), consisting of seven beds staffed by four CMU nurses and four case managers, to which patients diagnosed with one of four conditions—chest pain, heart failure, asthma, or hyperglycemia—are assigned. This dual CMU–ED structure allows for faster treatment and longer-term observation of nonemergent patients. Following their CMU stay, which lasts an average of 19 hours, 85 percent of patients are discharged, while 15 percent are admitted as inpatients. Prior to hospital discharge, CMU patients are assigned a case manager who provides disease-specific education, coordinates primary care follow-up (defined as occurring within 48–72 hours of discharge), and directs follow-up via telephone, as well as performing various data management chores. Among other benefits, the establishment of the Grady CMU has resulted in decreases in the number of short-stay admissions, admissions to telemetry beds, and patient relapse rates. The CMU also has resulted in improved patient satisfaction with Grady's ED services.

SOURCES: Grady Health System, 2005; Wilson et al., 2005.

of hospitals and two-thirds of teaching hospitals had opened or planned to open a CDU (Mace et al., 2003).

CDUs offer the potential to alleviate crowding in EDs and add elements of continuity to patient care. These units care for patients who would otherwise be admitted for inpatient stays two to three times as long. This frees up beds for other patients who would otherwise be boarded in the ED (Schneider et al., 2001), which in turn leads to a reduction in diversion hours (Dick et al., 2005). Use of CDUs may also allow ED staff to downgrade the type of bed required for those who still need admission after a CDU stay—instead of a telemetry or stepdown bed, admitting the patient to a regular medical-surgical bed.

Some units combine the concept of a CDU with the concept of case management. Such units employ case managers to focus on patients with exacerbations of chronic diseases that are known as "ambulatory care sensitive conditions" (e.g., asthma, diabetes, congestive heart failure). The

---

BOX 4-5
Case Study: St. John's Regional Health Center, Springfield, Missouri

St. John's Regional Health Center is an 866-bed, not-for-profit hospital and trauma center that serves as the dominant health care center in southwestern Missouri and parts of northwestern Arkansas. There were 74,000 visits to St. John's emergency department (ED) in fiscal year 2005, with approximately 22 percent of all ED patients requiring hospital admission. During the same time, ED-based admissions accounted for roughly 20 percent of the hospital's total surgical load.

In 2002, hospital leaders faced two significant patient flow–related problems. First, an inflexible process for scheduling elective surgeries had resulted in unpredictable and excessive use of overtime. Second, midweek peaks in surgery demands had resulted in admissions backups that were causing patients to be placed in beds on the wrong floors, jeopardizing the safe delivery of appropriate postsurgical care.

Seeking to resolve these issues, St. John's set aside a single operating room (OR) for elective and unplanned surgery overflow. This required the hospital's trauma surgeons to give up an OR that historically had been set aside in case they decided to schedule a surgery the day after their on-call period. The surgeons agreed on the condition that if no noticeable improvements were achieved during a 30-day trial period, the OR would be returned for their use. At the conclusion of the trial period, St. John's was able to increase the number of elective and unplanned surgeries by 5.1 percent, the number of OR rooms required after 3:00 PM dropped by 45 percent, and hospital trauma surgeons experienced a 4.6 percent increase in revenue. Based on this success, the OR change was made permanent.

---

assumption is that a diabetic with a blood sugar level of 700 mg/dL needs not only CDU care with the goal of avoiding hospitalization, but also case management, because the episode of hyperglycemia is a sentinel event for the failure of ambulatory care. While patients are getting hydrated or receiving an infusion of insulin, they are also being taught self-care skills and being reconnected with a primary care provider for close outpatient follow-up. Case managers can follow up with patients after discharge to make sure they keep their appointments. The goal is not only to prevent an expensive hospitalization, but also to reduce relapse rates and repeat visits to the ED due to another hyperglycemia/asthma/congestive heart failure episode by reconnecting the patient to primary care. In this way, the CDU aids the hospital in managing patient flow and reducing crowding while at the same time contributing to the smooth functioning of the ambulatory care system.

A second trial modified the elective surgery schedule, booking elective orthopedic surgeries evenly throughout the week. Although many surgeons initially objected to the plan and the physical therapy staff were required to adjust their work schedules, the change resulted in a 13 percent increase in the number of patients able to move to the appropriate floor for recovery. It also provided a number of surgical specialties, including orthopedics, with additional hours of OR block time. As with the OR change, modifications to the surgery schedule were made permanent following the successful trial period.

As a result of the above changes, the hospital was able to increase its surgical case volume by 7–11 percent annually with no capital investment over 3 years. The hospital administration attributes a number of recent operational, financial, and quality improvements to the continued success of the smoothing of elective surgeries for all surgical subspecialties (Personal communication, C. Dempsey, March 21, 2006):

- A 45 percent reduction in wait times for emergent and urgent surgical cases
- An increase in appropriate inpatient placement for orthopedic patients from 83 to 96 percent
- A 59 percent increase in inpatient capacity (excluding the intensive care unit) without the addition of a single staffed bed
- A 33 percent increase in surgical volume
- A 4.5 percent increase in revenues for surgeons who gave up block time
- A 2.9 percent reduction in OR overtime

SOURCE: Crute, 2005.

Hospitals can receive reimbursement for CDUs for three conditions: chest pain, asthma, and congestive heart failure. For other conditions, reimbursement for observation care is packaged or bundled into other ambulatory payment classification (APC) rates and not listed separately. Many groups, including the Society for Academic Emergency Medicine (SAEM) and the American College of Emergency Physicians (ACEP), have encouraged the Centers for Medicare and Medicaid Services (CMS) to expand separate payments for observation services beyond the three conditions currently allowed, claiming that the literature supports the effectiveness of observation services for many other conditions. Further, an APC advisory panel appointed by CMS unanimously recommended removing restrictions on diagnoses and conditions eligible for separate payment of observation; however, CMS has not enacted this change (Personal communication, M.B.

McClellan, July 8, 2005). While Medicare CDU payments would increase with the addition of eligible conditions, total costs of care should decline because of the reduction in the number of admissions. For Medicare, the change would be cost-saving.

On the basis of the foregoing evidence, the committee concludes that CDUs reduce the need for boarding and diversion, avoid expensive hospitalizations, and appear to contribute to improved management of common ambulatory care sensitive conditions. The committee believes CDU payments should be available for all clinical conditions for which observation is indicated, and therefore recommends that **the Centers for Medicare and Medicaid Services remove the current restrictions on the medical conditions that are eligible for separate clinical decision unit payment (4.1).**

Unit Assessment Tools

Unit assessment tools, based on the traffic light concept, can be used to determine and monitor the capacity of various units throughout the hospital system. The tool comprises graded, color-coded indicators that note the "workload tolerances" of each unit, based on a preset range of numerical scores. Under the system, green (go) indicates the unit is working at ≤85 percent of maximum capacity and therefore open for admissions; yellow (early caution) indicates the unit is working at >85 percent capacity and, though it is still able to accept admissions, alerts other units of current resource limitations; orange (late caution) indicates the unit is working immediately below its maximum capacity and suggests that capacity could be reached unless additional resources are made available; and red (stop) indicates the unit is at full capacity and cannot accept additional admissions without risking patient safety and staff burnout (JCAHO, 2004). Routine updates of the color grid allow staff to reallocate resources in response to status changes. This is accomplished most easily by a "resource czar," typically the nurse supervisor, with the authority to redirect staff or cap a unit as necessary. Using the unit assessment tool model, Luther Midelfort, a Mayo Health Systems hospital in Eau Claire, Wisconsin, saw steady declines in the number of red codes and steady increases in the number of green codes during a recent 6-month trial period (JCAHO, 2004).

Coordinated Patient Discharge

One of the most widely recognized bottlenecks in patient flow is the discharge process. By expediting discharge in a coordinated way, hospitals can better prepare patients for discharge, improve turnaround of vacant beds, and align vacancies with bed demands more accurately—all of which help alleviate crowding in the ED. Hospitals can alleviate discharge-related patient flow impediments through the creation of "discharge coordinator" positions and "discharge resource rooms." Much like a bed czar, a discharge coordinator can monitor charts to determine which patients are ready for discharge and work to expedite the disposition process. This coordinator, usually a nurse, also can provide or facilitate case management services. A discharge resource room is an area of the hospital where staff help patients prepare for their home care after discharge in a comfortable, central location. Upon arrival at the discharge room, patients are considered discharged from the hospital, making their bed available for rapid turnaround (JCAHO, 2004; Wilson and Nguyen, 2004; Wilson et al., 2005).

A number of hospitals have been able to reduce discharge delays and alleviate related ED crowding following establishment of a discharge coordinator or discharge resource room. For example, one Chicago-area facility was able to reduce the average length of stay for some patients from 5.7 to 4.3 days, with concurrent reductions in ED crowding rates (JCAHO, 2004). Short of adopting coordinated discharge approaches, simply requiring physicians to write discharge orders earlier in the day can also result in a substantial improvement in patient flow.

Techniques That Address Care of Patients in the ED

Fast Tracks

An ED fast track is a dedicated area in or next to the ED that is specifically designed and designated for patients with minor illnesses or injuries. It is typically staffed by midlevel providers, such as physician assistants and nurse practitioners working under the supervision of an emergency physician. Fast tracks can operate during regular business hours or during the ED's busiest times (e.g., evenings and weekends). Currently, fast tracks are in place at roughly 30 percent of all EDs, with approximately 30 percent of presenting patients being routed to these areas for care (JCAHO, 2004; Wilson and Nguyen, 2004). Identifying nonurgent patients and routing them to the fast track allows the ED to treat them more quickly. It also frees non–fast track ED resources to care for the most seriously ill and injured patients, moving them quickly into appropriate inpatient units. In this way, fast tracks can reduce delays in care for both urgent and nonurgent patients, thereby improving patient flow across the ED.

One example of the throughput time reductions associated with fast tracks is Grady Health Systems in Atlanta, Georgia (see Box 4-4). Using the fast-track approach, Grady was able to reduce the time from arrival to bed placement for nonurgent patients from 219 to 94 minutes, a 57 percent decrease (JCAHO, 2004; Wilson and Nguyen, 2004). It is important to note that fast-track capacity may vary widely for different hospitals and should be determined according to the specific circumstances of each ED, such as volume, patient mix, and severity-of-illness levels.

Zone Nursing

Based on the engineering concept of collocation, zone nursing ensures that all of a nurse's patients are located in one area, thereby eliminating the need for nurses to traverse a unit to provide care (JCAHO, 2004; Wilson and Nguyen, 2004). Explored by a number of hospitals nationwide, the zone approach has been found to reduce ED crowding. For example, as part of a pilot project at Boston Medical Center during which just one nurse received zone-approach assignments, the average patient throughput time was reduced by 70 minutes. Based on the success of the pilot, the approach was extended to the entire ED. A new version of the concept was recently initiated, involving zone collocation of both ED residents and nursing staff. Evaluation of this team approach is still under way (Wilson and Nguyen, 2004).

Bedside Registration

Bedside registration can help reduce long stays in the waiting room. Patients are quickly triaged in the reception area and immediately moved to a bed in the treatment area, where they can be seen immediately by a physician. In the treatment area, a computer on wheels allows staff to register the patient and collect insurance and other administrative information at the bedside, even after treatment has begun.

Triage

ED triage is typically performed by experienced emergency nurses, and sometimes by physicians. In crowded conditions, staff can feel pressure to perform triage quickly, creating opportunities for error. Some EDs are divided into separate areas—for example, pediatrics, obstetrics, and psychiatry—and triage is used to direct patients to the appropriate setting. Computer-enhanced triage is also being adopted by some hospitals to improve the reliability of triage decisions and expedite patient flow. These approaches are discussed in the next chapter.

Full-Capacity Protocols

Full-capacity protocols are plans put in place by hospitals to improve the treatment of patients and patient flow in conditions of extreme crowding due to full inpatient units. Rather than keeping patients in the ED, perhaps in hallways and unsafe areas, full-capacity protocols allocate patients to inpatient beds in alternative units on a temporary basis. The approach recognizes the systemwide nature of ED crowding and requires that all departments share the responsibility for addressing crowding. Allocating patients to several different departments greatly improves conditions in already understaffed EDs, while the addition of one or two hall patients to several inpatient units has a minimal impact on those units' staffing ratios. For example, adding two patients to a 30-bed unit with a 6- to 30-nurse staffing requirement yields a staffing ratio of 6.4—less than half a nurse below full staffing.

The State University of New York Stony Brook Hospital instituted this practice and found that a large percentage of patients never actually stayed in the hallway of the inpatient unit because staff were motivated to make beds available more quickly. Other patients spent less time in the inpatient unit than they would have had to spend in the ED. Early results showed that the average length of stay of ED hallway patients was 6.2 hours while that for unit hallway patients was 5.4 hours, and that patient satisfaction increased. A number of other institutions have adopted the practice, which is currently promoted by the New York State Department of Health.

Admission/Discharge Units

An admission/discharge unit separate from the ED area has the potential to improve coordination of emergency patients and enhance patient flow. Such a unit provides several advantages to an ED. It can respond rapidly to the needs of the ED since it will always have the physical capacity to add a patient to the expandable ward, and it is not dependent upon the location of a patient's physician for the writing of patient discharge orders. In addition, recently discharged patients remaining in the hospital are often poorly monitored and represent a liability exposure. Having a separate discharge unit greatly reduces this risk. Further, patients being staged for admission are conveniently located in one place for the staff to do their workups without taking resources (e.g., nursing, staff, space) from the ED.

Use of Information Technology

A number of approaches involving information technology can greatly enhance quality and efficiency in the ED. These include adoption of electronic health records with embedded error detection, patient tracking throughout the hospital system, "look-up" displays in critical care bays, health system–wide scheduling directly from the ED, and enhanced use of point-of-care testing and imaging. While many of these techniques are well established, others are in the early stages of development, and although they show promise, their effectiveness is unproven in many cases. Implementation of such techniques should be supported and informed by a robust clinical and health services research agenda.

Timely Support for Consults and Procedures

Just as patients often wait for laboratory results and pharmaceutical deliveries, excessive amounts of time can be required for staff physicians to arrive for consults or minor (nonoperative) procedures. There are myriad reasons for these delays, but the general cause in many cases is a simple lack of planning and coordination, for example, failure to anticipate and staff for periods of high demand. Arrangements for specialists who provide on-call services are also critical. Lack of adequate on-call coverage can cause serious delays and compromise patient care. This issue is dealt with extensively in Chapter 6.

Given the wide range of tools available to improve the efficiency of hospitals, their potential benefit in alleviating emergency and trauma care crowding and enhancing quality, and their limited application in these settings to date, the committee believes adoption of such tools is crucial to improving the delivery of emergency care services. The committee therefore recommends that **hospital chief executive officers adopt enterprisewide operations management and related strategies to improve the quality and efficiency of emergency care (4.2).**

OVERCOMING BARRIERS TO ENHANCED EFFICIENCY

Although a growing body of evidence supports a range of strategies for improving patient flow and efficiency of operations while reducing ED crowding, a number of barriers exist to the adoption and implementation of these strategies within the hospital setting. The challenges to improving the efficiency of hospital-based emergency care are multiple, and the demands on physicians and administrators should not be taken lightly, particularly in light of the many other demands they face—for example, interdepartmental battles for resources, cost and revenue management, community relations, and a bewildering assortment of potential threats and opportunities. Despite the best intentions, hospitals face an uphill battle to focus sufficient attention on emergency care in the face of these other demands. Some of the specific challenges are discussed below.

Hospital Leadership Issues

Hospitals are extremely complex, highly political environments that present numerous leadership challenges for chief executive officers (CEOs) and other executives. In many facilities, the clinical staff consists largely of independent agents working outside the traditional full-time staff structure (NAE and IOM, 2005). As a result, the vast majority of U.S. hospitals rely on clinicians who essentially serve as independent agents with distinct, and often disparate, agendas. Changes in the health care marketplace have resulted in many hospitals facing budget shortfalls, and the current reimbursement system offers little incentive for wholesale change. Added to these factors is the tenuous nature of most CEO appointments—data suggest the average hospital CEO tenure is just 6 years (American College of Healthcare Executives, 2004; Garman and Tyler, 2004)—and it is not surprising that many hospitals lack the leadership or support needed to embark on the systemwide analysis, innovation, and change necessary for improvements in patient flow.

Despite these challenges, it is clear that hospital leaders must be willing to lead if efforts to reduce ED crowding through improved patient flow and efficiency of operations are to succeed. Specifically, hospital leaders must recognize that ED crowding is a systemwide issue that must be addressed across hospital settings and is not limited to the ED itself. They must be willing to send a strong, consistent message that improving patient flow is a hospital priority. And they must back up those words with specific, demonstrable actions, including personal involvement in the development, implementation, and evaluation of patient flow improvement strategies.

Hospital executives, including both CEOs and midlevel managers, have an opportunity to provide visionary leadership in promoting patient flow and operations management approaches to improve hospital efficiency. The traditional paradigm of the ED as a safety valve for hospitalwide bottlenecks and inefficiencies is rapidly giving way to a modern view of the ED as an integrated component of a highly interconnected, organic system. Hospital leaders should be open to learning from the experiences of industries outside of health care and be bold and creative in applying these and other new ideas. The early evidence from The Robert Wood Johnson Foundation's Urgent Matters project, IHI, and other such efforts suggests that not only does this view make sense for patients and providers, but it also makes sense for the bottom line.

To foster the development of hospital leadership in improving hospital efficiency, the committee recommends that **training in operations management and related approaches be promoted by professional associations; accrediting organizations, such as the Joint Commission on Accreditation of Healthcare Organizations and the National Committee for Quality Assurance; and educational institutions that provide training in clinical, health care management, and public health disciplines (4.3).**

Staff Buy-In

Hospital clinicians, including those in the ED, tend to be conservative in nature and reluctant to embrace systemic change; efforts to identify and resolve barriers to patient flow through such strategies as those noted above are not likely to succeed without the early and strong support of hospital leaders, clinicians, and other staff. The recent failure of Cedars-Sinai Medical Center to implement a computerized provider order entry (CPOE) system demonstrates the magnitude and significance of this resistance. In November 2002, Cedars-Sinai began a 14-week, department-by-department rollout of its newly installed CPOE system. The rollout was called off and the system removed less than 2 months later following what has been characterized as a "staff revolt" (Chin, 2003; Cedars-Sinai Learns, 2004; Connolly, 2005).

The selection of a well-respected, highly regarded individual to serve as a champion for improved patient flow is an important step in ensuring the success of flow improvement strategies. Among other responsibilities, this individual can help sell the necessary changes to medical staff and executive managers. He/she can also help exert the constant pressure needed to reshape the policies, processes, relationships, and cultural norms that have historically impeded patient flow throughout the hospital.

Data Collection

The collection and analysis of reliable, comprehensive data concerning all aspects of patient flow is imperative if hospitals are to understand and resolve the factors contributing to crowding in their EDs. Currently, however, most hospital data systems do not adequately monitor or measure patient flow. For example, few systems distinguish between when a patient is ready to move to an ancillary location for care and when that move actually takes place—a limitation that prevents the capture and analysis of data on ED boarding, as well as other ED throughput delays.

Rigorous data collection and analysis is essential to the success of any patient flow improvement strategy. Using the I/T/O model, hospitals can identify key performance indicators for evaluating patient flow performance. Examples of such indicators used successfully by hospitals participating in the Urgent Matters initiative are time from inpatient bed assignment to bed placement, inpatient bed turnaround time, total ED throughput time, and time to thrombolysis for cardiac patients (Wilson et al., 2005). Other key performance indicators identified by the Government Accountability Office (GAO) as measures of ED crowding include the number of hours an ED is on ambulance diversion, the percentage of patients who board in the ED and for how many hours, and the number of patients who leave the ED after triage but before a medical evaluation as a percentage of ED visits (GAO, 2003).

Systems Approach

Research has shown that while the causes of ED crowding, boarding, and diversion are complex, the principal factors involved lie not in the ED itself but in inpatient departments to which ED patients are referred (Asplin et al., 2003). As a result, as noted earlier, it is increasingly understood that ED crowding is a systemwide issue that must be addressed across multiple hospital and acute care settings (Richardson et al., 2002; Asplin et al., 2003; Schafermeyer and Asplin, 2003; GAO, 2003; Magid et al., 2004). Thus it is not surprising that a key characteristic of successful patient flow improvement is the adoption of a systemwide approach to change. Such an approach includes, among other features, the development of a multidisciplinary, hospitalwide team that can work collaboratively to identify problems, propose solutions, and oversee the implementation and evaluation of various improvement strategies. (An example of a hospital team is shown in Figure 4-2.) Such an approach also includes timely collection and analysis of data at multiple points across several hospital settings to enable

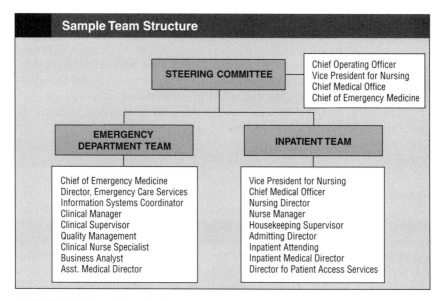

FIGURE 4-2 Sample hospital team structure.
SOURCE: Reprinted, with permission, from Wilson and Nguyen, 2004.

evaluation of patient flow and assess changes in operations. Results of these analyses and outcome measures should be shared within and outside the hospital setting. Such transparency increases ownership and accountability among hospital leaders and staff; it also improves patient understanding of the complex, multidisciplinary nature of emergency care.

Alignment of Incentives

The degree of crowding and boarding that occurs in the ED would not be tolerated in inpatient departments. The strategies discussed above have the potential to improve patient flow significantly; enhance the quality, safety, and timeliness of emergency care; and produce related cost savings. Yet history has demonstrated that little progress will be made toward achieving these goals unless hospitals are held accountable through regulatory and incentive-based policies. Without such policies, hospitals will continue to marginalize patient flow matters, relegating most of the related consequences to EDs and their patients through crowding, prolonged periods of boarding, and ambulance diversions. There are a number of steps that can be taken by hospital leaders to address these issues, as well as policy initiatives that should be considered to align payment incentives with the goals of enhanced efficiency and quality of care.

Positive Incentives

No major change in health care can take place without strong financial incentives, and today hospitals have almost no incentives to address the myriad problems associated with inefficient patient flow or ED crowding. Indeed, as detailed below, hospitals have a number of financial incentives to continue the practices that lead to these problems.

Financial incentives must be instituted to ensure that hospitals act aggressively to eliminate ED crowding, boarding, and ambulance diversions. Rewarding hospitals that demonstrate efficient delivery practices that appropriately manage patient flow should be a consideration in reimbursement. All payers, including Medicare, Medicaid, and private insurers, should develop contracts that reward hospitals for efficient ED operations and penalize them for delays in hospital admission, for ED crowding, and for ambulance diversions. Through its purchaser and regulatory power, CMS has the ability to drive hospitals to address and manage patient flow and ensure timely access to quality care for its clients. Current CMS payment policies should be revised to reward hospitals that manage patient flow appropriately; conversely, hospitals that fail to do so should be subject to penalties.

Finally, CMS should evaluate the potential effect of existing diagnosis-related group (DRG) payments on the relative priority assigned to elective patients and emergency admissions. Patients admitted from the ED are more likely to have a higher severity of illness, to be uninsured, or to have lower rates of reimbursement. Results of research undertaken at a small group of hospitals indicate that patients transferred to inpatient units and ICUs from the ED are more costly than elective patients for selected surgical DRGs (Munoz et al., 1985; Henry et al., 2003). A similar study found that patients transferred acutely to tertiary surgical ICUs were significantly more costly than elective admissions (Borlase et al., 1991). A disincentive to admit ED or transferred patients over elective patients may contribute to crowding and boarding in the ED. If such a disincentive exists, CMS should identify alternative payment methodologies to eliminate it.

Negative Incentives

Hospitals face virtually no reimbursement-related disincentives for operating a crowded ED. Indeed, they may benefit financially if this situation reduces Emergency Medical Treatment and Active Labor Act (EMTALA)-mandated admissions and preserves their capacity to admit elective patients. In 2004, JCAHO instituted new guidelines that would require accredited hospitals to take serious steps to reduce crowding, boarding, and diversion. This action followed a July 2002 alert that linked treatment delays to more than 50 deaths. Under pressure from the hospital industry, however, these requirements were withdrawn (Morrissey, 2004). They were replaced in January 2005 with a patient flow standard—Managing Patient Flow—that applies to the entire hospital. Among other things, this standard requires that hospitals develop plans and implement ways to monitor and manage patient flow that will reduce ED overcrowding and its consequences and ensure acceptable quality of care. Joint Commission Resources, an arm of JCAHO, has published a document aimed at educating hospital leadership about the new standard and providing guidance on how to comply with its provisions (JCAHO, 2004). While the new standard correctly acknowledges that patient flow is a system-level issue that must be addressed on a hospitalwide basis, it allows hospitals to continue using the ED as a holding area. Therefore, the committee recommends that **the Joint Commission on Accreditation of Healthcare Organizations reinstate strong standards designed to sharply reduce and ultimately eliminate emergency department crowding, boarding, and diversion (4.4).**

Not only do hospitals face no financial penalties for crowding and boarding, but there are several financial incentives that promote the practices that lead to these problems. First, a hospital benefits financially from increased volume (up to a point). Operating at high capacity is risky for any business because it means there is limited capacity available to deal with spikes in demand. But the ED provides a convenient escape valve for hospitals operating at or near capacity. During periods of peak demand, patients can be cared for in the ED in relative safety because of the highly skilled and interdisciplinary staff that are available to deal with any exigency, staff that are used to a high-volume, high-pressure environment.

Second, according to a recent GAO report, one reason patients back up in the ED is that, as noted earlier, elective admissions for surgery or other procedures tend to be more profitable than emergency admissions through the ED (GAO, 2003). While many hospitals may not intentionally favor scheduled over ED admissions, which would potentially constitute an EMTALA violation, the GAO report found that only a minority of hospitals that diverted ambulances took other measures, such as postponing or canceling elective admissions.

Third, as discussed previously, patients admitted through the ED are more likely to be uninsured—indeed in many private hospitals, the only way an uninsured patient can be admitted is through the ED—and ED crowding has the effect of slowing the influx of uninsured and underinsured patients admitted through the ED.

Fourth, when hospitals hold emergency admits in the ED and instead give an available bed to the next elective patient, they essentially receive two inpatient reimbursements for the price of one because ED staff (a fixed cost) provide inpatient care at no additional cost to the hospital, while the elective patient gets the bed. Giving the ED admission priority over the elective one forfeits that advantage. Also, if the elective admission does not get the bed, the patient's admitting physician may look to another hospital for admission. By contrast, ED admissions are "captive" in that they are already inside the facility and are too sick or injured to go elsewhere except in extreme circumstances.

Finally, when EDs are crowded in a community, especially if ambulances are being diverted and patients are walking away from the local public hospital or nonprofit equivalent, it can be financially perilous under EMTALA to have a "wide open" ED because uninsured and low-reimbursement patients are likely to flood the available ED. Although there is a paucity of data on the practice, some hospitals have been known to adopt "defensive diversion" to shield themselves from receiving diverted ambulance patients from the local public hospital. Further, some hospitals divert on a case-by-case basis—meaning they accept ambulances if the patient's doctor is on the medical staff and refuse otherwise. While this practice constitutes an EMTALA violation, it is difficult to identify and pursue. In the absence of external regulatory mechanisms, monitoring of diversion status, and independent verification of how crowded the ED and hospital really are, it is impossible to limit this sort of practice.

The committee would like to see improved monitoring of hospital admission patterns by CMS to ensure that hospitals are not regularly using diversion while continuing to accept elective admissions. Such a practice would be in violation of EMTALA, and its prohibition should be strictly enforced (Medical Advisory Committee and Pennsylvania Emergency Health Services Council, 2004). Furthermore, the committee concludes that the practices of boarding and diversion are so antithetical to quality medical care that the strongest possible measures must be taken to eliminate them. Therefore, the committee recommends that **hospitals end the practices of boarding patients in the emergency department and ambulance diversion, except in the most extreme cases, such as a community mass casualty event. The Centers for Medicare and Medicaid Services should convene a working group that includes experts in emergency care, inpatient critical care, hospital operations management, nursing, and other relevant disciplines to develop boarding and diversion standards, as well as guidelines, measures, and incentives for implementation, monitoring, and enforcement of these standards (4.5).**

Public Awareness

A final step in implementing the changes recommended by the committee is to make the public understand what is going on; appreciate the seriousness of the situation; know what questions to ask; and realize that the problem affects each individual, rich or poor, old or young, black or white, urban or rural. In short, the public needs to know what good performance is and understand who does and does not experience it. Hospitals should be required to measure key indicators of ED crowding and make those measures available to policy makers and the public. This could be accomplished through a variety of mechanisms, including patient flow performance report cards, public notices regarding diversion, and educational efforts focused on the unique and critical role served by safety net hospitals. For example, a community could provide "diversion alerts," similar to storm alerts, to inform the public about EDs unable to accept new patients.

The reliance of EDs on other hospital units to eliminate ED crowding and its consequences through the effective management of patient flow demands a systemwide approach supported by hospital leaders and staff, policy makers, and the American public. Without immediate intervention, the quality, safety, and timelines of emergency care will continue to experience strain under the pressures of ED crowding, boarding, and diversion. Eliminating these pressures is no longer just a matter of convenience; it is a matter of life and death.

SUMMARY OF RECOMMENDATIONS

4.1: The Centers for Medicare and Medicaid Services should remove the current restrictions on the medical conditions that are eligible for separate clinical decision unit payment.

4.2: Hospital chief executive officers should adopt enterprisewide operations management and related strategies to improve the quality and efficiency of emergency care.

4.3: Training in operations management and related approaches should be promoted by professional associations; accrediting organizations, such as the Joint Commission on Accreditation of Healthcare Organizations and the National Committee for Quality Assurance; and educational institutions that provide training in clinical, health care management, and public health disciplines.

4.4: The Joint Commission on Accreditation of Healthcare Organizations should reinstate strong standards designed to sharply reduce and ultimately eliminate emergency department crowding, boarding, and diversion.

4.5: Hospitals should end the practices of boarding patients in the emergency department and ambulance diversion, except in the most extreme cases, such as a community mass casualty event. The Centers for Medicare and Medicaid Services should convene a working group that includes experts in emergency care, inpatient critical care, hospital operations management, nursing, and other relevant disciplines to develop boarding and diversion standards, as well as guidelines, measures, and incentives for implementation, monitoring, and enforcement of these standards.

REFERENCES

AMA (American Medical Association). 2003. *National Physician Survey of Professional Medical Liability.* Chicago, IL: AMA.

American College of Healthcare Executives. 2004. *Hospital CEO Turnover: 1981–2004.* Chicago, IL: Health Administration Press.

Andrulis DP, Kellermann A, Hintz EA, Hackman BB, Weslowski VB. 1991. Emergency departments and crowding in United States teaching hospitals. *Annals of Emergency Medicine* 20(9):980–986.

Asplin BR, Magid DJ, Rhodes KV, Solberg LI, Lurie N, Camargo CA Jr. 2003. A conceptual model of emergency department crowding. *Annals of Emergency Medicine* 42(2):173–180.

Asplin BR, Rhodes KV, Levy H, Lurie N, Crain AL, Carlin BP, Kellermann AL. 2005. Insurance status and access to urgent ambulatory care follow-up appointments. *Journal of the American Medical Association* 294(10):1248–1254.

Begley CE, Chang YWRC, Weltge A. 2004. Emergency department diversion and trauma mortality: Evidence from Houston, Texas. *The Journal of Trauma Injury, Infection, and Critical Care* 57(6):1260–1265.

Berwick DM. 1996. A primer on leading the improvement of systems. *British Medical Journal* 312(7031):619–622.

Borlase BC, Baxter JK, Kenney PR, Forse RA, Benotti PN, Blackburn GL. 1991. Elective intrahospital admissions versus acute interhospital transfers to a surgical intensive care unit: Cost and outcome prediction. *Journal of Trauma-Injury Infection & Critical Care* 31(7):915–918; discussion 918–919.

Cedars-Sinai Learns from its CPOE Mistakes to Improve Workflow. 2004. [Online]. Available: http://www.bio-itworld.com/newsletters/healthit/2004/09/09/20040909_10115/ [accessed August 1, 2005].

Chin T. 2003, February 17. Doctors pull plug on paperless system. *AMNews.* [Online]. Available: http://www.ama-assn.org/amednews/2003-02/17/bil20217.htm [accessed May 20, 2006].

Chisholm CD, Collison EK, Nelson DR, Cordell WH. 2000. Emergency department workplace interruptions: Are emergency physicians "interrupt-driven" and "multitasking"? *Academic Emergency Medicine* 7(11):1239–1243.

Connolly C. 2005, March 21. Cedars-Sinai doctors cling to pen and paper. *The Washington Post.* P. A.01.

Crute S. 2005. *Quality Matters, Case Study: Flow Management at St. John's Regional Health Center.* New York: The Commonwealth Fund.

de Leon AC Jr, Farmer CA, King G, Manternach J, Ritter D. 1989. Chest pain evaluation unit: A cost-effective approach for ruling out acute myocardial infarction. *South Medical Journal* 82(9):1083–1089.

DeLia D. 2006, in press. Annual bed statistics give a misleading picture of hospital surge capacity. *Annals of Emergency Medicine.*

Derlet R, Richards J. 2000. Overcrowding in the nation's emergency departments: Complex causes and disturbing effects. *Annals of Emergency Medicine* 35(1):63–68.

Derlet R, Richards J, Kravitz R. 2001. Frequent overcrowding in U.S. emergency departments. *Academic Emergency Medicine* 8(2):151–155.

Dick RS, Schneider SM, Macdonald I. 2005. A cure for crowding: The impact of an emergency department observation unit on ambulance diversionary hours. *Academic Emergency Medicine* 12(5 Suppl. 1):10-a.

Eckstein M, Chan LS. 2004. The effect of emergency department crowding on paramedic ambulance availability. *Annals of Emergency Medicine* 43(1):100–105.

Epstein SK, Slate D. 2001. The Massachusetts College of Emergency Physicians ambulance diversion study. *Academic Emergency Medicine* 8(5):526–527.

Fineberg HV, Scadden D, Goldman L. 1984. Care of patients with a low probability of acute myocardial infarction. Cost effectiveness of alternatives to coronary-care-unit admission. *New England Journal of Medicine* 310(20):1301–1307.

Gabow P, Eisert S, Karkhanis A, Knight A, Dickson P. 2005. *A Toolkit for Redesign in Health Care, Final Report.* Rockville, MD: Agency for Healthcare Research and Quality.

Gallagher EJ, Lynn SG. 1990. The etiology of medical gridlock: Causes of emergency department overcrowding in New York City. *Journal of Emergency Medicine* 8(6):785–790.

GAO (U.S. Government Accountability Office). 2003. *Hospital Emergency Departments: Crowded Conditions Vary among Hospitals and Communities.* Washington, DC: GAO.

Garman AN, Tyler JL. 2004. *CEO Succession Planning in Freestanding U.S. Hospitals: Final Report.* Chicago, IL: Health Administration Press.

Gorunescu F, McClean SI, Millard PH. 2002. Using a queuing model to help plan bed allocation in a department of geriatric medicine. *Health Care Management Science* 5(4):307–312.

Grady Health System. 2005. *About Grady.* [Online]. Available: http://www.gradyhealthsystem. org/ [accessed July 1, 2005].

Graff LG, Dallara J, Ross MA, Joseph AJ, Itzcovitz J, Andelman RP, Emerman C, Turbiner S, Espinosa JA, Severance H. 1997. Impact on the Care of the Emergency Department Chest Pain Patient from the Chest Pain Evaluation Registry (CHEPER) Study. *American Journal of Cardiology* 80(5):563–568.

Graff LG, Prete M, Werdmann M, Monico E, Smothers K, Krivenko C, Maag R, Joseph A. 2000. Implementing emergency department observation units within a multihospital network. *Joint Commission Journal on Quality Improvement* 26(7):421–427.

Green LV, Soares J, Giglio JF, Green RA. 2006. Using queuing theory to increase the effectiveness of emergency department provider staffing. *Academic Emergency Medicine* 13(1):61–68.

Henneman PL, Marx JA, Cantrill SC, Mitchell M. 1989. The use of an emergency department observation unit in the management of abdominal trauma. *Annals of Emergency Medicine* 18(6):647–650.

Henry MC. 2001. Overcrowding in America's emergency departments: Inpatient wards replace emergency care. *Academic Emergency Medicine* 8(2):188–189.

Henry MC, Thode HCJ, Havasy SP. 2003. Financial effects of emergency department admissions compared to electives within surgical diagnosis related groups (DRGs) at 11 hospitals in Suffolk County, NY. *Academic Emergency Medicine* 10(5):532-a.

Hostetler B, Leikin JB, Timmons JA, Hanashiro PK, Kissane K. 2002. Patterns of use of an emergency department-based observation unit. *American Journal of Therapeutics* 9(6):499–502.

Huang XM. 1995. A planning model for requirement of emergency beds. *IMA Journal of Mathematics Applied in Medicine & Biology* 12(3–4):345–353.

IOM (Institute of Medicine). 2000. *To Err Is Human: Building a Safer Health System.* Washington, DC: National Academy Press.

IOM. 2001. *Crossing the Quality Chasm: A New Health System for the 21st Century.* Washington, DC: National Academy of Sciences.

JCAHO (Joint Commission on Accreditation of Healthcare Organizations). 2004. *Managing Patient Flow: Strategies and Solutions for Addressing Hospital Overcrowding.* Washington, DC: Joint Commission Resources, Inc.

Kennedy J, Rhodes K, Walls CA, Asplin BR. 2004. Access to emergency care: Restricted by long waiting times and cost and coverage concerns. *Annals of Emergency Medicine* 43(5):567–573.

Kleinke JD. 1998. *Bleeding Edge: The Business of Health Care in the New Century.* Gaithersburg, MD: Aspen Publishers, Inc.

The Lewin Group. 2002. *Emergency Department Overload: A Growing Crisis, the Results of the AHA Survey of Emergency Department (ED) and Hospital Capacity.* Washington, DC: American Hospital Association.

Litvak E. 2005. Optimizing patient flow by managing its variability. In: JCAHO, *From Front Office to Front Line: Essential Issues for Health Care Leaders.* Oakbrook Terrace, IL: Joint Commission Resources, Inc.

Litvak E, Long MC. 2000. Cost and quality under managed care: Irreconcilable differences? *American Journal of Managed Care* 6(3):305–312.

Lucas CE, Buechter KJ, Coscia RL, Hurst JM, Meredith JW, Middleton JD, Rinker CR, Tuggle D, Vlahos AL, Wilberger J. 2001. Mathematical modeling to define optimum operating room staffing needs for trauma centers. *Journal of the American College of Surgeons* 192(5):559–565.

Lynn SG, Kellermann AL. 1991. Critical decision making: Managing the emergency department in an overcrowded hospital. *Annals of Emergency Medicine* 20:287–292.

Mace SE, Graff L, Mikhail M, Ross M. 2003. A national survey of observation units in the U.S. *American Journal of Emergency Medicine* 21(7):529–533.

Magid DJ, Asplin BR, Wears RL. 2004. The quality gap: Searching for the consequences of emergency department crowding. *Annals of Emergency Medicine* 44(6):586–588.

McCaig LF, Burt CW. 2005. *National Hospital Ambulatory Medical Care Survey: 2003 Emergency Department Summary.* Hyattsville, MD: National Center for Health Statistics.

McKay JI. 1999. The emergency department of the future: The challenge is in changing how we operate! *Journal of Emergency Nursing* 25(6):480–488.

McManus ML, Long MC, Cooper A, Mandell J, Berwick DM, Pagano M, Litvak E. 2003. Variability in surgical caseload and access to intensive care services. *Anesthesiology* 98(6):1491–1496.

McManus ML, Long MC, Cooper A, Litvak E. 2004. Queuing theory accurately models the need for critical care resources. *Anesthesiology* 100(5):1271–1276.

Medical Advisory Committee, Pennsylvania Emergency Health Services Council. 2004. *Joint Position Statement: Guidelines for Hospital Ambulance-Diversion Policies.* Mechanicsburg, PA: Pennsylvania Emergency Health Services Council.

Mikhail MG, Smith FA, Gray M, Britton C, Frederiksen SM. 1997. Cost-effectiveness of mandatory stress testing in chest pain center patients. *Annals of Emergency Medicine* 29(1):88–98.

Morrissey J. 2004. Going with the (patient) flow. JCAHO's watered down' ER patient-management standard relieves hospital executives, disappoints docs. *Modern Healthcare* 34(6):1, 6–7.

Munoz E, Regan DM, Margolis IB, Wise L. 1985. Surgonomics: The identifier concept: Hospital charges in general surgery and surgical specialties under prospective payment systems. *Annals of Surgery* 202(1):119–125.

Murray M, Berwick DM. 2003. Advanced access: Reducing waiting and delays in primary care. *Journal of the American Medical Association* 289(8):1035–1040.

NAE, IOM (National Academy of Engineering, Institute of Medicine). 2005. *Building a Better Delivery System: A New Engineering/Health Care Partnership.* Washington, DC: The National Academies Press.

National Association of Public Hospitals, AHRQ. 2005. Presentation at the meeting of the Getting LEAN: Health care's challenge, Denver, CO.

Picker Institute. 2000. *Eye on Patients. A Report by the Picker Institute for the American Hospital Association.* Boston, MA: Picker Institute.

Reinus WR, Enyan A, Flanagan P, Pim B, Sallee DS, Segrist J. 2000. A proposed scheduling model to improve use of computed tomography facilities. *Journal of Medical Systems* 24(2):61–76.

Richardson LD, Asplin BR, Lowe RA. 2002. Emergency department crowding as a health policy issue: Past development, future directions. *Annals of Emergency Medicine* 40(4):388–393.

Ross MA, Compton S, Richardson D, Jones R, Nittis T, Wilson A. 2003. The use and effectiveness of an emergency department observation unit for elderly patients. *Annals of Emergency Medicine* 41(5):668–677.

Rydman RJ, Isola ML, Roberts RR, Zalenski RJ, McDermott MF, Murphy DG, McCarren MM, Kampe LM. 1998. Emergency department observation unit versus hospital inpatient care for a chronic asthmatic population: A randomized trial of health status outcome and cost. *Medical Care* 36(4):599–609.

Schafermeyer RW, Asplin BR. 2003. Hospital and emergency department crowding in the United States. *Emergency Medicine (Fremantle)* 15(1):22–27.

Schneider S, Zwemer F, Doniger A, Dick R, Czapranski T, Davis E. 2001. Rochester, New York: A decade of emergency department overcrowding. *Academic Emergency Medicine* 8(11):1044–1050.

Schull MJ, Lazier K, Vermeulen M, Mawhinney S, Morrison LJ. 2003. Emergency department contributors to ambulance diversion: A quantitative analysis. *Annals of Emergency Medicine* 41(4):467–476.

Siddharthan K, Jones WJ, Johnson JA. 1996. A priority queuing model to reduce waiting times in emergency care. *International Journal of Health Care Quality Assurance* 9(5):10–16.

Sinclair D, Green R. 1998. Emergency department observation unit: Can it be funded through reduced inpatient admission? *Annals of Emergency Medicine* 32(6):670–675.

Solberg LI, Asplin BR, Weinick RM, Magid DJ. 2003. Emergency department crowding: Consensus development of potential measures. *Annals of Emergency Medicine* 42(6):824–834.

Southard PA, Hedges JR, Hunter JG, Ungerleider RM. 2005. Impact of a transfer center on interhospital referrals and transfers to a tertiary care center. *Academic Emergency Medicine* 12(7):653–657.

Starfield B. 2000. Is U.S. health really the best in the world? *Journal of the American Medical Association* 284(4):483–485.

Talbot-Stern J, Richardson H, Tomlanovich MC, Obeid F, Nowak RM. 1986. Catheter aspiration for simple pneumothorax. *Journal of Emergency Medicine* 4(6):437–442.

Thorpe KE. 1990. The current hospital crisis in New York City and policy options for resolving it. *New York State Journal of Medicine* 90(5):247–252.

Vallee P, Sullivan M, Richardson H, Bivins B, Tomlanovich M. 1988. Sequential treatment of a simple pneumothorax. *Annals of Emergency Medicine* 17(9):936–942.

Viccellio P. 2001. Emergency department overcrowding: An action plan. *Academic Emergency Medicine* 8(2):185–187.

Wears RL, Perry SJ. 2002. Human factors and ergonomics in the emergency department. *Annals of Emergency Medicine* 40(2):206–212.

Weissert W, Chernew M, Hirth R. 2003. Titrating versus targeting home care services to frail elderly clients: An application of agency theory and cost–benefit analysis to home care policy. *Journal of Aging & Health* 15(1):99–123.

Wilson JW, Oyen LJ, Ou NN, McMahon MM, Thompson RL, Manahan JM, Graner KK, Lovely JK, Estes LL. 2005. Hospital rules-based system: The next generation of medical informatics for patient safety. *American Journal of Health-System Pharmacy* 62:499–504.

Wilson MJ, Nguyen K. 2004. *Bursting at the Seams: Improving Patient Flow to Help America's Emergency Departments*. Washington, DC: The George Washington University Medical Center.

Zwiche DL, Donohue JF, Wagner EH. 1982. Use of the emergency department observation unit in the treatment of acute asthma. *Annals of Emergency Medicine* 11:77–83.

5

Technology and Communications

Daniel Conway is a 65-year-old male who has a sudden on-set of excruciating back pain. He calls his primary caregiver, Dr. Thompson, who tells him to call an ambulance to bring him to the Eastern Hospital emergency department (ED).

Dr. Thompson clicks on a Web page for the Eastern Hospital Emergency call-in program. He imports his last progress note with Mr. Conway's history and adds a personal note describing his concerns that the patient's uncontrolled hypertension could have led to a ruptured abdominal aortic aneurysm.

The ED immediately receives the on-line submission and begins preparations for the patient's arrival while the ambulance is still en route. Paramedics, using interoperable communications systems that give them equal capability to communicate with fire and police agencies on one hand and hospitals on the other, inform the ED that Mr. Conway's vital signs are stable but he is in severe pain. The emergency physician advises them to administer a dose of intravenous morphine and carefully monitor his blood pressure, oxygenation, and respiratory rate. Upon arrival, Mr. Conway is rapidly transported to a preassigned room, where the emergency physician, Dr. Hendricks, and his team are waiting. While the nurses take his vital signs and the doctor examines him, a clerk arrives at the bedside with a wireless laptop. After the initial evaluation, she collects the information necessary to register him in the system without delay. The paramedics complete their run report on a tablet computer and use the wireless network to beam it into the hospital databases.

Mr. Conway is in too much pain to recall all of his medications accurately. Dr. Hendricks queries a clinical data-sharing network, which compiles a list from the computerized records of local pharmacies. The doctor has a question about which would be the best diagnostic test to order given the specifics of Mr. Conway's history. He consults the hospital's digital library, and with several mouse clicks he confirms that a computer-assisted tomography (CAT) scan is still the expert-recommended choice. He orders the study via the computerized physician order entry (CPOE) system and also orders some pain-relieving medication. The program alerts him that his choice could have a dangerous interaction with one of the medications Mr. Conway is taking. The computer suggests an alternative, which the doctor selects instead.

A few moments later, Dr. Hendricks sees that the patient is not in his room. He looks at the electronic dashboard, which is tracking the radio frequency identification (RFID) tag on Mr. Conway's wristband. He learns that the patient was transported to radiology 5 minutes ago and is currently undergoing the scan. Shortly thereafter, an alert on the dashboard warns him that the radiologist has reported an abnormality on the study. Luckily, the pain is being caused by a kidney stone instead of something more serious. With a single click the emergency physician is able to view the digital images and confirm the findings.

Looking for assistance in managing Mr. Conway's kidney stone, Dr. Hendricks pages a urologist. Instead of wasting time waiting by the phone, he immediately goes to see another patient. He knows that whenever his call is returned, it will be routed to the digital communication device he wears on his lapel.

Dr. Hendricks generates the documentation for the patient's ED visit through a wireless dictation or wireless tablet system that allows him to note historical and physical findings, order laboratory tests and radiographs, and submit orders via CPOE with integrated decision support. In either case, he does not have to search for a chart or wait for someone else to finish using it.

The dashboard is updated with Mr. Conway's pending discharge so the housekeeping manager can ensure that the resources required to clean the room will be available when needed. The triage nurse in the ED selects the next patient to use the room when it becomes available.

A short time later, Mr. Conway is feeling better and is ready to be discharged home. He receives a computer-generated instruc-

tion sheet with information about his diagnosis of a kidney stone, including what warning signs to watch for, as well as whom to follow up with and when. Upon discharge, the system sends the patient's primary care physician, Dr. Thompson, and the consulting urologist a secure e-mail summarizing the ED visit and the patient's discharge instructions. The e-prescribing module, having screened for potential drug interactions and provided dosage guidance, electronically routes Mr. Conway's prescriptions to the pharmacy near his home, saving time and reducing the risk of errors associated with legibility problems.

Mr. Conway uses his secure doctor–patient messaging application to communicate with Dr. Thompson 2 days later, letting him know he passed the stone and is feeling much better. He also mentions how pleased he was with his emergency visit. Even though the ED seemed to be incredibly busy, everything went smoothly and efficiently, and he feels he got great care.

Although the story of Mr. Conway's visit to the ED sounds futuristic, all of the technology described above exists today as both home-built and commercial products. But the diffusion of these technologies to date has been limited. The average community hospital and even some large medical centers lack basic information technology (IT) enhancements that have been shown to improve the efficiency of care and patient flow, inform clinical decision making, and enhance provider-to-provider and provider-to-patient communications. This chapter describes the current state of the art in health care IT and highlights several specific IT tools that have proven ability to improve emergency care in six key areas: management and coordination of patient flow and hospital patient care, linkage of the ED to the wider health care community, clinical decision support, clinical documentation, training and knowledge enhancement, and population health monitoring. The chapter also considers some of the new clinical technologies that are expected to impact emergency care within the coming decade. This is followed by a discussion of challenges and barriers hospitals may face in adopting these technologies. Finally, the chapter addresses the need for and approaches to prioritizing investments in technologies that can improve emergency care now and in the future.

INFORMATION TECHNOLOGY IN THE
HEALTH CARE DELIVERY SYSTEM

The early application of health care IT was limited almost exclusively to hospital accounting systems. As early as the 1960s, hospitals began to use various computer programs for business operations and financial management (Detmer, 2000; Shortliffe, 2005). By the mid-1970s, a small number of hospitals had equipped their programs to process data with medical content (Henley and Wiederhold, 1975; Hospital Financial Management Association, 1976). During the 1980s and 1990s, many hospitals further enhanced their systems to include electronic health records (EHRs), a trend that was also seen among a small percentage of private physician practices (IOM, 1991, 2003).

Despite these early advances, progress toward widespread adoption of health IT has been slow. This is especially true of applications aimed at improving the quality and timeliness of patient care, such as programs that assist with patient flow, clinical decision making, and medical communications. Today, it is estimated that fewer than one-third of hospitals and one-fifth of private physicians use EHRs. Use of CPOE systems is even less common, with only 12 percent of hospitals and 10 percent of private physicians using the technology (Brailer and Teresawa, 2003; Goldsmith et al., 2003; The Lewin Group, 2005; Healthcare Information and Management Systems Society, 2005; Burt and Hing, 2005; Bower, 2005). In comparison, more than one-half of primary care physicians in New Zealand and the United Kingdom have reported using both EHRs and CPOEs in their daily practices (Harris Interactive, 2001). Commonly cited barriers to the adoption of these and other IT tools include prohibitive costs, lack of standardization, and physician resistance to change; additional discussion of these barriers is provided later in this chapter.

While usage rates for specific IT applications remain low, data do suggest that American physicians are increasingly reliant on computer-based resources within their offices. According to a recent American Medical Association survey, 99 percent of private practices and 96 percent of physicians use computers in their offices, 84 percent have a computer network in place, and 75 percent have Internet access. At the same time, however, the interconnectedness of these resources with other points in the health care system, such as the ED, has been found to be lagging, with only 35 percent of physicians reporting a connection with a hospital or laboratory (Chin, 2002). The apparent isolation of this emerging IT usage raises significant concerns about the continuity of care, particularly for ED patients, for whom immediate access to medical records can mean the difference between lifesaving intervention and life-threatening medical errors.

Data also suggest providers' growing recognition of the potential of IT to significantly improve the quality of health care in the United States. For example, a majority of respondents to a 2005 survey conducted by the Healthcare Information Management and Systems Society (HIMSS) cited "reducing medical errors and improving patient safety" as their top IT priority. Of these respondents, nearly two-thirds indicated their next IT development would be the adoption of an EHR system. Other applications identified by respondents included CPOE and clinical decision support systems (CDSSs). The HIMSS survey respondents included hospitals, physician offices, mental/behavioral health facilities, long-term care facilities, and home health agencies with annual gross revenues ranging from $50 million or less to $1 billion or more (Healthcare Information and Management Systems Society, 2005).

Given that more providers recognize and are turning to IT as a tool to improve the safety and quality of care, one might expect to find significant IT investments occurring in the health care field. After all, the United States invests approximately $1.7 trillion, or 16 percent of its gross domestic product (GDP), on health care annually. Data reveal, however, that the expected level of investment simply has not occurred. In 2004, just $17–$42 billion, or 10–25 percent of all U.S. health care investments, was applied to health IT. Less than one-third of this amount, or approximately $7 billion, was invested in hospital clinical systems such as EHRs, CPOE, or CDSSs (Goldsmith et al., 2003; Bower, 2005; The Lewin Group, 2005).

The health care field has also failed to keep pace with IT investments as a percentage of industry revenue. While spending on health care IT as a percentage of revenue has increased slightly in recent years, rising from 1–2 percent in 1998 to 2–3 percent today, these figures are far below those for the IT and financial services industries, which invested 10 and 7 percent, respectively (The Lewin Group, 2005). This disparity becomes even more striking when one examines IT investment rates on a per worker basis; while most U.S. industries invested approximately $8,000 per worker for IT in 2004, the health care industry invested only about $1,000 (DHHS and ONCHIT, 2005).

The paucity of investments in health care IT has ramifications far beyond the financial. Without adequate resources for the coordinated development or implementation of proven IT systems, efforts to enhance safety, optimize workflow, and foster communication among and across health care settings have largely stalled. Further, where improvements have been made, they have occurred in relative isolation, resulting in islands of innovation rather than systemic repairs to a failing system.

Progress toward a highly integrated and coordinated emergency care system has been slow even though the value of such integration and coordination has long been recognized (NHTSA, 1996). Instead, multiple systems of varied quality have developed independently of one another. The resulting fragmentation undermines the quality, safety, and timeliness of emergency care; limits the application of proven health care IT; and prevents the aggregation of data for public health surveillance and research purposes (Halamka et al., 2005).

The federal government recently assumed a leadership role through the provision of funding and other support to develop a uniform national health information infrastructure capable of supporting integrated health IT (Taylor, 2004; Cunningham, 2005; Hillestad et al., 2005; Shortliffe, 2005). This initiative can lead to significant improvements in emergency care, as well as in other areas. Federal leadership is needed because of failures in the health IT marketplace, including asymmetrical risks and rewards for technological innovation and the inability to offer aggregated data comparisons (Taylor, 2004; Middleton, 2005). Moreover, such leadership is needed today to ensure that IT advances are made in a coordinated way that facilitates the necessary interoperability and communication.

The federal government has shown the ability to initiate essential industry innovation when market forces have failed to do so. The Hill-Burton Act, for example, is largely responsible for the nation's hospital infrastructure (Halvorson, 2005). Adopted in 1946, Hill-Burton provided federal grants to states for the construction of hospitals, requiring states to adopt plans ensuring that constructed facilities would meet a variety of minimum requirements. Over the course of the next 30 years, Hill-Burton subsidized the construction of 40 percent of all U.S. hospital beds. Other examples of federal leadership filling a market void include the Rural Electrification Act of 1936 and the Federal Aid Highway Act of 1956 (Halvorson, 2005).

A number of other industrial nations have already embraced the need for national leadership in and funding of health IT innovation. Britain's National Health Service (NHS), for example, recently embarked on the world's largest civilian IT project, planning to spend approximately $11 billion on a national system that will replace the existing hodgepodge of local systems and paper medical records (The Lewin Group, 2005). Among the IT tools to be featured in this effort are lifelong EHRs coordinated at the national level, integrated information sharing among all health care settings, and online communications and data access for patients and providers (Detmer, 2000).

Using a Regional Health Information Organization (RHIO) model that provides common elements across the full continuum of health care settings, the U.S. government has the potential to significantly improve the quality, safety, and timeliness of emergency care. While the direct costs associated with this effort are estimated at $276 billion over 10 years, a national health information infrastructure would generate direct savings amounting to $613 billion over the same period and $94 billion annually thereafter—this in addition to the many ancillary savings associated with such benefits as improved management of chronic disease (Kleinke, 2005).

INFORMATION TECHNOLOGY
IN THE EMERGENCY DEPARTMENT

The ED is a unique setting in modern medicine—a complex and chaotic environment that presents an increasing number of challenges. ED clinicians are frequently called upon to make crucial decisions under pressure with limited data while maintaining continual readiness for new arrivals, stressing available resources. Because ED providers must often make critical decisions without patient records or histories, it has been said that EDs operate on "information fumes." EDs are subject to increasing patient volumes and more complex conditions, yet over the last decade they have experienced a diminished capacity caused by decreasing resources. One solution to the serious challenges facing today's EDs may be found in IT, which can both facilitate analysis of the problems and support solutions.

All of the common medical tasks performed by doctors involve information processing: taking a history, examining a patient, ordering and interpreting test results, considering diagnoses, devising a treatment plan, and communicating with other providers about the appropriateness of admission or discharge. All of these are data management tasks. Information is generated when procedures are performed, and simply by the presence and flow of patients. Emergency providers are eager consumers of available past clinical data and are creators of information to be used during follow-up. The quality of information management determines how well providers manage the care of their patients.

Today, there is an especially urgent need to apply IT to the delivery of emergency care. Among other factors, this urgency stems from the life-and-death nature of emergency care, the myriad threats to such care posed by ED crowding, and the increasingly common role of the ED as the public's portal of choice for medical services.

Six key areas of emergency care could immediately benefit from an infusion of IT:

• **Management and coordination of patient flow and hospital patient care**—Technologies such as electronic dashboards, radio frequency tracking, and wireless communications systems can help ED staff manage patients and maintain control over department workflow.

• **Linkage of the ED to the wider health care community**—Enhanced communications among providers within a community can greatly improve the availability of useful clinical information for emergency care, coordination of care, and allocation of community health care resources. Computerized messaging between patients and doctors can ensure that all providers fully coordinate their care. And telemedicine enables advanced medical knowledge to improve the care of patients in remote areas.

- **Clinical decision support**—As stand-alone units or part of a broader system, CDSSs can help guide clinicians in choosing the optimal and most economical therapy and can enhance the safety and efficiency of triage. Clinical alerts and reminders can warn providers if a proposed treatment plan poses unrecognized risks.
- **Clinical documentation**—Electronic documentation of emergency services can facilitate the timely, accurate collection and storage of information regarding the course of patient care, serving as proof of services rendered for reimbursement purposes and supporting public health and research functions, among other benefits.
- **Training and knowledge enhancement**—Computerized education and training resources can make the most up-to-date medical knowledge rapidly available to clinicians so they can deliver quality care.
- **Population health monitoring**—Emerging IT applications can provide real-time population health monitoring, including syndromic surveillance and outbreak detection, necessary for many public health and homeland security priorities.

In each of these areas, IT has the potential to significantly enhance the timeliness, safety, and quality of emergency care, improving patient flow and reducing health costs in the process. The challenge for the future is to integrate these technologies effectively so that hospitals can invest in applications that address goals and objectives in all of the above six areas. For example, systems should be able to support clinical decisions as well as operations management. It should also be emphasized that the future development and advancement of IT applications must accommodate the special needs of pediatric patients.

Management and Coordination of Patient Flow and Hospital Patient Care

The case of Mr. Conway presented above illustrates the need for seamless communications among prehospital IT systems; hospital departmental systems, such as laboratory and radiology; and hospital patient-tracking systems. To meet the complex data needs of an ED clinician, data must be shared easily and securely between clinical and financial systems using widely accepted standards and protocols. Among the IT tools currently available to assist with the management and coordination of emergency care are those described below.

Electronic Dashboards

The pre-IT solution for managing ED flow was for staff to track patients on a centrally visible whiteboard. Commonly arranged in the form of a grid, this whiteboard contained a list of patients and their locations, current providers, the status of the visit, and orders to be completed. The information was updated manually when the staff noticed a change and had the time to update the board. Such a system provides a useful central source of individual data points. However, many management decisions are based on aggregate information that needs to be assembled in real time. Since information on whiteboards is updated only when someone notices a change and has time to enter the update, this manual process breaks down during the ED's busiest times, when the accuracy and timeliness of information are most critical. This problem tends to self-propagate: outdated data cause inefficiencies, further taxing a harried staff that then does not have time to update the whiteboard with further changes.

Computer technology transforms the manual whiteboard into an electronic "dashboard" that continuously displays updated information and integrates multiple data sources, such as laboratory, radiology, and admitting databases. Using a combination of colors or symbols to represent ongoing tasks and processes, many dashboards can present information in a tabular, grid-like format (similar to the manual whiteboard), while others arrange the screen as a graphical representation of the ED. Sometimes, the dashboard tracking function is used as a central point of an ED information system, providing links to other systems discussed in this chapter. At other times, the system is a stand-alone tool that can be modified to interface with other components of the hospital information system.

However they are configured, electronic dashboards allow providers to see the most recent information without the need for manual input. Computerized systems provide an excellent overview of the ED and patient flow for both clinicians in the ED and administrators in their offices. Bottlenecks become readily apparent, staff members are able to see developing problems, and action can be taken before operations are affected.

Long-term storage of the data tracked by a dashboard system, as with several other systems discussed in this chapter, is another useful tool that can aid in resource planning and error identification, analysis, and prevention. Given accurate models of patient flow and information on past bottlenecks, it becomes possible to anticipate future demands on staff and maximize the efficient deployment of resources (Cone et al., 2002). The complexity of the ED makes error identification a difficult process, and sole reliance on clinician reporting will likely be inadequate to effect change (Handler et al., 2000). Readily accessible data on all ED visits facilitates analysis of standard quality assurance measures, such as unplanned revisits, as well as the formulation of new metrics for quality care. In the case of an adverse event, analysis of stored dashboard parameters can allow reconstruction of the event, similar to the capability provided by an airplane's "black box" after a crash.

Further, allowing clinicians (especially trainees) to access stored tracking data to follow up on their patients encourages self-monitoring for errors and helps mitigate a key deficiency of the feedback system of the ED: that an unknown result of treatment has the same reinforcing effect as a positive outcome (Croskerry, 2000). Often, errors and near misses are caught during follow-up care but not reported back to the original treating clinician. Storage of visit data makes it easy for ED providers to review a list of patients they have seen in the past. That list could integrate data from the ED course with other information from the hospital system, allowing providers to follow up on whether their diagnoses were correct and their treatments appropriate.

While there have been only a few effectiveness studies concerning comprehensive ED dashboard systems, preliminary findings appear to support the benefits of their use. Among these benefits, hospitals with ED dashboards have reported reductions in lengths of stay, fewer patients leaving prior to treatment, and less time spent on diversion (Jensen, 2004). Providing emergency physicians with an updated display of the status of laboratory tests has been shown to improve their perceptions of efficiency and communication with patients (Marinakis and Zwemer, 2003). And the ability to better communicate estimated wait times to patients using dashboard technology has been found to improve patient satisfaction with emergency care (Thompson et al., 1996).

Radio Frequency Identification Tracking

Effective workflow in the ED requires knowledge of the locations of patients, caregivers, and equipment. New tracking technologies, such as radio frequency identification (RFID), can show the exact locations of people and resources, enabling caregivers to optimize workflow and empowering administrators to understand how people move through the department.

Such tracking systems are available in two basic forms: (1) passive systems that require the use of RFID scanners to read unpowered RFID tags and (2) active systems that use existing hospital wireless networks to track battery-operated RFID transmitters. Using hardware and software, active RFID systems then track the position of these transmitters with enough accuracy to identify the room in which they are located.

Several pilot studies of RFID tracking in the ED offer insight regarding the potential of this technology to improve the quality, timeliness, and efficiency of emergency care. At Beth Israel Deaconess Medical Center in Boston, for example, RFID is being used to track equipment and key staff members. At Summa Health System in Akron, Ohio, RFID is being used to optimize patient flow and track patient location. Finally, an ED in Memphis is using RFID as a means to reduce patient waiting times by providing real-time notification of bed availability.

Digital Voice Communications

While the ED dashboard provides complete integration of all hospital data in a single location, there is still a need for real-time discussion of patient care issues among caregivers. Cellular technologies appear to be an obvious answer to this real-time need given the ubiquity of such devices, but pose a number of challenges for hospitals, including electronic interference, varied reception, and germ transfer (Tri et al., 2001; Shaw et al., 2004). One means of addressing these issues is hands-free Voice over Internet Protocol (VoIP) devices for voice communications over existing hospital wireless data networks. Newer VoIP devices provide dual capability—automatic use of the hospital network when indoors and automatic use of the standard cellular network when outdoors. Of note, users of such technology must remain cognizant of their surroundings to ensure that patient confidentiality is protected and that ambient noise does not degrade voice recognition.

Wireless Registration

In a typical ED, several components of emergency care occur simultaneously. A patient having a heart attack, for example, may require a physician performing an exam, a nurse inserting an intravenous tube, and a medical technician performing an electrocardiogram (EKG). At the same time, the laboratory will be processing blood tests, while radiology is developing an x-ray and the catheterization laboratory is being instructed to prepare for a new arrival. In most EDs, however, there is a critical point of failure in the simultaneous nature of this response: the ED registration clerk.

Currently at most facilities, ED registration represents a significant bottleneck in what should be a serial process. For patients who have been triaged with a high severity of illness, one strategy for improvement is to move the formal registration process to the bedside via a wireless network. Such an approach would make the registration process more flexible as it would remove the need to tie the registration process to a single physical space (Smith and Feied, 1998).

Mobile Computing

Mobile computing (MC) technology, such as specialized wireless laptop carts equipped with 24-hour batteries or specialized tablet PCs, are being increasingly well received by ED physicians and their patients (Bullard et al., 2004). Among their other applications, MC technology can provide ED staff with bedside access to patient EHRs and CDSSs. Tablets can also enable physicians and nurses to document their findings and care in real time rather than dictating later, and provide the clinician with feedback to ensure proper documentation for coding and billing purposes. These devices also help clinicians remember the relevant questions to ask, findings to check, and checklists to review before administering hazardous treatments, such as thrombolytic therapy. In addition, MC technology can enhance the capability of the ED to deploy a fully functional system to any location at a moment's notice, as might be required during severe crowding or a mass casualty event.

Handheld Wireless Devices

Handheld computers and multifunction wireless devices, such as Blackberries, are increasingly popular with physicians who use them in their clinical practice (ACP and ASIM, 2005). Numerous published reports describe their utility for medical education (Bertling et al., 2003), dissemination of new medical practice guidelines (Strok et al., 2003), and documentation of patient care and procedures in the ED (Bird et al., 2001). When integrated with wireless communications devices, handheld computers can be used to view patient data (Duncan and Shabot, 2000), record and transmit real-time patient vital signs during intrahospital transport (Lin et al., 2004), and serve as triage and screening tools for large public events (Chang et al., 2004). These devices also can be used to enhance patient safety by alerting physicians to abnormal test results (Bates and Gawande, 2003).

Digital Radiography and Picture Archiving and Communications Systems

In recent years, many hospitals have migrated from film to digital capture and display of x-ray, magnetic resonance imaging (MRI), computed tomography (CT), angiography, and ultrasound images. These images are then stored in a picture archiving and communications systems (PACS). Both digital radiography and PACS have been shown to provide interpretations that are as reliable as traditional film-based methods (Kundel et al., 2001). With respect to emergency care in particular, a number of benefits are associated with these technologies, such as reduction of the time required to capture images (Redfern et al., 2002). PACS offer instantaneous sharing of images with multiple clinicians, reduce the risk of films being irrevocably lost or misplaced, and eliminate all delays associated with retrieving films from archives and record rooms. And both technologies facilitate remote interpretation of films, a service especially important in rural or community ED settings, which may not have access to 24-hour radiologist coverage. In addition, PACS enable on-call specialists to view films from home, office, or another hospital, thereby expediting care.

Electronic Health Records

Whether implemented as stand-alone systems or part of a more comprehensive IT array, each of the coordination and management tools discussed here has the potential to significantly improve patient flow and enhance the quality, timeliness, and safety of care in the ED. This is particularly true when these tools are complemented by an integrated system of EHRs.

The ED operates in a relative data vacuum with respect to information on patients and their conditions. Typically, there is no medical record for ED patients, who may be uncommunicative or unconscious upon arrival. Moreover, extreme urgency of treatment is paramount as life-threatening illnesses or injuries have occurred. Under such circumstances, accurate diagnosis is made more difficult, drug allergies can be missed, and important comorbidities can go undetected. Fortunately, EHRs offer a solution to this information void.

The potential of EHRs to improve patient care in all health care settings has been well recognized for more than a decade, with the Institute of Medicine (IOM) having called for the complete elimination of paper-based medical records as early as 1991 (IOM, 1991). As currently defined by the IOM, an EHR system consists of four key elements: (1) longitudinal collection of electronic health information for and about patients, defined as including information pertaining to the health of an individual or health care provided to an individual; (2) immediate electronic access to patient- and population-based information for those with designated authority; (3) provision of knowledge and decision support to enhance the quality, safety, and efficiency of patient care; and (4) support for efficient processes of health care delivery (IOM, 2003).

Over the last 15 years, numerous studies have documented the advantages of EHR systems over traditional paper-based medical records. Among these advantages, EHRs improve the reliability of chart access, allow multiple individuals to access the record simultaneously, and facilitate electronic communication between health care providers. They enhance the quality and completeness of medical data and facilitate the integration of clinical decision support for providers. They also provide efficient access to medical references and assist with the collection of population health measures (Holbrook et al., 2003). Studies examining the use of EHR systems in EDs have yielded similar findings, concluding that the systems can improve documentation, patient care, and patient satisfaction without detracting from direct patient care or resident education or supervision (Buller-Close et al., 2003).

Linkage of the ED to the Wider Health Care Community

A number of IT tools are available to improve provider-to-provider and provider-to-patient communications during the course of ED care and beyond.

Prehospital Communications

The potential for IT to improve patient flow and enhance the quality, timeliness, and safety of emergency care begins even before the patient reaches the hospital. Prehospital EMS units often are the first caregivers to acquire medical information about patients en route to the ED. The ability of these units to accurately capture and transmit vital signs, patient history, and early treatment information to receiving hospitals can be enhanced by several IT applications. For example, prehospital 12-lead electrocardiography has been shown to be safe, to improve times to reperfusion therapy, and to decrease patient morbidity and mortality (Urban et al., 2002). Also, the rapid diffusion of messaging and data transmission through commercial cellular telephones suggests a significant potential for the development of cell-based prehospital–hospital communications. It is critically important that the design and implementation of these systems support full interoperability, that is, allow EMS personnel to "talk" to each other, the police, emergency management personnel, fire departments, and EDs.

Emergency Management

A number of cities have begun to eliminate communication barriers by purchasing equipment that enables officials from public safety and public health to communicate in real time (GAO, 2004). Some cities have also begun to address disaster preparedness communication issues with the help of the Health Alert Network, a nationwide communication network designed to facilitate communications through high-speed Internet connectivity, broadcast capabilities, and training.

In addition, the real-time capture and transmission of EMS dispatch data can improve the coordination of prehospital and emergency care for critically ill patients (Teich et al., 2002). Such data exchange allows EMS teams to quickly determine the best location to which they should deliver patients. This capability not only minimizes delays caused by routine ambulance diversions, but also significantly strengthens a community's ability to respond to mass casualty events. Retrospective analysis of EMS dispatch data also suggests that the monitoring of EMS data is a viable approach to public health monitoring and surveillance (Mostashari et al., 2003).

Regional Health Information Organizations

The development of RHIOs holds significant promise for connecting emergency medical services (EMS), EDs, and other providers within regions (Koval, 2005). Regional health systems can link providers who serve the safety net so they can coordinate emergency and other community care. Many communities already have primary care networks that integrate hospital EDs into their planning and coordination efforts. A rapidly growing number of communities, such as San Francisco and Boston, have developed RHIOs that coordinate the development of information systems to facilitate patient referrals and tracking and the sharing of medical information between providers to optimize the patient's care across settings. The San Francisco Community Clinic Consortium, for example, brings together primary care, specialty care, and EDs in a planning and communications network that closely coordinates the care of safety net patients throughout the city.

The development of these networks is a centerpiece of the federal government's strategic plan for health care IT (Thompson and Brailer, 2004). The Agency for Healthcare Research and Quality (AHRQ) has provided seed money through grants to a number of RHIO startups.

Telemedicine

Telemedicine has a number of important applications for improving the delivery of emergency and trauma services in remote locations, including emergency patient care, education, research, and patient follow-up. A recent IOM study, *Quality Through Collaboration: The Future of Rural Health*, highlighted the growing application of telemedicine to emergency and trauma care (IOM, 2004b). The use of two-way videoconferencing, available since the 1960s, has begun to increase as a result of the accelerated development of telecommunications infrastructure in the last decade, the introduction of digital communications, and the improved capabilities and cost value of computer hardware and applications. Videoconferencing has facilitated specialty consultation in a number of critical areas, including trauma, radiology, cardiology, and orthopedics.

Cost and outcome studies on the role of telemedicine in rural areas are limited and warrant further attention. Studies have shown telemedicine to be effective in the delivery of acute care to victims of trauma in remote locations (Marcin et al., 2004). Teleradiology has been found to have a significant impact on diagnosis and treatment decisions (Lee et al., 1998). Studies have also indicated high levels of patient and provider satisfaction with these technologies (Boulanger et al., 2001).

Automated Discharge Systems

For many patients who enter the health care system through the ED, treatment concludes with discharge instructions on self-care and on when to return for follow-up care. Unfortunately, patient recall of these instructions is often quite poor, a problem exacerbated by the frequent use of medical jargon and difficult-to-read handwriting (Vukmir et al., 1993). Further, patients' noncompliance with instructions for follow-up services often hampers recovery, thereby contributing to return ED visits. These problems are compounded for non-English-speaking patients. Good communication between patient and clinician is essential to quality care and good outcomes. The IOM report *Health Literacy: A Prescription to End Confusion* documented the poor state of health literacy, even among English-speaking patients, and the serious consequences this can have for health outcomes (IOM, 2004a). For non-English-speaking patients, the problem is clearly more critical. As the number of non-English-proficient U.S. residents increases, the need for IT solutions will grow.

A number of IT tools available today can assist with the discharge process. These include automated discharge programs that produce clear, concise, legibly written instructions proven to enhance patients' understanding of their condition and their adherence to treatment plans (Vukmir et al., 1993; Jolly et al., 1995). In addition, discharge communication programs allow ED physicians to establish a primary care appointment for follow-up care, a service that has been shown to markedly improve patient show rates at follow-up appointments, providing an additional opportunity to offer important preventive services (O'Brien et al., 1999).

Automated Referral Systems

A common frustration facing ED staff today is how best to receive information on patients who are referred to the ED by their primary care physician. In an effort to streamline care, referring physicians often wish to share insights and suggestions about the patient they are referring. In large EDs, however, it is often impractical and interruptive to have a busy ED physician stop patient care to take a call from a referring physician. To solve this problem, some EDs make fax or phone transcription options available to callers. Yet at the busiest times, a large number of patient referrals can pile up by the triage desk, and matching them up accurately as patients arrive becomes a challenging and time-consuming task.

To address this challenge, many hospitals are adopting automated referral systems to facilitate information transfer. Beth Israel Deaconess Medical Center in Boston, for example, developed a system that allows physicians to access a secure Web page and input or import the patient's information.

Once the information has been submitted, the system prints out a summary report and attaches an electronic copy of the report to the patient's EHR. Thus even if the triage staff is unable to match the paper referral to the appropriate patient chart, clinical staff can still see and act on the information via the dashboard display. Prior to the system's implementation, ED administration at Beth Israel Deaconess Medical Center received several complaints per week related to this problem; now such complaints are almost nonexistent.

Electronic Prescribing

Electronic prescribing, or the electronic transfer of prescription data from clinicians to pharmacies, is an increasingly common method of ensuring that providers, pharmacists, and patients have timely access to accurate prescription and medication information. ED clinicians can use electronic prescribing technology to send discharge medication prescriptions automatically to a pharmacy that is convenient for their patients. This capability improves the timeliness and accuracy of prescriptions and eliminates risks due to poor handwriting or inaccurate transcription (Bizovi et al., 2002). It also improves enforcement of formularies and enhances communication among providers. Electronic prescribing technology can be implemented alone or integrated with other discharge programs, such as those as described above.

Electronic Communications

The complexity of modern medicine has made the sharing of information a critical function in health care. Failures of communication between health care providers are among the most common factors contributing to adverse events (Bates and Gawande, 2003). Health care IT can facilitate communication between physicians, as well as between patients and providers. It can also help make the dissemination of information more efficient by ensuring that the information is received and handled with appropriate priority.

There are currently two common approaches to secure electronic communications. The first is Secure/Multipurpose Internet Mail Extensions (S/MIME) gateways. With this approach, organizations obtain digital certificates that are used to encrypt e-mail as it travels over the Internet. Thus, the organization-to-organization transmission of e-mail is protected. Once the electronic message has arrived at the destination organization, it is treated as secure internal e-mail. The second approach involves storing all messages in a secure database accessible only via a password-protected encrypted website. Doctors and patients communicate via this website, but reminders are sent to their regular e-mail accounts informing them that they have new messages pending. In this way, no patient-identified information is sent via regular, unsecured e-mail technologies. This secure website approach enables discharge summaries, admission notification, and other clinical correspondence to be transmitted electronically between doctors. Additionally, patients and doctors can use the system to exchange clinical results and clinical messages.

With both of these approaches, efforts must be made to facilitate use of the system in ways that make both providers and patients more comfortable with the technology. A recent study found that while 45 percent of on-line consumers wished to communicate with their physicians using e-mail, only 6 percent had done so (Manhattan Research, 2002). The adoption of privacy standards and other protections is needed to encourage use of electronic communications at both ends of the care spectrum. An example of a system linking patients and providers is described in Box 5-1.

Clinical Decision Support

Adverse events can often be prevented if additional information is known at the time critical decisions are made. Sometimes the pivotal facts are available, but because of information overload, they are not readily apparent among a large volume of less important data. Computers can be programmed to use guidelines to alert physicians of unexpected results or remind them of important information at the time decisions are being made. Numerous studies have shown that alerts and reminders are an effective means of changing physician behavior and improving the quality of care (McDonald, 1976; Kuperman et al., 1999; Kilpatrick and Holding, 2001). Specific examples of clinical decision-support tools currently available to improve emergency care are described below.

Automated Triage Systems

Automated triage systems are commonly used to refer patients to the appropriate levels of medical care. For example, nurse call centers routinely use protocols and guidelines to triage patients to self-care, primary care, or emergency care. Initial attempts at the development and implementation of such systems for use in the ED have achieved variable levels of success (Brillman et al., 1996; Haukoos et al., 2002; Dale et al., 2003). While additional research on the potential of triage systems to enhance ED patient flow and improve the quality of emergency care is needed, there is at least one tool available to assist with ED triage efforts—the Emergency Severity Index (ESI).

Consisting of a five-level triage system, the ESI has been shown to correlate reliably with resource utilization, the need for hospitalization, and

---

BOX 5-1
The PatientSite Project

CareGroup HealthCare Systems is an integrated health care delivery system based in Boston consisting of five hospitals, including its flagship facility, the Beth Israel Deaconess Medical Center. The system employs approximately 1,700 medical staff who provide care to more than 1 million patients at CareGroup centers and through numerous affiliated practices. CareGroup implemented the world's first clinical computer system and on-line medical record program.

In 1999, CareGroup and Beth Israel staff began discussing how best to involve patients in their care and meet the demands of on-line patients. Using a variety of information servers and databases, including some developed by project authors, the team established an independent clinical platform that could display patient information on a secure website accessible through a number of web browsers. Known as PatientSite, this system features secure messaging among patients, providers, and staff; it allows patients to perform routine tasks, such as requesting appointments, obtaining prescription refills, or requesting primary care referrals, on-line; and it supports patient homepages that can be customized with a range of health education links, as well as messages from identified providers.

Patients registered with PatientSite have access to a comprehensive medical file, including medical records, established at the time of their registration. They also can maintain personal medical records, recording such information as medication problems, allergies, and other pertinent notes. Numerous security measures are in place to ensure that patients have access only to their own files. Physicians registered with PatientSite, by contrast, have access to information on all of their patients.

In early 2003, PatientSite claimed more than 120 participating providers representing 40 CareGroup centers and practices. It had more than 11,000 active patients, defined as those who had logged on at least once following their registration. Participation rates for both providers and patients have steadily increased since the program's inception in 2000. Additional information about PatientSite, including a demonstration page, is available at http://www.patientsite.org.

SOURCE: Sands and Halamka, 2004.

---

length of stay (Wuerz et al., 2000). It has excellent interrater reliability and a high correlation with the need for intensive care unit (ICU) admission (Tanabe et al., 2004). The ESI also has been validated in pediatric populations (Baumann and Strout, 2005). Integrating the ESI into automated triage systems in the ED could assist in the accurate and rapid assignment of severity scores, and immediate capture of the results could help expedite care and provide real-time data on departmental workload. Further, when combined with metrics of throughput and capacity, ESI data could be used to plan staffing and bed requirements, helping to avoid the need for ambulance diversion and minimizing the impact of ED overcrowding.

The University of Alberta's eTRIAGE system, developed in conjunction with the Alberta provincial government, uses the five-level Canadian Triage Acuity Scale (CTAS). It has been prospectively validated and found to have a high level of interrater reliability (Dong et al., 2005). Existing computer triage systems can also be modified to support syndromic surveillance. Even more promising is the notion of modifying eTRIAGE and similar systems to alert the triage nurse automatically whenever a patient presents with a history, symptoms, or clinical signs that suggest exposure to a bioterrorism agent or other public health threat.

Electronic and even manual triage systems can be designed to facilitate advance ordering of diagnostic tests (e.g., urinalysis, pregnancy test, ankle x-rays) in accordance with evidence-based clinical algorithms. This enables testing to begin before the patient is even seen by the physician.

Computerized Physician Order Entry

Recent efforts to decrease the incidence of adverse drug events have focused on providing clinical alerts at the time of ordering. CPOE systems force the entry of key information and provide suggestions for changes or additional orders as appropriate. Many CPOE systems prevent errors by checking that safe and effective doses have been prescribed, while others add checks for allergies or interactions with other prescribed medications. Adverse reactions to medications occur even when prescribers follow dosing recommendations and safety checks are performed; a detailed audit from CPOE systems and automated dispensing machines (discussed below) can assist with the identification of these rare events.

Over the last decade, CPOE systems have been shown to save time (Tierney et al., 1993), improve resource utilization (Tierney et al., 1988; Bates et al., 1999), improve adherence to clinical guidelines (Overhage et al., 1997; Teich et al., 2000), and decrease medication errors (Bates et al., 1998, 1999). They also have been found to enhance patient safety by providing extra safeguards for high-risk situations (Kuperman et al., 2001). These advantages have been shown only for custom-written CPOE software, however, and may not be replicable with commercial systems (Kaushal and Bates, 2001). It should also be noted that although efforts to implement CPOE in the ED are just beginning—as of 2003, only 18 percent of emergency medicine residency–affiliated EDs reported having medication order entry systems, and only 7 percent reported having systems that could check for errors (Pallin et al., 2003)—results of preliminary studies suggest that these systems have the potential to introduce inefficiencies (Shu et al., 2001; Field, 2004). A process change in a busy ED that slows care not only would be frustrating, but also could cause more harm than a CPOE system would prevent. As a result, it is especially important that CPOE systems for the ED be specifically designed for use in that setting and that their impacts on the quality, timeliness, and safety of emergency care be carefully monitored (Handler et al., 2004).

Automated Dispensing Machines

Automated dispensing machines (ADMs) are another patient-safety technology that has been gaining acceptance among health care providers. These devices are cabinets that contain multiple drawers filled with medications. They process medication orders and restrict the user's access to those medicines that have been prescribed, helping to ensure that the correct drug is chosen. The ADM maintains an audit trail that records which provider had access to each medication, facilitating investigation of adverse events. The machines are usually networked with a central pharmacy that keeps track of inventory and proactively replenishes stocks when they are running low.

While ADMs appear to have the potential to promote safety and improve patient flow, further study is needed to determine whether their benefits outweigh their negative aspects (Murray, 2001; Oren et al., 2003). For example, if the number of machines installed is inadequate, efficiency may be compromised as staff wait in line instead of caring for patients. Further, certain classes of medications (e.g., those used in case of cardiac arrest) need to be accessed immediately, and therefore are not appropriate for storage in ADMs in the ED.

Clinical Decision Support Systems

CDSSs integrate information on the characteristics of individual patients with a computerized knowledge base for the purpose of generating patient-specific assessments or recommendations designed to aid clinicians and/or patients in making clinical decisions in three areas: prevention and monitoring tasks, prescribing of drugs, and diagnosis and management (IOM, 2001). Use of CDSSs has been found to improve clinician compliance with a number of prevention and monitoring guidelines, including vaccinations, breast cancer screening, colorectal cancer screening, and cardiovascular risk reduction (Shea et al., 1996; Balas et al., 2000). Studies examining CDSS usage for drug selection, screening for interactions, and monitoring and documenting of adverse side effects similarly suggest some positive effect (Classen et al., 1992; Evans et al., 1998; Hunt et al., 1998). However, serious questions have emerged regarding the systems' ability to have a meaningful role in diagnosis or to improve patient outcomes (Wexler et al., 1975; Chase et al., 1983; Pozen et al., 1984; Wellwood et al., 1992; Hunt et al., 1998; Gallagher, 2002). If the time needed to consult a CDSS inadvertently slowed the delivery of emergency care, for example, the system's implementation would result in far more negative consequences than the benefits its use could offer. Additional research concerning the effectiveness and safety of CDSSs for diagnosis and management, particularly in the ED, is therefore warranted.

Clinical Documentation

All emergency encounters require documentation of the salient details of the visit. This information is maintained to fulfill a number of important goals: it serves as a record to assist in the care of the patient, it serves as proof of services rendered for reimbursement purposes, it records the provider's thoughts for use in defense against a potential negligence claim, and it supports public health and research functions. Creating documentation that is legible and meets these goals is a time-consuming task. Physicians overwhelmingly prefer to spend their time caring for patients rather than documenting the visit. The result has been a number of programs aimed at making the documentation process as efficient as possible.

Among the clinical documentation programs available, some require entering information in a structured manner, forcing the user to choose from provided options by selecting findings from rows of checkboxes, traversing a nested hierarchical tree of options, or clicking on symbols on a diagram of a human body. Others permit unstructured input, allowing users to type free text or dictate with minimal or no restrictions on what they can enter. A third technology is computer-assisted dictation, whereby a computer voice-recognition program makes a first pass at understanding the words, and a human "correctionist" then verifies the accuracy of the results.

Free-text and unstructured entry options permit rapid input. Because of limitations in computer understanding of human language, however, they do not provide much more capability than computer-assisted storage and transmission. Structured systems usually involve a more cumbersome and time-consuming data entry process, but they store information in a way that programs can easily understand, allowing them to serve as the basis for many other computer-assisted functions. Often, the increased time spent entering the data is compensated by increases in efficiency elsewhere. Human factors play a key role in the choice among these technologies, and the ways clinicians actually use and interact with different systems will ultimately determine the best approach. A well-designed tablet may turn out to be more efficient than dictation.

For example, fully computerized ED charts can support automated error surveillance (Schenkel, 2000) and help monitor the quality of ED care. Computer algorithms that search for the presence or absence of certain physical examination findings can lead to increases in the sensitivity of biosurveillance algorithms (Teich et al., 2002). CDSSs use programmed rules to promote safer health care; with a structured computerized chart, these rules can be written to handle a much wider range of less common clinical scenarios without the inefficiency or annoyance of asking the user too many questions.

The user-interface and data-entry modules of clinical documentation systems should be rigorously crafted to promote high-quality data entry and efficiency. Although there are many potential benefits to electronic clinical documentation, carelessly designed interfaces will slow the charting task and leave clinicians with two bad choices: allow the system to delay care in the ED, or batch the charting for completion at a later time (Davidson et al., 2004). These systems often necessitate a trade-off between obtaining more accurate and detailed information on patients and increasing the amount of time required to input the information.

Training and Knowledge Enhancement

IT can provide ED and associated staff with a number of informational and educational tools. Examples of these technologies are described below.

Integrated Information Resources

With the increasing complexity of medical care, emergency providers may care for patients who have conditions that were unheard of during their training or who are being treated with medications just recently approved. It is impossible for anyone with patient care responsibilities to memorize current information on every possible pathology, medication, or therapy that he or she could potentially encounter. Given the rapidly expanding volume of medical information and the wide variety of conditions that present to an ED, easy access to electronic references is key to improving patient safety (Bates et al., 1999).

Through new IT tools, the medical reference industry is now able to bring medical knowledge to the point of care in the ED and beyond. For example, textbook websites offer on-line versions of key medical texts and publications, a format that facilitates remote viewing, subject searches, and routine errata and addendums. Likewise, medication websites provide ED physicians and other staff with quick access to monographs on all prescription, nonprescription, and herbal preparations, as well as information on drug interactions and prescription costs. Many of these services are evolving to provide an increased level of integration into the clinical information system so that, for example, a provider who encountered an unfamiliar diagnosis in a patient record could read a summary simply by clicking on its name.

In addition, IT translation and visual communication tools can help providers deal with the dozens of languages that are heard in the ED. Important applications include the gathering of information for triage and diagnosis, communication regarding treatment decisions and care in the hospital, and provision of written information to patients for subsequent compliance and follow-up.

Training and Simulation

The nature of emergency medicine requires clinicians to rapidly assess a situation and execute an intervention plan, often with incomplete information. Extensive training can help prepare future emergency medicine staff for these types of challenging situations. Just as with the training of commercial airline pilots, computer-driven simulators can provide valuable educational experiences for both the development and evaluation of emergency practitioners' knowledge (Gordon et al., 2004). Simulation also can be especially useful for training emergency medicine residents in invasive procedures (Vozenilek et al., 2004). The potential of IT-based training and simulation recently led the Society of Academic Emergency Medicine to issue the following recommendation:

> EM residency programs should consider the use of high-fidelity patient simulators to enhance the teaching and evaluation of core competencies among trainees. . . . The impact of patient simulation on emergency medicine resident training is believed to be so significant that, were it not mindful of administrative and cost burdens for individual programs, the consensus panel would have advised that all emergency residency programs obtain access to a simulator. (Vozenilek et al., 2004, P. 1153)

Population Health Monitoring

Real-time population health monitoring is an emerging technology in emergency and public health informatics. Initial efforts have focused largely on regional monitoring of disease among ED patients. Interest and funding in this area were propelled in 2000 and 2001 by concerns about bioterrorism.

Public health agencies have long used surveillance—the systematic monitoring of health conditions of importance within populations—to measure the incidence of disease, identify outbreaks, and evaluate the impact of prevention programs (Buehler et al., 2004). Active surveillance using traditional methods such as postcards, telephone lines, faxed forms, and even e-mail is erratic because clinicians may forget to report a case when they see one or assume someone else is doing so. This can be true whether the condition involves an infectious disease such as tuberculosis or a high-impact injury, such as a gunshot wound (Kellermann et al., 2001). Electronic monitoring of key triage complaints and/or discharge diagnoses would greatly facilitate ED compliance with this traditional public health obligation.

A relatively recent development in population health monitoring is the notion of syndromic surveillance (Mandl et al., 2004)—methods relying on the detection of individual and population health indicators that are discernible before confirmed diagnoses are made. Before there is laboratory confirmation of an infectious disease, ill persons may behave according to identifiable patterns or have symptoms, signs, or laboratory findings that can be tracked through mining of data sources, including ED chief complaints (Fleischauer et al., 2004), International Classification of Diseases (ICD)-9 codes (Espino and Wagner, 2001), laboratory data, and pharmaceutical data (Tsui et al., 2003).

The goal of outbreak detection is to generate an alert whenever observed data depart sufficiently from an expected baseline. To this end, the system must be able to detect a signal (i.e., disease outbreak) against background noise (i.e., normally varying baseline disease in the region). A number of syndromic surveillance systems are currently being developed regionally as well as nationally. These include the Automated Epidemiologic Geotemporal Integrated Surveillance System (AEGIS) in Massachusetts (Mandl et al., 2004; Children's Hospital Informatics Program, 2005), the Real Time Outbreak Disease Surveillance System (RODS) in Pittsburgh (Tsui et al., 2003), the Electronic Surveillance System for the Early Notification of Community-based Epidemics (ESSENCE) system in the National Capital Area (Lombardo et al., 2003), and the national BioSense system being developed by the Centers for Disease Control and Prevention (Loonsk and CDC, 2004).

As such systems become more advanced, the need for standard protocols for alerting appropriate personnel of abnormal conditions becomes more pressing. One model may be AEGIS, which fully automates population health monitoring from end to end and interfaces with a statewide health alert network. This network, a comprehensive communication and alert messaging switch that provides message content and routing, is an example of a communications technology that helps unite clinical and public health entities.

NEW CLINICAL TECHNOLOGIES

New clinical technologies can be expected to alter the way care is delivered in the ED, but in ways that are difficult to predict. In general, however, a wide range of technologies that provide faster and more mobile diagnostic capabilities can be anticipated. Such technologies can be expected to diffuse gradually from the hospital to the prehospital environment. For example, strategically locating advanced imaging equipment in the ED would shorten patient wait times and improve throughput by accelerating diagnosis. Among the technologies positioned to do just that are 16-slice or higher CT scanners and high-field magnetic resonance (MR) systems, cardiac CT angiography (CTA), portable ultrasound systems, rapid diagnostics, and laboratory automation. As with all medical technologies, well-designed, controlled studies should be used to assess their efficacy and cost-effectiveness in general and for ED applications in particular.

Multislice Computed Tomography Scanners and High-Field Magnetic Resonance Systems

The improved temporal resolution and ever-increasing thin-slice imaging ability of these systems will have a significant impact on ED imaging. The performance of 16-slice CT is the proven standard for general whole-body clinical utility in the ED. However, 64-slice scanners offer a full complement of applications for both radiology and cardiology. In between, there are 32- and 40-slice systems that are less costly than 64-slice systems and are upgradable.

Manufacturers are redefining "open" MR by improving the performance of these systems with stronger magnets or redefining the term to include wider-bore, short-cylinder systems with traditional high-field image quality. With some of these systems, such as the Siemens Magnetom Espree, the patient's head frequently remains outside the gantry. The combination of a patient table with lateral movements and wide offset capability makes these systems well suited to orthopedic studies.

Although 1.5-tesla MR imaging systems continue to offer the broadest range of applications and clinical utility, the newer very-high-field (3.0-tesla) MR systems offer improved performance, particularly for neurologic, orthopedic, and spinal studies. Body imaging techniques continue to improve with new surface coils and software designed to reduce motion artifacts. The 3.0-tesla MR imaging systems show promise for cardiac imaging with cardiac sequences that are near-real-time and do not require patients to hold their breath. Adoption of very-high-field MR is currently limited but will expand as more sequence development work using these systems is done.

A promising new imaging system developed in South Africa is currently being evaluated at a handful of medical centers around the country. It allows the trauma team to obtain a quick, low-dose "total body x-ray" to evaluate the entire patient in under 30 seconds.

Cardiac Computed Tomography Angiography

Over the next decade, CTA will become part of routine clinical practice in the ED, where its high negative predictive value for coronary artery disease will provide efficient triage of patients with chest pain. In cases where the diagnosis for chest pain is not clear after more basic tests have been completed, CTA offers a rapid evaluation of three possible causes of the pain—abdominal aortic aneurysm, pulmonary embolism, and coronary artery obstruction. Although a 16-slice scanner is the minimum performance level for cardiac imaging, the newer 64-slice scanners have better image quality, particularly for very small vessels. Scanners with dedicated cardiac application packages provide CTA for the heart, great vessels, and peripherals, as well as calcium scoring and other functional cardiology tools.

Portable Ultrasound Systems

Ultrasound systems have become increasingly compact and mobile. The size of a laptop computer, these portable units come equipped with linear probes for vascular and small-parts imaging for use in echocardiography. These ultrasound systems will become a mainstay in the ED as they allow the emergency physician to perform focused echocardiography and vascular studies, resulting in earlier diagnosis and treatment. Several manufacturers offer portable systems that can be used at the bedside. An example is Zonare's US system, which features the ability to remove the handheld data processing unit and probe from the cart, complete an exam, then return the system to the cart to review the results. ED ultrasound is for focused identification of time-critical events, such as focused abdominal sonography for trauma (FAST) scans or right upper quadrant ultrasounds to look for gallstones, or a scan to identify the internal jugular vein for placement of a central line. The technology is not intended to replace the precision of comprehensive ultrasound exams by radiologists at a later time—a qualifier radiologists would insist on emphasizing.

Rapid Diagnostics

Current methods for rapid diagnosis of disease in the ED are limited. As an example, 90 percent of aseptic meningitis cases are caused by enteroviruses that result in benign disease. Only 10 percent of patients need to be admitted and given intravenous antibiotics, but many are unnecessarily hospitalized because of the difficulty of distinguishing aseptic meningitis from more severe bacterial meningitis. Currently, when a patient suspected of having meningitis presents to the ED, he or she is admitted and prescribed prophylactic antibiotics while awaiting results from the laboratory culture, a process that takes 3 to 10 days. Given that infections of various types and fevers of unknown origin are among the top 20 diagnoses sending patients to the ED, technologies that can speed diagnosis will have an important benefit in improving ED workflow.

For example, real-time polymerase chain reaction (PCR) tests designed to identify enterovirus (EV) infection can diagnose EV-positive patients within 5 hours. The patient remains in the ED and is admitted only after the results have identified the cause as bacterial or of unknown origin. Rapid diagnostic tests are available for an increasing number of conditions seen in the emergency setting, including *Streptococcus pneumoniae* infection, meningitis, bloody diarrhea, and septicemia. Emerging real-time PCR tests will replace laboratory evaluations for occult bacteremia and with their rapid, accurate test results may sharply decrease the use of antibiotics. Early targeted disease detection not only expedites diagnosis and improves the accuracy of clinical decision making, but also speeds recovery by identifying causative organisms and allowing for optimal antibiotic selection.

At least initially, most molecular tests that will impact the ED will be offered through centralized molecular diagnostics laboratories. As the technology advances over the next 2 to 5 years, however, real-time PCR will allow decentralization to rapid-response laboratories with even faster test turnaround times. Recent advances in real-time PCR improve its speed. The traditional PCR requires three steps, real-time PCR requires two steps, and the next generation of real-time PCR will require one step. This translates into samples that can be extracted, amplified, and detected in less than 25 minutes, significantly reducing patient wait times and expediting diagnosis.

An added benefit is that rapid diagnostics can be used to determine whether a patient is a carrier of a disease that could potentially harm other patients and health care workers. For example, rapid bedside testing could help EDs identify difficult-to-reach patients who are at risk of HIV infection and refer them for treatment. A substantial subgroup of patients come to the ED for care but are unlikely ever to seek HIV testing at a health department. Provision of rapid bedside screening with an oral swab rather than a blood draw might allow ED personnel to detect HIV-infected patients, advise them to modify high-risk activity, and refer them for treatment, although evaluations are needed to validate the social and clinical feasibility of this strategy.

Laboratory Automation

The automation of laboratory services will have a significant impact on care provided in the ED. As laboratory testing devices become smaller and easier to use, it will become possible to perform laboratory tests more frequently at the point of care. Laboratory information systems allow for the rapid transfer of test results to the ED and in some circumstances can even provide real-time information, as in the case of PCR-based tests.

In the ED, point-of-care testing will improve patient throughput. To reduce lengthy ED stays, Massachusetts General Hospital established a point-of-care satellite testing laboratory in the ED to perform urinalysis, glucose tests, rapid strep tests, pregnancy tests, tests for cardiac markers, and influenza tests. As a result, test turnaround times were reduced by 87 percent, ED lengths of stay declined by 41 minutes per patient, and ED diversions decreased. Also, emergency physicians' satisfaction with the laboratory's turnaround time increased by 50 percent (Lee-Lewandrowski et al., 2003).

Laboratory automation can also eliminate ED bottlenecks by providing test results in a timely manner. Northwestern Memorial Hospital in Chicago improved its ED performance through the use of an automated centralized laboratory. Northwestern found that 18 percent of the average 4.5-hour ED visit was attributed to waiting for laboratory results (Personal communication, K. Clarke, 2004). The hospital developed a system to better connect its laboratory services to the ED, using an early draw process to reduce wait times. Now when a patient presents to the ED, the nurse screens the patient and, whenever possible, orders laboratory tests based on standing physician orders. After the nurse draws the patient's blood, an ED laboratory technician orders the tests on the laboratory information system and labels tubes with bar codes. The tubes are transported pneumatically to the automated laboratory. The results are available by the time the physician performs the initial patient examination. If additional tests are necessary, their results are available within 5 to 20 minutes. As a result of the use of automation in the centralized laboratory, patient throughput and room utilization increased by 20 percent, patient wait times were reduced by 40 percent, and Press-Ganey patient satisfaction survey scores rose to the 80th percentile.

A number of hospital IT tools have been demonstrated to be effective in improving patient flow and efficiency, and to have a direct and substantial impact on ED crowding and the quality of emergency care. Given the sporadic adoption of these IT tools to date, the committee believes hospitals should increase their efforts to enhance their IT capabilities that impact emergency and trauma care. The committee therefore recommends that **hospitals adopt robust information and communications systems to improve the safety and quality of emergency care and enhance hospital efficiency (5.1).**

BARRIERS TO THE ADOPTION
OF INFORMATION TECHNOLOGY

Given the array of IT tools available to improve patient flow and enhance the quality, safety, and timeliness of emergency care, the argument for the widespread adoption of such tools appears clear. From prehospital care to ED and ancillary services to recovery and rehabilitation, IT has the potential to address many of the challenges currently facing the U.S. emergency care system. Nonetheless, health care IT has not been widely implemented in the ED or other health care settings, and significant barriers to its implementation remain. It would be difficult to exaggerate the daunting challenges hospital face in implementing state-of-the-art IT systems. Limited resources—financial, physical, and intellectual—often stand in the way of even modest goals. The need to win the acceptance of older physicians and to deal with the existence of (often inadequate) hardware and software already in place compounds the problems involved. The investment required to achieve the goals described in this chapter is substantial, and must be addressed through public policy if the adoption of health care IT is to move forward rapidly. Five specific barriers to the adoption of health care IT in the ED are described below.

Financial Requirements

For most health care facilities, the lack of financial support continues to be the most significant barrier to IT implementation (Healthcare Information and Management Systems Society, 2005). Not only is capital needed to purchase and install new technology, a process that is often associated with sizable short-term transition costs, but specialized training and education costs also must be incurred to help physicians and other staff adapt to the new high-tech environment. Adding to these challenges is the fact that access to capital may be particularly limited for certain types of health care organizations, including the nonprofit hospitals that provide much of the nation's safety net emergency care. Further, while large for-profit hospitals and health plans may have ready capital to invest, they may lack the leverage and incentives needed to implement various IT tools (IOM, 2001).

While there are few published estimates of the costs of widespread implementation of health care IT, there are a number of estimates regarding specific IT applications. For example, the RAND Corporation recently projected that the cumulative cost for 90 percent of hospitals to adopt EHR systems would be $98 billion, assuming that 20 percent of these hospitals currently have such systems in place. Average yearly costs for hospitals across a 15-year adoption period would be $6.5 billion. For physicians, the cumulative costs for 90 percent adoption would be $172 billion, with average yearly costs of approximately $1.1 billion (Hillestad et al., 2005).

Efforts to quantify the return on investment of these costs suggest that short- and long-term returns would far exceed initial outlays. At 90 percent adoption of EHRs, for example, the RAND study projected average annual savings of more than $77 billion, with $42 billion saved each year on average during the 15-year adoption period. Related improvements in prevention and chronic disease management could result in an additional $147 billion in savings annually, while transaction improvements could yield up to $10 billion in savings annually (Hillestad et al., 2005). Estimated net potential savings associated with EHRs are shown in Figure 5-1.

Beyond EHRs, Kaiser Permanente of northern California estimates that it will break even on its systemwide $1.2 billion IT investment in 6.5 years, with a 200 percent return on investment to be achieved in 10 years (Detmer, 2000). Similarly, with IT-related improvements in quality and efficiency and reductions in medical errors, it is estimated that Medicare could save up to 30 percent of its annual spending (The Lewin Group, 2005). Altogether, at the national level, the federal government estimates that the nation would save $140 billion annually, or 20 percent of health care costs, through improved use of health care IT (DHHS and ONCHIT,

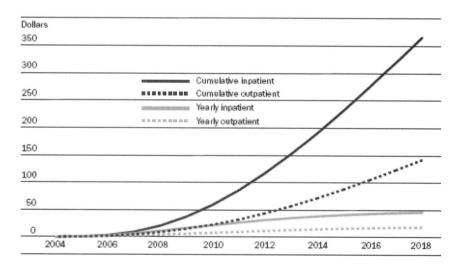

FIGURE 5-1 Net potential savings (efficiency benefits over adoption costs) for hospitals and physicians adopting electronic health record systems during a 15-year adoption period (2004–2018).
NOTE: Dollar figures are billions.
SOURCE: Reprinted from Hillestad et al., 2005, with permission from PROJECT HOPE via Copyright Clearance Center.

2005). Improved interoperability and shared diffusion would likely result in even more substantial savings.

Clinical technologies are somewhat different in that their adoption is linked more directly to reimbursement than to cost savings as in the case of other information technologies. There is a robust market for the development of new medical technologies. These and other changes will occur whether or not there is an active policy to promote their development and utilization or government support for their diffusion.

Lack of Interoperability Standards

A key factor inhibiting the rate of adoption of new health care technologies is the lack of development of common health care IT standards (Goldsmith et al., 2003). Data communication standards are sets of rules that allow disparate computer systems to exchange information without requiring custom programming for each new connection. Without such standards in place, a number of factors discourage the effective integration of multiple data sources into one useful whole. For example, data may be stored in isolated locations; they may be collected and stored using different internal systems, structures, or coding; and they may be generated in ways that do not match the expectations of clinical providers, researchers, or health care managers (McDonald et al., 2001). Widespread adoption of shared standards is necessary to overcome these barriers and permit the creation of clinical data-sharing networks that can build bridges between the various islands of information.

> We have people showing up at emergency rooms all the time and their data is not there. We've never stopped to ask, What are the standards that we need to get someone's data to the emergency room?
> —David Brailer, National Health Information
> Technology Coordinator (Cunningham, 2005)

The health care industry is just starting to realize the improvements in efficiency, safety, and quality that shared data systems can offer. Providers participating in the Massachusetts Healthcare Data Consortium, for example, have access to pharmacy prescription databases for treatment purposes. Such information is critical in emergency care as many patients arriving in the ED are unable to tell staff exactly which medicines they take, whether because of alterations to their mental status, forgetfulness, or the sheer number of different pills involved. Data communication standards also facilitate the sharing of clinical information, such as past medical histories, allergies, and EKG results. With standards in place, data sharing has already been proven effective within and among various health care systems (Halamka et al., 1997; Overhage et al., 2002).

In an article in the *New England Journal of Medicine*, Senate Majority Leader William H. Frist (R-Tennessee) recently described his vision for how interoperability standards allowing the sharing of clinical data could be used to save the life of a patient having a heart attack (Frist, 2005). Senator Frist, along with Senator Hillary Rodham Clinton (D-New York) and Representatives Nancy L. Johnson (R-Connecticut) and Patrick J. Kennedy (D-Rhode Island), is currently leading congressional efforts to promote the development and implementation of interoperability standards for health care IT. At the same time, President George W. Bush has called for federal action, establishing the Office of the National Coordinator for Health Information Technology (ONC) to provide "leadership for the development and nationwide implementation of an interoperable health information technology infrastructure to improve the quality and efficiency of health care and the ability of consumers to manage their care and safety" (DHHS and Office of the Secretary, 2005). ONC recently established the Healthcare Information Technology Standards Panel to harmonize health care data standards for the nation.

Limited IT Knowledge

With new technology comes the need for new expertise. Just as the purchase of health care IT tools requires significant investments of financial capital, human capital (e.g., professional time and knowledge) is needed if the tools are to be implemented and maintained successfully. Whereas many larger hospitals and health care systems may have dedicated IT staff able to oversee the adoption of new technologies, smaller organizations often lack such resources. Moreover, while IT staff is an essential part of the equation, failed attempts to launch new IT tools suggest that clinical staff must also be comfortable and conversant with the technology if its potential is to be realized.

Resource sharing, such as that offered by Beth Israel Deaconess Medical Center and the Veterans Health Administration (VHA), is one way to help ensure that all health care settings have access to the knowledge and expertise needed to adopt proven IT solutions. The VHA's Veterans Health Information Systems and Technology Architecture (VistA) program is described in Box 5-2. Comprehensive IT training modules, such as those supported by AHRQ, are another approach.

BOX 5-2
Veterans Health Information Systems
and Technology Architecture (VistA)

The Veterans Health Administration (VHA) is the nation's largest integrated health care system. With a staff of nearly 200,000, VHA provides care to more than 5.1 million veterans and other enrollees annually. It operates over 1,300 facilities nationwide, including 157 medical centers, with one in every state, Puerto Rico, and Washington, DC. It also oversees the nation's largest medical education and health professions training program, turning out approximately 83,000 health professionals each year.

A critical component of VHA operations is the Veterans Health Information Systems and Technology Architecture (VistA). Key aspects of VistA include the Computerized Patient Record System (CPRS), which offers providers a single interface through which they can review and update patients' medical records, as well as place orders for medications, laboratory tests, and other services. In its next-generation system, HealtheVet, VistA also implements standard functions for health data repository systems, registration systems, provider systems, management and financial systems, and information and educational systems.

VHA has shared both its health information and health IT resources—including software and staff expertise—with other federal agencies through the Health Information Technology Sharing (HITS) program since the late 1990s. The HITS program was expanded to include some nongovernmental and international organizations in 2001. Through the recent HealthyPeople Initiative, VistA software and expertise are now available as well at minimal or no cost to public- and private-sector organizations that serve the poor and near-poor.

SOURCE: Department of Veterans Affairs, 2005.

Human Factors

Some of the most challenging barriers to the adoption of IT in health care involve human factors. Currently there are more than 780,000 physicians and 2.2 million nurses, as well as many other health care providers, involved in the delivery of patient care in the United States (HRSA, 2003). These individuals possess highly varied levels of IT-related knowledge and experience. Further, clinicians tend to be conservative and reluctant to adopt new automated approaches, especially if previous attempts at IT solutions failed to prove useful in solving diagnostic, therapeutic, or workflow problems (Kassirer, 2000; IOM, 2001).

An important potential hurdle for institutions planning major IT enhancements is the 6- to 12-month learning curve for physicians. Implementation of such systems must be carefully executed and supported, and products must be tailored to each institution through use and modification over time. No system is fully applicable directly off the shelf. Unless the system brings demonstrable value to its users, the potential for physician dissatisfaction and indirect patient dissatisfaction is substantial.

Human factors research deals with human–computer interaction and has developed methods for testing and improving the usability of software. Used by the aviation industry for more than a decade, human factors research is largely credited with minimizing pilot error and improving the safety of air travel (Vincente, 2004). Many of the actual and perceived problems with health care IT in the ED could be overcome by employing human factors techniques (Helmreich, 2000; Wears and Perry, 2002).

For example, the "usability" of software is based on its perceived usefulness as well as its perceived ease of use. A useful program enhances the performance of its users; it makes them more efficient or improves the quality of their work. A program's ease of use is judged by the amount of effort required to accomplish tasks. Studied barriers to program use include accessibility (whether there are enough computers for all users), availability (whether the system crashes when people wish to use it), start–stop times (whether it takes too long to begin/resume a task or save work to be continued later), system dynamics (whether the response time is too slow), training barriers (whether it takes too many hours to learn to use the program effectively), and lack of consistency (whether various components of a system work together in the same way).

Several examples can be found to demonstrate the inefficiencies and reductions in patient safety that accompany poor implementation of health care IT (Ash et al., 2004). As noted earlier, for example, Cedars-Sinai Medical Center removed its CPOE system after less than 6 months as a result of significant resistance by doctors and nurses who claimed the system was difficult to use. Such resistance may be less pronounced among emergency clinicians as IT adoption typically occurs more rapidly in ED than other settings (Healthcare Information and Management Systems Society, 2005).

While the barriers to IT adoption are significant, research demonstrates that they are hardly insurmountable. In fact, as was so clearly stated in *Crossing the Quality Chasm: A New Health System for the 21st Century*, "solutions to these barriers can and must be found given the critical importance of the judicious application of IT to addressing the nation's health care quality concerns" (IOM, 2001, p. 166). An essential step in realizing the potential of health care IT to improve patient flow and enhance the quality, safety, and timeliness of patient care is the creation of a national health information infrastructure, discussed earlier.

Confidentiality

One of the biggest challenges to the development of electronic systems for tracking patients, documenting care, and communicating among clinicians is protecting the confidentiality of patient information. As quickly as systems are developed, protections against security breaches and new methods of attack are devised. While technical solutions exist, there must also be trade-offs between the capabilities of systems and the requirements for confidentiality.

PRIORITIZING INVESTMENTS IN EMERGENCY CARE INFORMATION TECHNOLOGY

The specific costs and benefits of many of the technologies described above to individual hospitals are largely unknown, and can be expected to vary according to the individual circumstances and the technology infra-

---

BOX 5-3
Roadmap for the Implementation of
Health Information Technologies

In an ideal world, where all hospitals and health care systems were equally flush with capital and similarly motivated to invest in new health care information technologies, the IT tools known to improve the quality, safety, and timeliness of emergency care would be immediately adopted and embraced by staff and patients alike. In the real world, however, financial and other limitations temper the pace at which IT improvements can be implemented. This is particularly true among the nation's small, rural, and safety net hospitals, which typically have less revenue and more limited IT systems at their disposal.

Given these real-world constraints, it is important that IT investments in the ED be made strategically, with close attention paid to such issues as total costs, staff education and training requirements, and the time needed to complete workplace transitions. For example, automated discharge systems represent a relatively inexpensive, easy-to-use technology that many hospitals could turn to as a first step in modernizing their care delivery. While significantly more expensive than automated discharge systems, electronic dashboards are also a priority because they have the potential to improve so many aspects of patient care management. Dashboards also can serve as a launching pad for future IT investments, such as clinical decision support systems (CDSSs) and computerized physician order entry (CPOE).

structure and readiness of each institution. For example, adopting advanced systems in a hospital that has a limited existing IT platform would probably not be cost-effective; on the other hand, in a hospital with a sophisticated platform, adoption of such systems could be highly cost-effective as the marginal costs associated with their addition would be very small. Given these inherent variations, it would be difficult to prioritize the many technologies in a way that could be generalized to all hospitals. However, the committee identified categories of technologies that would have a substantial impact on emergency care and that could feasibly be adopted by many institutions within 3–5 years:

• Technologies that facilitate patient flow management, such as electronic dashboards and tracking systems
• Technologies that improve the continuity of care across the continuum of care, particularly EMS–hospital system linkages and RHIOs that enhance the information available to clinicians across settings

Clinical documentation programs are the next logical choice for many hospitals and health care systems seeking to improve patient flow and enhance quality and safety. Wireless registration, radio frequency identification (RFID) tracking, and digital hands-free Voice over Internet Protocol (VoIP) communications can facilitate more seamless care with fewer interruptions and more time for direct patient care. These programs also can capitalize on existing hospital wireless networks or dashboard programs, further reducing costs and encouraging coordination.

Finally, hospitals may look to CPOE systems to reduce errors, improve safety, and save time in the ED. Efforts should be made to ensure that applied CPOE systems are customized for use in the ED, a task that will require additional expenditures. Further, the impact of such systems on the quality, timeliness, and safety of emergency care should be carefully monitored.

Several organizations are moving to make their IT tools more widely available through resource sharing and discounted pricing. For example, the Veterans Health Administration routinely shares its health information and health IT resources—including software and staff expertise—through the Health Information Technology Sharing Program at no or minimal cost. Further, through its Center for Healthcare Information Technology, the American Academy of Family Physicians is making low-cost, standards-based IT more available to family physicians nationwide. In many rural hospitals, it is family physicians who represent the bulk of ED staff.

• Decision-support tools, such as automated triage, that facilitate optimal use of resources
• Systems that reduce the likelihood of errors in the ED, such as CPOE
• Systems that facilitate public health surveillance

Some specific strategies for the cost-effective adoption of these technologies are described in Box 5-3. The committee also believes the ED should be a priority site for the early development of enterprisewide IT systems. For example, the development of EHRs is important throughout the hospital and across the health care delivery system. The ED has a particular need for this technology, especially since 43 percent of inpatients are admitted to the hospital through the ED (Merrill and Elixhauser, 2005).

SUMMARY OF RECOMMENDATIONS

5.1: Hospitals should adopt robust information and communications systems to improve the safety and quality of emergency care and enhance hospital efficiency.

REFERENCES

ACP, ASIM (American College of Physicians, American Society of Internal Medicine). *ACP-ASIM Survey Finds Nearly Half of U.S. Members Use Handheld Computers.* [Online]. Available: http://www.acponline.org/college/pressroom/handheld_survey.htm [accessed July 1, 2005].
Ash JS, Berg M, Coiera E. 2004. Some unintended consequences of information technology in health care: The nature of patient care information system-related errors. *Journal of the American Medical Informatics Association* 11(2):104–112.
Balas EA, Weingarten S, Garb CT, Blumenthal D, Boren SA, Brown GD. 2000. Improving preventive care by prompting physicians. *Archives of Internal Medicine* 160(3):301–308.
Bates DW, Gawande AA. 2003. Improving safety with information technology. *New England Journal of Medicine* 348(25):2526–2534.
Bates DW, Leape LL, Cullen DJ, Laird N, Petersen LA, Teich JM, Burdick E, Hickey M, Kleefield S, Shea B, Vander Vliet M, Seger DL. 1998. Effect of computerized physician order entry and a team intervention on prevention of serious medication errors. *Journal of the American Medical Association* 280(15):1311–1316.
Bates DW, Teich JM, Lee J, Seger D, Kuperman GJ, Ma'Luf N, Boyle D, Leape L. 1999. The impact of computerized physician order entry on medication error prevention. *Journal of the American Medical Informatics Association* 6(4):313–321.
Baumann MR, Strout TD. 2005. Evaluation of the emergency severity index (version 3) triage algorithm in pediatric patients. *Academic Emergency Medicine* 12(3):219–224.
Bertling CJ, Simpson DE, Hayes AM, Torre D, Brown DL, Schubot DB. 2003. Personal digital assistants herald new approaches to teaching and evaluation in medical education. *WMJ: Official Publication of the State Medical Society of Wisconsin* 102(2):46–50.
Bird SB, Zarum RS, Renzi FP. 2001. Emergency medicine resident patient care documentation using a hand-held computerized device. *Academic Emergency Medicine* 8(12):1200–1203.

Bizovi KE, Beckley BE, McDade MC, Adams AL, Lowe RA, Zechnich AD, Hedges JR. 2002. The effect of computer-assisted prescription writing on emergency department prescription errors. *Academic Emergency Medicine* 9(11):1168–1175.

Boulanger B, Kearney P, Ochoa J, Tsuei B, Sands F. 2001. Telemedicine: A solution to the followup of rural trauma patients? *Journal of the American College of Surgeons* 192(4):447–452.

Bower AG. 2005. *The Diffusion and Value of Healthcare Information Technology.* Santa Monica, CA: Rand Corporation.

Brailer DJ, Teresawa EL. 2003. *Use and Adoption of Computer-Based Patient Records.* Oakland, CA: California HealthCare Foundation.

Brillman JC, Doezema D, Tandberg D, Sklar DP, Davis KD, Simms S, Skipper BJ. 1996. Triage: Limitations in predicting need for emergent care and hospital admission. *Annals of Emergency Medicine* 27(4):493–500.

Buehler JW, Hopkins RS, Overhage JM, Sosin DM, Tong V. 2004. Framework for evaluating public health surveillance systems for early detection of outbreaks: Recommendations from the CDC Working Group. *Morbidity and Mortality Weekly Report* 53(RR05):1–11.

Bullard MJ, Meurer DP, Colman I, Holroyd BR, Rowe BH. 2004. Supporting clinical practice at the bedside using wireless technology. *Academic Emergency Medicine* 11(11):1186–1192.

Buller-Close K, Schriger DL, Baraff LJ. 2003. Heterogeneous effect of an emergency department expert charting system. *Annals of Emergency Medicine* 41(5):644–652.

Burt CW, Hing E. 2005. Use of computerized clinical support systems in medical settings: United States, 2001–03. *Advance Data* (353):1–8.

Chang P, Hsu YS, Tzeng YM, Sang YY, Hou IC, Kao WF. 2004. The development of intelligent, triage-based, mass-gathering emergency medical service PDA support systems. *Journal of Nursing Research: JNR* 12(3):227–236.

Chase CR, Vacek PM, Shinozaki T, Giard AM, Ashikaga T. 1983. Medical information management: Improving the transfer of research results to presurgical evaluation. *Medical Care* 21(4):410–424.

Children's Hospital Informatics Program. 2005. *Research.* [Online]. Available: http://www.chip.org/research.cgi [accessed December 1, 2005].

Chin T. 2002, December 2. Have physician offices become more wired? *American Medical News.*

Classen DC, Evans RS, Pestotnik SL, Horn SD, Menlove RL, Burke JP. 1992. The timing of prophylactic administration of antibiotics and the risk of surgical-wound infection. *New England Journal of Medicine* 326(5):281–286.

Cone DC, Nedza SM, Augustine JJ, Davidson SJ. 2002. Quality in clinical practice. *Academic Emergency Medicine* 9(11):1085–1090.

Croskerry P. 2000. The feedback sanction. *Academic Emergency Medicine* 7(11):1232–1238.

Cunningham R. 2005. Action through collaboration: A conversation with David Brailer. *Health Affairs* 24(5).

Dale J, Higgins J, Williams S, Foster T, Snooks H, Crouch R, Hartley-Sharpe C, Glucksman E, Hooper R, George S. 2003. Computer assisted assessment and advice for "non-serious" 999 ambulance service callers: The potential impact on ambulance dispatch. *Emergency Medicine Journal* 20(2):178–183.

Davidson SJ, Zwemer FL Jr, Nathanson LA, Sable KN, Khan AN. 2004. Where's the beef? The promise and the reality of clinical documentation. *Academic Emergency Medicine* 11(11):1127–1134.

Department of Veterans Affairs. 2005. *Facts about the Department of Veterans Affairs.* [Online]. Available: http://www1.va.gov/opa/fact/vafacts.html [accessed September 1, 2005].

Detmer DE. 2000. Information technology for quality health care: A summary of United Kingdom and United States experiences. *Quality in Health Care* 9(3):181–189.

DHHS, Office of the Secretary (Department of Health and Human Services, Office of the Secretary). 2005. *Office of the National Coordinator for Health Information Technology; Statement of Organization, Functions, and Delegations of Authority.* [Online]. Available: http://a257.g.akamaitech.net/7/257/2422/01jan20051800/edocket.access.gpo.gov/2005/05-16446.htm [accessed May 20, 2006].

DHHS, ONCHIT (Department of Health and Human Services, Office of the National Coordinator for Health Information Technology). 2005. *Value of HIT.* [Online]. Available: http://www.hhs.gov/healthit/valueHIT.html [accessed July 1, 2005].

Dong SL, Bullard MJ, Meurer DP, Colman I, Blitz S, Holroyd BR, Rowe BH. 2005. Emergency triage: Comparing a novel computer triage program with standard triage. *Academic Emergency Medicine* 12(6):502–507.

Duncan RG, Shabot MM. 2000. Secure remote access to a clinical data repository using a wireless personal digital assistant (PDA). *American Medical Informatics Association Annual Symposium Proceedings* 210–214.

Espino JU, Wagner MM. 2001. Accuracy of ICD-9-coded chief complaints and diagnoses for the detection of acute respiratory illness. *American Medical Informatics Association Annual Symposium Proceedings* 164–168.

Evans RS, Pestotnik SL, Classen DC, Clemmer TP, Weaver LK, Orme JF Jr, Lloyd JF, Burke JP. 1998. A computer-assisted management program for antibiotics and other antiinfective agents. *New England Journal of Medicine* 338(4):232–238.

Field MH. 2004. The perils of CPOE. *Lancet* 363(9402):86.

Fleischauer AT, Silk BJ, Schumacher M, Komatsu K, Santana S, Vaz V, Wolfe M, Hutwagner L, Cono J, Berkelman R, Treadwell T. 2004. The validity of chief complaint and discharge diagnosis in emergency department-based syndromic surveillance. *Academic Emergency Medicine* 11(12):1262–1267.

Frist WH. 2005. Shattuck lecture: Health care in the 21st century. *New England Journal of Medicine* 352(3):267–272.

Gallagher EJ. 2002. How well do clinical practice guidelines guide clinical practice? *Annals of Emergency Medicine* 40(4):394–398.

GAO (U.S. Government Accountability Office). 2004. *Homeland Security: Effective Regional Coordination Can Enhance Emergency Preparedness.* Washington, DC: Government Printing Office.

Goldsmith J, Blumenthal D, Rishel W. 2003. Federal health information policy: A case of arrested development. *Health Affairs* 22(4):44–55.

Gordon JA, McLaughlin S, Shapiro M, Spillane L, Bond W. 2004. *Simulation in Emergency Medicine.* Loyd GE, Lake CL, Greenberg R, eds. Philadelphia, PA: Hanley and Belfus.

Halamka J, Overhage JM, Ricciardi L, Rishel W, Shirky C, Diamond C. 2005. Exchanging health information: Local distribution, national coordination. As more communities develop information-sharing networks, a coordinated approach is essential for linking these networks. *Health Affairs* 24(5):1170–1179.

Halamka JD, Szolovits P, Rind D, Safran C. 1997. A WWW implementation of national recommendations for protecting electronic health information. *Journal of the American Medical Informatics Association* 4(6):458–464.

Halvorson GC. 2005. Wiring health care. Healthcare cannot be reengineered without data. *Health Affairs* 24(5):1266–1268.

Handler JA, Gillam M, Sanders AB, Klasco R. 2000. Defining, identifying, and measuring error in emergency medicine. *Academic Emergency Medicine* 7(11):1183–1188.

Handler JA, Feied CF, Coonan K, Vozenilek J, Gillam M, Peacock PR Jr, Sinert R, Smith MS. 2004. Computerized physician order entry and online decision support. *Academic Emergency Medicine* 11(11):1135–1141.

Harris Interactive. 2001. *U.S. Trails Other English Speaking Countries in Use of Electronic Medical Records and Electronic Prescribing.* [Online]. Available: http://www.harrisinteractive.com/news/allnewsbydate.asp?NewsID=367 [accessed July 1, 2005].

Haukoos JS, Witt MD, Zeumer CM, Lee TJ, Halamka JD, Lewis RJ. 2002. Emergency department triage of patients infected with HIV. *Academic Emergency Medicine* 9(9): 880–888.

HRSA (Health Resources and Services Administration). 2003. *United States Health Workforce Personnel Factbook.* Washington, DC: Bureau of Health Professions.

Healthcare Information and Management Systems Society. 2005. *16th Annual HIMMS Leadership Survey, February 2005.* [Online]. Available: http://www.himms.org/2005survey/ [accessed July 1, 2005].

Helmreich RL. 2000. On error management: Lessons from aviation. *British Medical Journal* 320(7237):781–785.

Henley RR, Wiederhold G. 1975. *An Analysis of Automated Ambulatory Medical Record Systems.* San Francisco, CA: AARMS Study Group, University of California-San Francisco.

Hillestad R, Bigelow J, Bower A, Girosi F, Meili R, Scoville R, Taylor R. 2005. Can electronic medical record systems transform health care? Potential health benefits, savings, and costs. The adoption of interoperable EMR systems could produce efficiency and safety savings of $142–$371 billion. *Health Affairs* 24(5):1103–1117.

Holbrook A, Keshavjee K, Troyan S, Pray M, Ford PT, COMPETE Investigators. 2003. Applying methodology to electronic medical record selection. *International Journal of Medical Informatics* 71(1):43–50.

Hospital Financial Management Association. 1976. *State of Information Processing in the Health Care Industry.* Chicago, IL: Hospital Financial Management Association.

Hunt DL, Haynes RB, Hanna SE, Smith K. 1998. Effects of computer-based clinical decision support systems on physician performance and patient outcomes: A systematic review. *Journal of the American Medical Association* 280(15):1339–1346.

IOM (Institute of Medicine). 1991. *The Computer-Based Patient Record: An Essential Technology for Health Care.* Washington, DC: National Academy Press.

IOM. 2001. *Crossing the Quality Chasm: A New Health System for the 21st Century.* Washington, DC: National Academy Press.

IOM. 2003. *Patient Safety: Achieving a New Standard for Care.* Washington, DC: The National Academies Press.

IOM. 2004a. *Health Literacy: A Prescription to End Confusion.* Washington, DC: The National Academies Press.

IOM. 2004b. *Quality Through Collaboration: The Future of Rural Health.* Washington, DC: The National Academies Press.

Jensen J. 2004. United hospital increases capacity usage, efficiency with patient-flow management system. *Journal of Healthcare Information Management* 18(3):26–31.

Jolly BT, Scott JL, Sanford SM. 1995. Simplification of emergency department discharge instructions improves patient comprehension. *Annals of Emergency Medicine* 26(4): 443–446.

Kassirer JP. 2000. Patients, physicians, and the internet. *Health Affairs* 19(6):115–123.

Kaushal R, Bates DW. 2001. Computerized physician order entry (CPOE) with clinical decision support systems (CDSSs). In: Shojania KG, Bradford DW, McDonald KM, Wachter RM, eds. *Evidence Report/Technology Assessment.* Vol. 43 (AHRQ Publication No. 01-E058). Rockville, MD: Agency for Healthcare Research and Quality.

Kellermann AL, Bartolomeos K, Fuqua-Whitley D, Sampson TR, Parramore CS. 2001. Community-level firearm injury surveillance: Local data for local action. *Annals of Emergency Medicine* 38(4):423–429.

Kilpatrick ES, Holding S. 2001. Use of computer terminals on wards to access emergency test results: A retrospective audit. *British Medical Journal* 322(7294):1101–1103.

Kleinke JD. 2005. Dot-Gov: Market failure and the creation of a national health information technology system. The market has failed to produce a viable health information technology system; we need government intervention instead. *Health Affairs* 24(5):1246–1262.

Koval D. 2005. Real-world RHIO. A regional health information organization blazes a trail in upstate New York. *Journal of American Health Information Management Association* 76(3):44–48.

Kundel HL, Polansky M, Dalinka MK, Choplin RH, Gefter WB, Kneelend JB, Miller WT Sr, Miller WT Jr. 2001. Reliability of soft-copy versus hard-copy interpretation of emergency department radiographs: A prototype study. *American Journal of Roentgenology* 177(3):525–528.

Kuperman GJ, Teich JM, Tanasijevic MJ, Ma'Luf N, Rittenberg E, Jha A, Fiskio J, Winkelman J, Bates DW. 1999. Improving response to critical laboratory results with automation: Results of a randomized controlled trial. *Journal of the American Medical Informatics Association* 6(6):512–522.

Kuperman GJ, Teich JM, Gandhi TK, Bates DW. 2001. Patient safety and computerized medication ordering at Brigham and Women's Hospital. *Joint Commission Journal on Quality Improvement* 27(10):509–521.

Lee JK, Renner JB, Saunders BF, Stamford PP, Bickford TR, Johnston RE, Hsaio HS, Phillips ML. 1998. Effect of real-time teleradiology on the practice of the emergency department physician in a rural setting: Initial experience. *Academic Radiology* 5(8):533–538.

Lee-Lewandrowski E, Corboy D, Lewandrowski K, Sinclair J, McDermot S, Benzer TI. 2003. Implementation of a point-of-care satellite laboratory in the emergency department of an academic medical center. Impact on test turnaround time and patient emergency department length of stay. *Archives of Pathology & Laboratory Medicine* 127(4):456–460.

The Lewin Group. 2005. *Health Information Technology Leadership Panel, Final Report.* Falls Church, VA: The Lewin Group.

Lin YH, Jan IC, Ko PC, Chen YY, Wong JM, Jan GJ. 2004. A wireless PDA-based physiological monitoring system for patient transport. *IEEE Transactions on Information Technology in Biomedicine* 8(4):439–447.

Lombardo J, Burkom H, Elbert E, Magruder S, Lewis SH, Loschen W, Sari J, Sniegoski C, Wojcik R, Pavlin J. 2003. A systems overview of the electronic surveillance system for the early notification of community-based epidemics (Essence II). *Journal of Urban Health* 80(2 Suppl. 1):i32–i42.

Loonsk JW, CDC (Centers for Disease Control and Prevention). 2004. Biosense: A national initiative for early detection and quantification of public health emergencies. *Morbidity & Mortality Weekly Report* 53(Suppl.):53–55.

Mandl KD, Overhage JM, Wagner MM, Lober WB, Sebastiani P, Mostashari F, Pavlin JA, Gesteland PH, Treadwell T, Koski E, Hutwagner L, Buckeridge DL, Aller RD, Grannis S. 2004. Implementing syndromic surveillance: A practical guide informed by the early experience. *Journal of the American Medical Informatics Association* 11(2):141–150.

Manhattan Research. 2002. *CyberCitizen Health V2.0.* New York: Manhattan Research.

Marcin JP, Schepps DE, Page KA, Struve SN, Nagrampa E, Dimand RJ. 2004. The use of telemedicine to provide pediatric critical care consultations to pediatric trauma patients admitted to a remote trauma intensive care unit: A preliminary report. *Pediatric Critical Care Medicine* 5(3):251–256.

Marinakis HA, Zwemer FL Jr. 2003. An inexpensive modification of the laboratory computer display changes emergency physicians' work habits and perceptions. *Annals of Emergency Medicine* 41(2):186–190.

McDonald CJ. 1976. Protocol-based computer reminders, the quality of care and the non-perfectability of man. *New England Journal of Medicine* 295(24):1351–1355.

McDonald CJ, Schadow G, Suico J, Overhage JM. 2001. Data standards in health care. *Annals of Emergency Medicine* 38(3):303–311.

Merrill CT, Elixhauser A. 2005. *Hospitalization in the United States, 2002* (HCUP Fact Book No. 6, AHRQ Publication No. 05-0056). Rockville, MD: Agency for Healthcare Research and Quality.

Middleton B. 2005. Achieving U.S. health information technology adoption: The need for a third hand government intervention, judiciously and gently applied, can give the extra assistance needed to boost hit adoption nationwide. *Health Affairs* 24(5):1269–1272.

Mostashari F, Fine A, Das D, Adams J, Layton M. 2003. Use of ambulance dispatch data as an early warning system for communitywide influenzalike illness, New York City. *Journal of Urban Health* 80(2 Suppl. 1):i43–i49.

Murray MD. 2001. Automated medication dispensing devices. In: Shojania KG, Bradford DW, McDonald KM, Wachter RM, eds. *Evidence Report/Technology Assessment*. Vol. 43 (AHRQ Publication No. 01-E058). Rockville, MD: Agency for Healthcare Research and Quality.

NHTSA (National Highway and Traffic Safety Administration). 1996. *Emergency Medical Services Agenda for the Future*. Washington, DC: Government Printing Office.

O'Brien GM, Stein MD, Fagan MJ, Shapiro MJ, Nasta A. 1999. Enhanced emergency department referral improves primary care access. *American Journal of Managed Care* 5(10):1265–1269.

Oren E, Shaffer ER, Guglielmo BJ. 2003. Impact of emerging technologies on medication errors and adverse drug events. *American Journal of Health-System Pharmacy* 60(14):1447–1458.

Overhage JM, Tierney WM, Zhou XH, McDonald CJ. 1997. A randomized trial of "corollary orders" to prevent errors of omission. *Journal of the American Medical Informatics Association* 4(5):364–375.

Overhage JM, Dexter PR, Perkins SM, Cordell WH, McGoff J, McGrath R, McDonald CJ. 2002. A randomized, controlled trial of clinical information shared from another institution. *Annals of Emergency Medicine* 39(1):14–23.

Pallin D, Lahman M, Baumlin K. 2003. Information technology in emergency medicine residency-affiliated emergency departments. *Academic Emergency Medicine* 10(8): 848–852.

Pozen MW, D'Agostino RB, Selker HP, Sytkowski PA, Hood WB Jr. 1984. A predictive instrument to improve coronary-care-unit admission practices in acute ischemic heart disease. A prospective multicenter clinical trial. *New England Journal of Medicine* 310(20):1273–1278.

Redfern RO, Langlotz CP, Abbuhl SB, Polansky M, Horii SC, Kundel HL. 2002. The effect of PACS on the time required for technologists to produce radiographic images in the emergency department radiology suite. *Journal of Digital Imaging* 15(3):153–160.

Sands DZ, Halamka JD. 2004. PatientSite: Patient-centered communication, services, and access to information. In: Nelson R, Ball MJ, eds. *Consumer Informatics: Applications and Strategies in Cyber Health Care*. New York: Springer-Verlag. Pp. 20–32.

Schenkel S. 2000. Promoting patient safety and preventing medical error in emergency departments. *Academic Emergency Medicine* 7(11):1204–1222.

Shaw CI, Kacmarek RM, Hampton RL, Riggi V, Masry AE, Cooper JB, Hurford WE. 2004. Cellular phone interference with the operation of mechanical ventilators. *Critical Care Medicine* 32(4):928–931.

Shea S, DuMouchel W, Bahamonde L. 1996. A meta-analysis of 16 randomized controlled trials to evaluate computer-based clinical reminder systems for preventive care in the ambulatory setting. *Journal of the American Medical Informatics Association* 3(6):399–409.

Shortliffe EH. 2005. CPOE and the facilitation of medication errors. *Journal of Biomedical Informatics* 38(4):257–258.

Shu K, Boyle D, Spurr C, Horsky J, Heiman H, O'Connor P, Lepore J, Bates DW. 2001. Comparison of time spent writing orders on paper with computerized physician order entry. *Medical Informatics* 10(Pt. 2):1207–1211.

Smith MS, Feied CF. 1998. The next-generation emergency department. *Annals of Emergency Medicine* 32(1):65–74.

Strok B, Speedie SM, Ratner ER. 2003. A novel way of distributing medical practice guidelines using personal digital assistants (PDA). *American Medical Informatics Association Annual Symposium Proceedings* 1021.

Tanabe P, Gimbel R, Yarnold PR, Kyriacou DN, Adams JG. 2004. Reliability and validity of scores on the emergency severity index version 3. *Academic Emergency Medicine* 11(1):59–65.

Taylor TB. 2004. Information management in the emergency department. *Emergency Medicine Clinics of North America* 22(1):241–257.

Teich JM, Merchia PR, Schmiz JL, Kuperman GJ, Spurr CD, Bates DW. 2000. Effects of computerized physician order entry on prescribing practices. *Archives of Internal Medicine* 160(18):2741–2747.

Teich JM, Wagner MM, Mackenzie CF, Schafer KO. 2002. The informatics response in disaster, terrorism, and war. *Journal of the American Medical Informatics Association* 9(2):97–104.

Thompson DA, Yarnold PR, Williams DR, Adams SL. 1996. Effects of actual waiting time, perceived waiting time, information delivery, and expressive quality on patient satisfaction in the emergency department. *Annals of Emergency Medicine* 28(6):657–665.

Thompson TG, Brailer DJ. 2004. *The Decade of Health Information Technology: Delivering Consumer-Centric and Information-Rich Health Care, Framework for Strategic Action.* Washington, DC: U.S. DHHS.

Tierney WM, Miller ME, Overhage JM, McDonald CJ. 1993. Physician inpatient order writing on microcomputer workstations. Effects on resource utilization. *Journal of the American Medical Association* 269(3):379–383.

Tierney WM, McDonald CJ, Hui SL, Martin DK. 1988. Computer predictions of abnormal test results. Effects on outpatient testing. *Journal of the American Medical Association* 259(8):1194–1198.

Tri JL, Hayes DL, Smith TT, Severson RP. 2001. Cellular phone interference with external cardiopulmonary monitoring devices. *Mayo Clinic Proceedings* 76(1):11–15.

Tsui FC, Espino JU, Dato VM, Gesteland PH, Hutman J, Wagner MM. 2003. Technical description of rods: A real-time public health surveillance system. *Journal of the American Medical Informatics Association* 10(5):399–408.

Urban MJ, Edmondson DA, Aufderheide TP. 2002. Prehospital 12-lead ECG diagnostic programs. *Emergency Medicine Clinics of North America* 20(4):825–841.

Vincente K. 2004. *The Human Factor: Revolutionizing the Way People Live with Technology.* New York: Taylor and Francis.

Vozenilek J, Huff JS, Reznek M, Gordon JA. 2004. See one, do one, teach one: Advanced technology in medical education. *Academic Emergency Medicine* 11(11):1149–1154.

Vukmir RB, Kremen R, Ellis GL, DeHart DA, Plewa MC, Menegazzi J. 1993. Compliance with emergency department referral: The effect of computerized discharge instructions. *Annals of Emergency Medicine* 22(5):819–823.

Wears RL, Perry SJ. 2002. Human factors and ergonomics in the emergency department. *Annals of Emergency Medicine* 40(2):206–212.

Wellwood J, Johannessen S, Spiegelhalter DJ. 1992. How does computer-aided diagnosis improve the management of acute abdominal pain? *Annals of the Royal College of Surgeons of England* 74(1):40–46.

Wexler JR, Swender PT, Tunnessen WW Jr, Oski FA. 1975. Impact of a system of computer-assisted diagnosis. Initial evaluation of the hospitalized patient. *American Journal of Diseases of Children* 129(2):203–205.

Wuerz RC, Milne LW, Eitel DR, Travers D, Gilboy N. 2000. Reliability and validity of a new five-level triage instrument. *Academic Emergency Medicine* 7(3):236–242.

6

The Emergency Care Workforce

Emergency care is delivered in an inherently challenging environment, often requiring providers to make quick life-and-death decisions based on minimal information. Many who enter the emergency care profession enjoy the challenging work and the high-pressure environment, and take satisfaction in providing care to patients in urgent need. But providers on the front lines of emergency care increasingly express frustration with the deteriorating state of the emergency care system and the health care safety net. They experience the imbalance between demand and capacity described in earlier chapters on a daily basis, and find themselves spending an increasing proportion of their time on such tasks as getting patients admitted to crowded inpatient units; finding specialists willing to come in during the middle of the night; and finding psychiatric centers, skilled nursing facilities, or specialists who are willing to accept referrals. They also face a rigid regulatory environment that can make it difficult to address patients' needs in the most efficient, effective, and patient-centered manner.

This chapter describes the professionals working in the emergency department (ED) and addresses the unique challenges hospitals face in staffing EDs. A wide range of professionals deliver care in the ED, including physicians from multiple specialties, nurses, physician assistants, emergency medical technicians (EMTs), social workers, pharmacists, and technicians. The chapter begins with an overview of the roles and responsibilities, training, and demographic characteristics of these workers. The rest of the chapter addresses the committee's concerns with regard to the size, competency, effectiveness, and safety of the ED workforce.

PHYSICIANS

Several different types of physicians work in the ED extensively. With the exception of many rural hospitals, most hospitals have full-time coverage by emergency physicians, although the training and background of those physicians can vary considerably. Larger hospitals, particularly those designated as trauma centers, also have a host of other types of physicians on staff who can respond in the event a patient needs specialized medical care beyond what emergency physicians are trained to provide.

Emergency Physicians

Emergency physicians evaluate the presenting problems of patients, make diagnoses, and initiate treatment. They must be prepared for a wide variety of medical emergencies, and for this reason must be well versed in the emergency care aspects of such diverse subjects as anesthesia, cardiology, critical care, environmental illness, neurosciences, obstetrics/gynecology, ophthalmology, pediatrics, psychiatry, resuscitation, toxicology, trauma, disaster management, and wound management. In addition, because they often represent the sole source of primary care for patients whose only access to care is through EDs, they must be expert at delivering care for minor illnesses and injuries, providing care for chronic conditions, and delivering primary and preventive care. Emergency physicians also have specialized responsibilities beyond their scheduled clinical duties. A survey by Moorhead and colleagues (2002) found that physicians spend several hours per week performing unscheduled clinical duties; administrative work, such as ED quality improvement; medical direction of emergency medical services (EMS); supervision of midlevel providers, such as physician assistants (PAs) and nurse practitioners (NPs); teaching; and research. Many ED physicians also must serve on call for the ED (Moorhead et al., 2002).

Emergency physician staffing models are quite different from those seen in most other specialties. The Physician Socioeconomic Statistics Survey (AMA, 2003) found that 32 percent of emergency medicine physicians are self-employed, 19.8 percent are independent contractors, and 48.2 percent are employees. Of the employees, 29.6 percent are employed by freestanding centers or group practices and 66.8 percent by hospitals, medical schools, or state and local governments. These figures suggest that approximately 14 percent (29.6 percent of 48.2 percent) of emergency physicians are employed by contract management groups (CMGs), although there are conflicting data on this point. One survey of board-certified emergency physicians estimated only 18 percent to be employed by a multihospital contract company (Plantz et al., 1998). However, this study did not survey physicians who staffed the ED but were not board certified and was limited by its relatively small size (465 responses out of 1,050 surveyed). The

American Academy of Emergency Medicine estimates that approximately half of all EDs are staffed by large, national CMGs with majority ownership by non-physicians (Scaletta, 2003). Many of these are small, rural EDs that are unable to attract board certified emergency physicians. Penetration of CMGs is generally lower among large and urban hospitals.

A specialty in emergency medicine exists for physicians wishing to practice in the ED. Emergency medicine residency training involves 3–4 years of specialized training after medical school (see Box 6-1). Approximately 62 percent of physicians who identify their primary site of practice as a hospital ED are board certified in emergency medicine. Academic medical centers and large private hospitals in urban areas are much more likely than other types of hospitals to have residency-trained and board-certified emergency medicine physicians (Moorhead et al., 2002).

Physicians Not Board Certified in Emergency Medicine

Approximately 38 percent of practicing ED physicians are neither board certified nor residency trained in emergency medicine. EDs in suburban and rural locations are more likely to be staffed by emergency physicians that are not residency trained or board certified in emergency medicine than are academic medical centers and large urban hospitals (Moorhead et al., 2002). The majority (84 percent) of these physicians have completed a residency in another specialty, most commonly family practice or internal medicine (Moorhead et al., 2002).

The supply of board-certified emergency physicians is not sufficient to staff all ED physician positions, and in the absence of a large-scale expansion of training in the field will not be sufficient for several decades (Holliman et al., 1997). Therefore, physicians from other disciplines (e.g., internal medicine, family practice, pediatrics) are currently filling positions in EDs. Although they lack board certification, these physicians represent an essential component of the ED workforce at many hospitals, especially smaller facilities in suburban and rural settings. Many acquire a high level of competency in emergency care through a combination of postresidency education, directed skills training, and on-the-job experience.

Demographics

It is difficult to determine precisely how many ED physicians practice in the United States. A 2002 study of the emergency physician workforce in 1999 estimated that approximately 32,000 physicians were working in EDs in 1999, a figure that includes both board-certified and non-board-certified emergency medicine physicians (Moorhead et al., 2002). In a 2004 American Medical Association (AMA) physician survey, however, 25,500 physi-

BOX 6-1
The Specialty of Emergency Medicine

The specialty of emergency medicine began to organize in the mid-1960s in response to the growing demand by hospitals for full-time emergency room physicians. The American College of Emergency Physicians (ACEP) was founded in 1968 (Danzl and Munger, 2000). In 1970, leaders in emergency medicine established an educational curriculum for residency training, and the first emergency medicine residency program began at the University of Cincinnati. By 1975 there were 23 approved residency programs in the United States. In 1976, a Section on Emergency Medicine was formed at the American Medical Association, and pressure grew for the American Board of Medical Specialties (ABMS) to recognize the specialty. The American Board on Emergency Medicine (ABEM) was established in 1976, but the ABMS did not formally recognize it. The development of the specialty was initially resisted by physicians who believed that training in another discipline, such as internal medicine or family practice, was sufficient to practice emergency medicine (Rosen, 1995). Moreover, emergency medicine represented competition for "adjacent" specialties, such as trauma surgery, cardiology, and primary care. After 3 years of negotiations, however, the ABEM was accepted as a modified-conjoint board, making emergency medicine the twenty-third medical specialty (Rosen, 1995). The ABMS finally granted primary board status to the ABEM in 1989.

In 1980, 600 emergency physicians sat for the first certification exam. Emergency medicine developed a critical mass of specialists by allowing experienced practitioners to sit for the certifying exam until 1988, when the "practice track" to board certification was phased out (Marx, 2005). Approximately 20 percent of emergency physicians are board certified as emergency medicine physicians but not residency trained in emergency medicine (Moorhead et al., 2002). Since this "grandfather" track is no longer open, the number of physicians certified through this pathway will decrease over time and eventually disappear. Board certification has also been granted by the American Osteopathic Board of Emergency Medicine (AOBEM) since 1980, and now includes additional certifications in toxicology and sports medicine. In addition to ACEP, another small but growing emergency medicine specialty practice group is the American Academy of Emergency Medicine (AAEM). The

cians self-identified themselves as having an emergency medicine specialty (AMA, 2004); this number likely includes some physicians not board certified in emergency medicine but practicing in an ED on a full-time basis.

The AMA survey also provided some basic demographic information on those physicians. The composition of practicing self-identified emergency

AAEM was formed in 1993 as an organization limited to those emergency physicians with ABEM/ABOEM certification or eligibility for such certification. It has a particular focus on issues related to fair business practices (e.g., open books, physician practice ownership, contract negotiations) with respect to contract management companies.

Residency training requirements for emergency medicine physicians were established by the Accreditation Council for Graduate Medical Education, and since then, accredited emergency medicine residency programs have been growing at a rapid rate—from 1 in 1970 to 43 in 1980, 81 in 1990, and 132 in 2005. A recent report cites 3,909 new emergency medicine physicians being trained in accredited residency programs (ACEP Research Committee, 2005). In 2003, board-certified emergency physicians and pediatric emergency physicians were available at 63.5 percent and 18.1 percent of emergency departments, respectively (McCaig and Burt, 2005). Emergency medicine has demonstrated a regular increase in the percentage of U.S. medical students entering the specialty, growing from 2 percent in 1987 to 4 percent in 2002. There are now several subspecialties within emergency medicine: pediatric emergency medicine, medical toxicology, sports medicine, and undersea and hyperbaric medicine. There are also a number of nonaccredited fellowships not funded by Medicare's Graduate Medical Education (GME) funding that emergency medicine physicians may pursue. These include disaster medicine, medical direction of emergency medical services, ultrasound, health services research, and international emergency medicine.

A small number of emergency physicians hold Board Certification in Emergency Medicine (BCEM) from the American Board of Physician Specialties. This certification, which requires completion of a residency in some field plus 5 years of clinical practice in emergency medicine, is recognized only in Florida (ABPS, 2005).

While residency programs have grown at a rapid pace, academic departments in emergency medicine have progressed more gradually. The Society of Academic Emergency Medicine (SAEM) was formed in 1989 through the merger of the University Association for Emergency Medicine (UAEM) and the Society of Teachers of Emergency Medicine (STEM) to foster the development of academic emergency medicine and promote research in the field. Today there are 64 autonomous departments of emergency medicine at U.S. medical schools and 135 emergency medicine residency programs.

medicine physicians is less diverse than that of the general physician population. Eighty-three percent of self-identified emergency physicians are non-Hispanic white, compared with 75 percent of physicians overall. The primary difference, however, appears to be the lower number of Asians in emergency medicine: in 2002, Asians represented 13 percent of all physicians but only

214

HOSPITAL-BASED EMERGENCY CARE

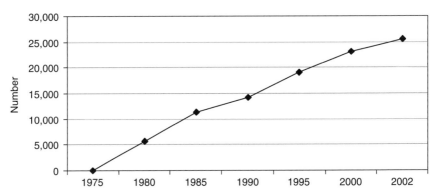

FIGURE 6-1 Number of nonfederal emergency medicine physicians in the United States, 1975 to 2002.
SOURCE: AMA, 2004.

7 percent of emergency medicine physicians. Additionally, only 20 percent of emergency medicine physicians are women, compared with 25 percent of all physicians. Emergency medicine physicians also tend to be younger than other physicians. Nearly one-quarter were under the age of 35 in 2002, and fully half were under the age of 45; among the overall physician population, 59 percent of physicians were aged 45 and older (AMA, 2004).

The number of self-identified emergency physicians in the United States has increased substantially since 1979, when emergency medicine was first recognized as a specialty (see Figure 6-1). Growth in emergency medicine has been much stronger than that in medicine overall. Since 1990, the number of self-identified emergency physicians in the United States has increased from 14,000 to more than 25,500—an increase of 79 percent compared with a 39 percent increase in the number of all physicians. One of the key reasons for the rapid growth in emergency medicine residency programs is that academic medical centers find these programs quite useful for staffing their own EDs. The "fill rate" of emergency medicine residency positions is quite high, reflecting the fact that the field is a popular career choice for U.S. medical students.

Physician Payment

ED physicians often are not hospital employees and are reimbursed separately from the hospital. Medicare physician payment is based on a resource-based relative value scale (RBRVS). The provider reports to the payer the service's Current Procedural Terminology (CPT) evaluation/management (E/M) code, which describes the intensity of the physician service given. Over 80 percent of ED care falls under the five emergency care CPT E/M codes (ACEP, 2004). The codes are converted by the Centers for Medicare and Medicaid Services (CMS) into relative value units (RVUs) and modified by area factors. There are three RVU categories: physician work, practice expense, and professional liability. Each of these RVUs is multiplied by a corresponding geographical practice cost index (GPCI). Medicare then pays the physician 80 percent of the charge, and the patient is responsible for the other 20 percent. An anomaly of reimbursement for emergency physicians is that they are sometimes not credited for some of the tasks they perform. In many cases, the emergency physician is the first to read a patient's electrocardiogram (EKG) or x-ray and use it to make the relevant clinical decisions. Hospital radiologists and cardiologists sometimes read these results and dictate interpretations hours or even days after treatment has been rendered, and then bill for the service. CMS will reimburse only one physician for each interpretation, and payment often goes to whoever rereads the study at a later time rather than to the emergency physician who applies his or her own interpretation to real-time patient care decisions.

Medicaid programs use similar systems that have different rates and details (Kaiser Commission on Medicaid and the Uninsured, 2003). In fact, over 70 percent of all ED physician payments for both public and private care are derived from an RBRVS (ACEP, 2004).

Uncompensated Care

The American College of Emergency Physicians (ACEP) has been active in an effort to increase the practice expense RVU, including a push to count uncompensated care mandated by the 1986 Emergency Medical Treatment and Active Labor Act (EMTALA) toward that RVU. An AMA survey of physicians in 2000 estimated that emergency physicians incurred an annual average of $138,000 in bad debt by providing care mandated by EMTALA (Kane, 2003). Actual foregone income is probably substantially less than this on average, since the $138,000 is based on charges and not actual payments. Nonetheless, a reimbursement rate of 50 percent suggests significant foregone income that has not been remediated through changes in the CMS practice expense RVU. It should be noted that other specialties that provide emergency care also deliver substantial amounts of uncompensated care and face similar economic problems. Reimbursement of on-call physicians is discussed later in this chapter.

Contract Management Groups

CMGs provide hospitals with ED physicians who work on a contract basis, allowing hospitals to staff their EDs around the clock, and they often provide contract management services, including coding and billing (McNamara, 2006). About 16 percent of emergency physicians are employed by a CMG company. If independent contractors are included, however, this figure rises to close to 40 percent of emergency physicians (AMA, 2004).

Contracting with a CMG is an attractive option for some rural hospitals because it guarantees full-time physician coverage of the ED (Williams et al., 2001). The availability of an ED staff also helps attract physicians from other specialties, who are relieved of the need to staff the ED on a rotating basis. CMGs may be an attractive option for physicians as well as they handle many of the business details of practice, such as billing, and provide health and other benefits. These advantages may come at a price, however. In some areas of the country, CMG companies represent such a large share of emergency physician practices that it may be difficult for a physician to practice emergency medicine unless employed by a CMG, which may require physicians to sign noncompete agreements.

Moonlighting

The pressing need for ED physicians frequently leads hospitals to augment their staffs with emergency medicine residents, known as "moonlighters," often to cover evening and weekend shifts. While typically emergency medicine residents, these moonlighters may also include nonemergency physicians and residents training in other specialties, who usually have no specific training or qualifications in emergency medicine (Kellermann, 1995). More than half of all emergency residents reported moonlighting in one survey, though not all in EDs (Li et al., 2000); they cited a variety of reasons for doing so, including supplementing their income and enhancing their educational experience. The practice is discouraged by the emergency medicine specialty organizations because it may place both the resident and the patient at risk, especially when there is no experienced backup in the ED (Keim and Chisholm, 2000). In addition to moonlighters, some physicians working in EDs are provided by "locum tenens" firms that supply physicians to hospital EDs to fill staffing gaps on an as-needed basis.

Trauma Surgeons

The other specialty of particular relevance to emergency care is the surgical subspecialty of trauma/critical care surgery. Trauma is defined as any bodily injury severe enough to pose a threat to life and limb. It requires an organized emergency response that guarantees immediate intervention, including, if needed, the immediate commencement of surgery. Trauma is a major national health problem and remains the leading cause of death for all Americans under age 44. In addition, it takes a huge economic toll on society as it accounts for the greatest loss of productive life in the nation. Trauma care requires a systemic approach that mandates coordination of all prehospital and hospital-based services to optimize care and outcomes. Trauma often occurs during off hours, and trauma centers are therefore busier at night and on weekends and holidays. This requires a 24-hour-a-day operational status that is costly in terms of both facility and human resources.

Most severe trauma care is directed by trauma surgeons who are general surgeons with a special commitment to the provision, management, and organization of trauma care within their hospital and region. The term "trauma surgeon" usually refers to a person trained in general surgery who has an additional 1 to 2 years of training in trauma surgery and critical care. These surgeons focus their practice and expertise on trauma surgery and care management, surgical critical care, and recently all emergency general and vascular surgery. They generally complete a minimum of 7 years of residency training—a complete 5-year general surgery residency, followed by 2 years of fellowship training in trauma surgery and surgical critical care. The American College of Surgeons estimates that there are currently about 3,000 trauma surgeons practicing in the United States (Personal communication, C. Williams, February 17, 2006).

Trauma surgeons tend to focus their practice in specially designated units known as trauma centers. Indeed, a key component of the trauma center designation process is documentation of continuous coverage by trauma surgeons. For level I designation, a trauma surgeon must be available 24 hours a day, 7 days a week. Most level I and some level II trauma centers have trauma surgeons in house 24 hours a day, 7 days a week, who are responsible for all aspects of care of the trauma patient. Trauma care is also provided by emergency physicians, especially in some level II, III, and IV trauma centers. Subspecialists in anesthesia, emergency medicine, orthopedics, neurosurgery, radiology, and, in some states, rehabilitation medicine are required for all level I and II trauma center accreditation.

In the last 30 years, the development of trauma centers and trauma systems has been recognized as a key factor in improving outcomes from injuries, especially those involving vehicular crashes. In addition, trauma centers are a critical component of the safety net system and play a vital role in preparations for potential disasters, both natural and man-made, as well as for acts of terrorism. Trauma that is treated at trauma centers and within an established system has the best outcomes, with significantly lower mortality rates than those seen in non–trauma center hospitals (MacKenzie et al., 2006). The development of trauma systems and trauma surgery practice has been largely directed and codified through a series of reports by the

American College of Surgeons and its Committee on Trauma, including, most recently, the so-called "Gold Book," *The Optimal Care of the Injured Patient* (Committee on Trauma, ACS, 1998).

Currently, hospitals face a decline in the numbers of trauma surgeons due to large amounts of uncompensated care, high levels of medical malpractice risk, and the burden placed by trauma practice on family life. A key factor is the low number of general surgeon trainees electing to go into trauma surgery. Today the majority of fellowships in trauma and surgical critical care are not filled. A national shortage of these specialists will become critical as trauma surgeons now in their late fifties and sixties retire. Furthermore, the trauma capacity in certain cities and regions has declined as trauma centers have closed because of high costs and high levels of uncompensated care.

Specialists Who Provide On-Call Emergency and Trauma Care Services

Hospitals that offer specialist services for inpatients, such as neurosurgery and vascular surgery, must make the same services available to patients who present at the ED (Glabman, 2005). ED physicians rely on and consult these specialists for a range of services—clinical consultation, surgical follow-up, inpatient care, and postdischarge care (Macasaet and Zun, 2005). The limited availability of certain specialists, however, is a well-documented problem that is concerning for both consumers and emergency care providers. Over the past several years, hospitals have found it increasingly difficult to secure specialists for their ED patients. In a 2004 survey by ACEP, two-thirds of ED medical directors reported shortages of on-call specialists at their hospitals (ACEP, 2004). An update to this survey found that the situation is growing worse. In 2005, 73 percent of EDs reported problems with on-call coverage, in contrast to 67 percent the year before (ACEP, 2006). Numerous other studies and surveys have investigated the shortage of on-call specialists, finding that the problem extends across many different specialties and all regions of the country and that it appears to be worsening (Green et al., 2005; O'Malley et al., 2005).

Consider the experience of a patient in San Antonio in his twenties who came to the ED with a vascular injury to his leg artery, the result of a gunshot wound. The vascular circulation needed to be repaired within 6 hours or the patient would risk losing his leg. When the patient arrived at the hospital, ED staff attempted to contact the specialist on call, but he was in surgery and could not respond. Another on-call surgeon was also unavailable because he was performing surgery. The ED staff ultimately decided to transfer the patient hundreds of miles away to a hospital with the expertise to treat him. By the time the patient arrived, however, too much time had elapsed for his leg to be saved (Glabman, 2005). EMTALA currently requires hospitals to have contingency plans for such situations, but unfortunately many do not.

The experience of this patient in San Antonio is not uncommon, yet it is remarkable. One would expect the city to have adequate specialty resources to care for a patient with such an injury. Another reason why the shortage of on-call specialists is remarkable is because it affects all patients, regardless of income or insurance status; insured patients are at the same risk as uninsured patients of not having a specialist available when needed.

Surveys of hospital administrators, ED staff, and specialists indicate that there are at least five underlying factors affecting the availability of emergency and trauma care specialists: (1) the supply of specialists, (2) compensation for providing emergency services, (3) quality-of-life issues, (4) liability concerns, and (5) relaxed EMTALA requirements for on-call panels (Yoo et al., 2001; California Healthcare Association, 2003; Taheri and Butz, 2004; Green et al., 2005; Salsberg, 2005). Each of these factors is discussed in turn below.

Supply of Specialists

Hospital by-laws often require physicians to take ED call for a certain period of time (e.g., 15 years) in exchange for admitting privileges. Historically, this arrangement worked well; it allowed hospitals to fill their on-call panel and gave young specialists an opportunity to build up their practices. But with the movement of specialists to large, multispecialty groups, younger physicians no longer need to rely on ED call to supply patients. Hospitals have less leverage to tie admitting privileges to ED call, and many groups discourage their members from taking ED call (Taheri and Butz, 2004).

The availability of on-call specialists is also dependent upon the local supply of specialists. If there are many specialists in the market, they may be more likely to serve on emergency call panels to draw new patients into their practices, assuming that some of these patients are insured. On the other hand, if there are shortages of certain specialists in a market, those specialists will likely be able to fill their practices without taking call. Indeed, in many areas of the country there is a shortage of certain specialists needed to cover the ED (GAO, 2003a). One reason is that medical school enrollment has not kept pace with the growing population. Neurosurgery is a good example of this point. Despite substantial increases in the U.S. population and in the number of trauma visits, there were fewer practicing neurosurgeons in 2002 (3,050) than there were 12 years earlier. There are far fewer neurosurgeons in the United States than the number of EDs (4,900) (Couldwell et al., 2003). The specialty attributes this decline largely to medical liability problems (discussed below).

The shortage of available on-call specialists is a serious and complex dilemma that appears to defy simple resolution. It reflects long-term trends in professional practice and physician supply that would take years to address even if the solution were clear. There are two approaches, however, that the committee believes warrant special consideration: regionalization of specialty services and development of an emergency surgery subspecialty.

Regionalization of specialty services   Much like the regionalization of trauma services, regionalization of certain specialty services would direct patients to those hospitals having access to the needed specialists and having demonstrated superior outcomes. The intent of regionalizing specialists would be to rationalize the limited supply of specialists by facilitating agreements that would ensure coverage at the key tertiary and secondary locations based on actual need. This arrangement would replace the current haphazard approach that is based on many factors other than patient need. Without such a regional arrangement, some hospitals may have an overabundance of certain specialists while others face a constant shortage. These patterns may be based on physician practice preferences, academic affiliations, reimbursement issues, contractual arrangements, or myriad other factors. They may also be due to simple ignorance of communitywide needs. Regionalization would provide a framework for recognizing and addressing these needs and imbalances through the collection of information on specialist demand and supply and the use of that information to reallocate specialist services through various arrangements, including payment incentives.

While there is limited direct evidence regarding regionalization of on-call specialty services, the approach has proven effective in other contexts and is consistent with the committee's broader vision of a regionalized emergency care system. There are few examples of regionalization with specific reference to emergency and trauma care specialty on-call services. One such effort is Palm Beach County's nascent attempt to regionalize the services of certain on-call specialists through a communitywide cooperative that will contract collectively for their services (described more fully in Chapter 3). Despite the current lack of direct evidence, however, the committee believes the approach holds promise and should be encouraged and evaluated. Therefore, the committee recommends that **hospitals, physician organizations, and public health agencies collaborate to regionalize critical specialty care on-call services (6.1).**

Emergency surgery subspecialization   To expand the pool of surgeons available to emergency and trauma patients, a new specialty designation of emergency surgeon has been proposed. The emergency surgeon would receive broad training in elective and emergency general surgery, trauma surgery, and surgical critical care. In addition to performing what is conventionally considered general trauma surgery (for neck, thoracic, and abdominal injuries), the emergency surgeon could also perform selected and limited neurosurgical and orthopedic procedures, with support from fellow surgical specialists (The Committee to Develop the Reorganized Specialty of Trauma, Surgical Critical Care and Emergency Surgery, 2005). The intent is not for this new specialist to perform major neurosurgical or orthopedic procedures, but only those procedures that can safely be performed without the direct intervention of those other specialists, thus enabling them to concentrate their efforts on more difficult cases.

In the traditional surgical practice model, surgeons may end up working all night operating or covering the intensive care unit (ICU) and then spend the following day seeing their own admitted patients, a physically stressful approach. Under the proposed new model, emergency surgical services would be shared by the emergency surgery group. Each surgeon would work 8–12 hours at a stretch and then be off until the next shift, with another member of the group assuming responsibility.

There has been some controversy about the inclusion of emergent neurological and orthopedic surgical procedures in this new training curriculum. However, the need for the new emergency surgeon to perform these procedures would come into play only when neurological and orthopedic surgical specialists were not available in emergent situations. This might occur in urban facilities where the latter specialists were on staff but unwilling to provide the coverage or in rural areas where the emergency surgeon might be the only surgeon available to provide this care.

Compensation

Another reason specialists may be unwilling to take emergency call is that they often receive little or no compensation for these services because of the large numbers of uninsured and underinsured patients that present in the ED. Yoo and colleagues (2001) reported the results of a 2000 California Medical Association survey on reimbursement for on-call emergency services. Nearly 80 percent of the respondents reported difficulty in obtaining payment for their services, regardless of insurance type. Fully 54 percent responded that they received no payment for on-call services, though the frequency of nonpayment is unclear. Another 42 percent reported underpayment and payment delay. Forty percent of the physicians who took voluntary call stated that lack of payment had forced them to reduce call, while 20 percent said they would be unable to continue voluntary call under the present circumstances.

Perhaps the most common strategy has been for hospitals to provide a stipend or extra payment for physicians to take call. According to a 2004 American Hospital Association (AHA) survey, approximately 40 percent of hospitals pay some specialists for ED call, with a median stipend of $1,000 per night (Glabman, 2005). Stipends have helped individual hospitals secure the availability of certain specialists, but the long-term viability of this strategy is questionable as the stipends are quite large for some specialists, and not all hospitals have funding to support such stipends. For example, one hospital in Miami is reportedly spending $13 million annually to compensate physicians for taking call in the ED (Mays et al., 2005). A Phoenix-area hospital reported paying each of its neurosurgical groups $10,000 per week in exchange for taking call (Hurley et al., 2005). These payments are in addition to any patient revenue the specialists may collect. Moreover, the practice of paying physicians to be on call is controversial. With many hospitals operating at a deficit, the AHA claims that hospitals cannot make these stipends a permanent feature of emergency call (Maguire, 2001). Additionally, the question of which specialists should receive payment may incite controversy across specialties.

An alternative model that may have advantages over paying stipends has been implemented successfully at Scripps Health in San Diego. This model uses an exclusive contract to secure neurosurgery coverage for the trauma center. It involves combining all emergency neurosurgery and trauma cases and issuing a request for proposals for exclusive rights to providing care for these patients. Substantial competition for the contract resulted in a qualified and committed group of neurosurgeons providing services for emergent and trauma care. The contract requires prompt response, participation in all process improvement and educational programs, and leadership in neurosurgical quality improvement. This model is likely to be more successful in areas where stipends for on-call staff are used and are rising quickly (Scheck, 2004).

Quality-of-Life Issues

The new generation of specialists appear to be less inclined to take call than their older colleagues because of quality-of-life issues. There is no question that the demands of on-call coverage are substantial. When on call, specialists may be summoned in the middle of the night and required to perform complex surgeries, diagnoses, or other services. It is not unusual for a surgeon on call to work through the night and then see a full day's worth of patients in the office. Specialists taking daytime call may be interrupted in the middle of a busy day of seeing patients in the office, forcing patients to reschedule. Furthermore, as the availability of specialists taking emergency call declines, the burden on those who continue to take call grows. In 2003, the Accreditation Council for Graduate Medical Education (ACGME), following the earlier lead of the New York State Bell Commission, placed strict limits on resident work hours, including the number of consecutive hours doctors in training can be required to work on call without a period of intervening sleep. The same limits do not apply to practicing physicians, and are routinely exceeded by surgical specialists and others who take overnight emergency call.

Younger physicians are assigning greater importance to the balance among work, marriage, and family time and are therefore demanding greater control over their work schedules, fewer absolute work hours, and more time devoted to their private practice (Salsberg, 2005). Further, many do not view ED call as a professional obligation to the degree that previous generations of specialists did, particularly when market factors enable them to build a successful practice without the addition of emergency patients (Taheri and Butz, 2004).

Liability Concerns

The high risk of being sued and the high costs of professional liability insurance premiums further discourage specialists from providing on-call services. Procedures performed on emergency patients are inherently risky and expose specialists to an increased likelihood of litigation. There are several reasons for this: emergency and trauma patients are often sicker than other patients and may have serious comorbidities, and the on-call physician usually has no preexisting relationship with the patient or his/her family.

Primary care physicians often refer patients with serious or complex medical problems to hospital EDs to shield themselves from liability during diagnostic workups (Berenson et al., 2003). Safety net hospitals are especially affected by the liability problem. As panels diminish at community hospitals, they increasingly transfer patients to the large safety net hospitals, which have no choice but to accept them; the result is even higher concentrations of uninsured, high-risk patients. Several reports have documented closings of trauma centers, at least temporarily, or downgrading of their status because of staffing shortages associated with liability concerns (Whaley, 2002). In the current environment of high liability risk, safety net hospitals are at risk of becoming the dumping ground for the liability crisis.

A 2004 nationwide survey of neurosurgeons conducted by the American Academy of Neurological Surgeons found that 35.8 percent of respondents had been sued by patients seen through the hospital ED (Perception Solutions, Inc., 2004). For this reason, specialists who regularly take ED call pay more for liability coverage than those who do not. An analysis of premiums paid by specialists in Palm Beach County, Florida, revealed that orthopedists who take regular ED call pay 75 percent more for malpractice insurance than orthopedists who do not take call (Taheri and Butz, 2004). One neurosurgeon reported being told by his insurance company that he must limit coverage of the ED to 10 nights per month or his premiums would be increased to prohibitive levels (Byrne and Bagan, 2004).

Liability premiums for specialists in general have been rising at an increasing rate. Data from the Medical Liability Monitor show that premiums for general surgeons grew approximately 1 percent in 1998 and 1999, but 7 percent in 2000, 12 percent in 2001, and 21 percent in 2002 (Thorpe, 2004). The result is burdensome premiums for specialists in many areas of the country. For example, the largest underwriter of professional liability insurance in Illinois reported that the average premium in 2005 for neurosurgeons in the Chicago area was $235,000 per year for only $1 million in coverage. While $1 million may appear to be adequate coverage, nearly half of settlements in the Chicago area exceeded $1 million in 2003, and more than 10 settlements exceeded $10 million (Byrne and Bagan, 2004). Growth in physician liability premiums has not been offset by growth in revenues. In fact, patient revenues, which are often set to the Medicare payment schedule, have actually been declining, making the burden of increased premium payments even greater (Valadka, 2004).

The specific effects of liability premiums on emergency and trauma care specialists were addressed in a 2003 report by the U.S. Government Accountability Office (GAO, 2003b). The report was based on a study that compared experiences in five states having reported medical malpractice problems (crisis states) with experiences in four states not having such problems. The GAO found that in the crisis states, access to emergency care was reduced, particularly for trauma and obstetrical services; transfers of patients were increased; and the availability of on-call specialists to EDs was reduced, especially for critical specialties such as orthopedic and neurological surgery. The study further documented that reduced on-call coverage resulted in frequent delays in care and transfers of patients to alternative facilities up to 100 miles away to receive specialist care. A section of West Virginia lost all neurosurgical coverage for 2 years, requiring all emergency patients needing neurosurgical consults to be transferred more than 60 miles away. The report noted, however, that confirmed problems in access frequently involved hospitals, often rural, with long-standing problems in maintaining the availability of services.

Trauma services were affected in every state in the study. The effects included temporary trauma center closings due to loss of on-call specialist services for trauma care in West Virginia, Pennsylvania, and Nevada. In each of these cases, the state had to resolve the crisis by either providing liability coverage or making the specialists state employees, thus limiting their exposure.

The effect of placing caps on malpractice awards at the state level to ameliorate access problems has been the subject of numerous research efforts over the past few years. The growing consensus is that state liability reforms have helped reduce physician liability premiums to some extent (Thorpe, 2004) and have led to some small increases in physician supply (Hellinger and Encinosa, 2005), particularly in rural areas (Encinosa and Hellinger, 2005; Matsa, 2005). However, the direct impact of these reforms on the delivery of emergency services has not been adequately examined.

A number of additional approaches could be used to protect emergency care specialists without compromising patient safety. One would be to provide "conditional immunity" for emergency physicians and specialists while seeing patients on call. Another promising approach is a public no-fault system modeled on the National Vaccine Injury Compensation System. In such a system, malpractice in emergency care would be compensated through a fund that would be supported by hospitals and physicians. Such an approach would provide much more rapid and certain compensation than the current tort system while encouraging hospitals and individual providers to address patient safety issues in a transparent and energetic manner. Alternatively, caps on noneconomic damage awards, which have been effective in some states, could be placed on emergency services (Thorpe, 2004).

Whatever liability reform strategies are used to ease the crisis in availability of emergency providers, they must be balanced by protections for patient safety. One proposed mechanism is the establishment of a national emergency care patient safety initiative. This initiative would include reporting systems for sentinel events, with penalties for failure to report incidents; a national database of patient safety events; development of standards of care; monitoring and reporting of performance standards; and corrective measures to be taken in instances of repeated problems. An additional feature that might be considered is tying protections from liability exposure to demonstrated performance on quality-of-care indicators.

Many states have enacted some form of liability reform, though the types of reforms undertaken have varied. These reforms have created a "natural experiment" through which researchers can investigate their impact. Congressional policy makers, with advice from health services researchers, should monitor the impact of these reforms at the state level and consider federal liability reform.

Because of the critical nature of the on-call specialty crisis and the substantial role that liability appears to play in creating and sustaining this crisis, the committee believes it is of crucial importance to the nation to understand more clearly the true impact of liability on specialty services, to identify the range of public policy and private initiatives that can make a significant difference in resolving the problem, and to take urgent actions based on these findings. Therefore, the committee recommends that **Congress appoint a commission to examine the impact of medical malpractice lawsuits on the declining availability of providers in high-risk emergency** and trauma care specialties, and to recommend appropriate state and federal actions to mitigate the adverse impact of these lawsuits and ensure quality of care (6.2).

The committee recognizes that medical malpractice is a national issue that affects all areas of medicine, not just emergency care. But it also recognizes that the issue represents a unique and urgent challenge in emergency care that cannot wait for long-term national or state solutions. Special consideration is warranted not only because of the crisis facing emergency care, but also because of emergency care's unique public-good characteristics. Medical emergencies are unpredictable events, and the emergency care system must maintain a state of readiness to handle them as they arise. Because individuals cannot know when they will need emergency services, they will underconsume the readiness aspect of emergency care. Government intervention is warranted to maintain an efficient level of readiness. Liability protections for emergency providers could be a stop-gap measure until broad, national legislation addressing medical malpractice reform is enacted.

Relaxed Requirements of the Emergency Medical Treatment and Active Labor Act

The responsibility of hospitals to ensure the availability of on-call staff was revisited by CMS in guidance published in September 2003. Prior to the 2003 amendment, there was considerable confusion surrounding hospitals' on-call list responsibilities. Afraid of violating EMTALA, many hospitals adopted a "rule of three" policy, which states that if a hospital has more than three physicians in a specialty, it must provide continuous ED coverage for that specialty. Struggling to maintain their on-call lists, some hospitals required specialists to be on call 24 hours a day, 7 days a week (Russell, 2004). Complaints by on-call physicians and hospitals led to a clarification of the policy in 2003. CMS stated that EMTALA does not require hospitals to follow the "rule of three" and changed its statutory language as follows: "Each hospital must maintain an on-call list of physicians on its medical staff in a manner that best meets the needs of the hospital's patients who are receiving services required under this section in accordance with the resources available to the hospital, including the availability of on-call physicians" (42 Code of Federal Regulations §489.24). CMS also clarified that physicians could be on call at more than one hospital simultaneously (hospitals must have procedures in place for when a physician is on call at another hospital and is unable to respond) and that surgeons could perform elective surgery while on call (Russell, 2004).

The impact of the EMTALA amendment on the supply of and access to on-call specialists is not clear. Many believe that access to on-call specialists has worsened as a result. In the example cited earlier of the patient from San Antonio, the local on-call surgeons would not have been allowed to perform elective surgeries while on call prior to the 2003 EMTALA guidance. Though it is unclear in the above example whether the on-call specialists were performing elective or emergency surgery, it is easy to see how the change to EMTALA potentially makes access to on-call specialists more difficult. But others argue that the amendment has been beneficial. Had CMS not loosened on-call requirements, they argue, more specialists might have refused to take call in the ED altogether.

As an alternative, some have advanced the idea of a more direct approach in which CMS would hold specialists rather than hospitals accountable for providing on-call services. One variation on this approach would be to require specialists to take call as a condition for Medicare participation. While the directness of this approach has some appeal, it fails to address the underlying problems, such as the declining numbers of specialists, and is indeed likely to contribute to that decline.

Hospitalists and Critical Care Specialists

Hospitalists

In 2003 more than 8,000 hospitalists—physicians who focus exclusively on managing hospital inpatients—were practicing in U.S. hospitals according to the Society of Hospital Medicine (Society of Hospital Medicine, 2006). That number is expected to reach 30,000 in the next decade. The use of hospitalists will increase as hospitals seek to reduce costs, streamline patient flow, and improve patient safety (Pham et al., 2005).

Hospitalists have traditionally been used to care for inpatients, and their service has been shown to decrease lengths of stay and reduce morbidity. Adding them to a hospital's medical staff is an attractive option because they are generally more willing to accept emergency admissions after hours or at night, avoiding the need to involve the patient's office-based physician. Faster acceptance by the admitting physician can help an ED maintain patient flow and reduce the risks of crowding and ambulance diversion. In some hospitals, hospitalists may provide backup when the ED is particularly busy by assisting with the disposition of patients who clearly need to be admitted. Hospitalists can also staff observation units in EDs (Dresnick, 1997).

On the other hand, hospitalists sometimes utilize ED resources (e.g., space and staff) in conducting workups of patients they are admitting, placing a drain on crowded EDs. This situation is alleviated in some hospitals by admissions units that are separate from the ED. Because hospitalists focus on inpatient care rather than traveling back and forth from their office, they are often more efficient than office-based practitioners. One hospital found that by using hospitalists to coordinate care immediately following the admission decision, the hospital cut the average length of stay for patients admitted through the ED by 2 days, increasing bed availability (Brewster and Felland, 2004). Many hospitalists are being asked to become more involved in ED triage decisions. The theory is that hospitalists may have more time than emergency physicians to fully evaluate patients, and may also be more familiar with home care or skilled nursing facilities (Wachter, 2004). However, this strategy is not without its drawbacks. Hospitalists may refuse to be the physician of record for unassigned patients in communities with large uninsured populations, and many hospitals do not have the funding to hire hospitalists (Maguire, 2001).

Hospitalists may also help alleviate some problems with the availability of on-call staff. Hospitalists in the ED can assess the status of unassigned patients and make a determination as to whether a specialist is needed. According to a survey for the California Healthcare Foundation, emergency physicians appreciate the availability of hospitalists as timesavers, and specialists value fewer calls and fewer late-night trips to the ED. In fact, more survey respondents favored using hospitalists to address the on-call problem than favored mandating on-call coverage or contracting with a third party for call coverage. However, hospitalists are best used for medical patients and are unlikely to help alleviate problems with on-call subspecialists and surgeons (Green et al., 2005).

Critical Care Specialists/Intensivists

Critical care specialists are an essential component of emergency and trauma care in addressing the needs of severely ill and injured patients. The use of intensivists has been associated with a 30 percent reduction in hospital mortality and a 40 percent reduction in ICU mortality (Pronovost et al., 2002). Greater use of intensivists has also led to significantly reduced hospital and ICU lengths of stay (Pronovost et al., 1999). The Leapfrog Group is promoting the use of a full-time intensivist model to meet its ICU Physician Staffing standard. Currently only 10 percent of ICUs actually meet this standard (The Leapfrog Group, 2004).

As discussed earlier, because inpatient units are becoming increasingly crowded, critically ill patients are boarding in the ED for longer periods of time. This is a challenge for EDs because critically ill patients require an intensive amount of resources, including medical attention, monitoring equipment, and medications (Church, 2003). This situation has led some hospitals to use intensivists in the ED. The committee recognizes the importance of providing critical care services quickly to admitted patients but does not endorse the practice of using intensivists as a way to accommodate the practice of boarding. Instead, the committee encourages hospitals to address the root causes of boarding so that critically ill patients are moved quickly to intensive care beds.

There is currently a severe national shortage of critical care physicians—so much so that the critical care societies have petitioned Congress to increase the number of foreign medical graduates with critical care training. Emergency physicians with subspecialty certification in critical care medicine could help address this shortage, provide a margin of safety for ED boarders, and provide extra capability in community hospitals that cannot afford to keep both types of providers on staff every night (Osborn and Scalea, 2002). However, the American Board of Medical Specialties (ABMS) currently blocks residency-trained, board-certified emergency physicians and other acute and primary care specialists from obtaining subspecialty certification in critical care. To increase the pool of well-trained intensivists in both adult and pediatric practice, the committee recommends that **the American Board of Medical Specialties and its constituent boards extend eligibility for certification in critical care medicine to all acute care and primary care physicians who complete an accredited critical care fellowship program (6.3).**

NURSES AND OTHER CRITICAL PROVIDERS

Nurses

There are approximately 90,000 nurses working in EDs (NHT, 2006). According to the Emergency Nurses Association (ENA), emergency registered nurses (RNs) perform the following tasks: assessment, analysis, nursing diagnosis, planning, implementation of interventions, outcome identification, evaluation of responses, triage and prioritization, emergency operations preparedness, stabilization and resuscitation, and crisis intervention for unique patient populations (e.g., sexual assault survivors) (Cole et al., 1999). In a 2000 national survey of nurses commissioned by the Department of Health and Human Services (DHHS), nurses working in EDs overwhelmingly reported that their dominant function was direct patient care (83 percent). Smaller numbers of ED nurses reported working in supervision (3.5 percent) or administration (2.5 percent).

To become a nurse, an individual can either pursue an associate's degree in nursing (ADN) or a bachelor of science in nursing (BSN). The ADN course is typically a 2-year degree program and is focused on the practical applications of nursing. The BSN is a 4-year course of study that expands into the theoretical realms of patient care. A third course of study is the diploma, which was common prior to the 1970s. The diploma program is a 2- to 3-year course of study that is located in a hospital and prepares students for hospital positions. There are fewer than 100 diploma programs in existence today (All Nursing Schools, 2005). In recent years, national nursing organizations have pushed to mandate that the BSN be a minimum requirement for being a professional nurse. After graduation from one of these programs, nurses must take the state board examination to become an RN.

Emergency Nurses

The Emergency Department Nurses Association was formed in 1970. The name of the organization was changed to the Emergency Nurses Association in 1975 to reflect that emergency nurses may work in a variety of settings (ENA, 2005a). In the late 1970s, a committee was convened to write a certification examination, and the ENA helped establish a Board of Certification for Emergency Nursing. The first certification examination was administered in 1980, and 902 emergency nurses passed the exam. In the early 1990s, the board also assisted with the development of the certification program for flight nurses (ENA, 2005b).

In 2004, 13,115 RNs nationwide were credentialed as certified emergency nurses (CENs). There are also other advanced degree options for nurses, including master's and doctoral degree programs with various areas of specialization and practice. Many nursing management positions require advanced degrees. Some ED nurses specialize in caring for children and may work in pediatric EDs, but no certification is available in pediatric emergency nursing, and there is a paucity of data available regarding these nurses. State boards of nursing may require training in pediatric advanced life support for nurses providing conscious sedation. Pediatric EDs are likely to require advanced pediatric courses and may even require advanced training in neonatal resuscitation for nurses.

According to DHHS's National Center for Health Workforce Analysis, ED nurses are overwhelmingly non-Hispanic white (88.5 percent). All racial/ethnic groups are severely underrepresented in the ED nursing population relative to the U.S. population. ED nurses are predominantly female (86 percent) and are younger on average than nurses that work in other settings, with a median age of 40 compared with 43 for other nurses. But ED nurses are aging at approximately the same rate as other nurses, with the median age increasing by 3 years (from 37 to 40) between 1988 and 2000. ED nurses generally have less experience than nurses in other settings. Thirty percent reported graduating in the last 5 years, compared with 20.6 percent of other nurses. Only 11.4 percent of ED nurses reported graduating 26 or more years ago, compared with 22.6 percent of all nurses. ED nurses were more likely than other nurses to report an associate's degree as their highest level of education (45.6 versus 36.6 percent) and were less likely to have attained a master's degree (5.8 versus 10.6 percent) (DHHS, 2000).

Advanced Practice Nurses

Advanced practice nurses (APNs) are masters-prepared RNs who provide significant medical care to patients, often with supervision by a physician depending upon their role and scope of practice. APNs include nurse
practitioners (NPs), clinical nurse specialists (CNSs), certified registered
nurse anesthetists (CRNAs), and certified nurse midwives (CNMs). APNs
are required to have a defined scope-of-practice statement for their role,
approved by the state board of nursing.

There is no national certification for APNs in emergency care, but
NPs and other APNs may obtain training in emergency care skills through
university-based programs, continuing education, and work experiences
(Cole et al., 1999). In a recent survey sponsored by the ENA, APNs in
emergency settings were most likely to report specialties in family NP (43
percent), acute care NP (13 percent), adult care NP (12 percent), critical care
CNS (9 percent), or pediatric NP (7 percent) (Cole et al., 2002).

National data are not available on the demographic characteristics of
APNs in EDs. However, data collected on licensed NPs in New York State
in 2000 allow examination of some of these characteristics in this one state.
NPs in EDs were somewhat less likely to be female than other NPs. Despite
being younger, ED NPs had spent slightly more years on average as an NP
than other NPs (5.5 versus 5) and had also been in their current position for
a longer period of time (3 years versus 2 for other NPs). NPs in EDs were
more likely than other NPs to hold a Drug Enforcement Administration
(DEA) certification, which is required to prescribe controlled substances
(86.3 versus 66.3 percent), although they were less likely than other NPs
to have hospital admission privileges (4.5 versus 7.3 percent) (Center for
Health Workforce Studies, 2000).

Nursing Supply Issues

The nursing shortage in both hospital and nonhospital settings has been
the subject of press reports and research articles for years (DHHS, 2002). Although shortages of nurses persist, and the average age of practicing nurses
continues to grow, the pipeline of new nursing graduates has been very
favorable for the last several years. Enrollments in undergraduate nursing
programs increased by 20.8 percent in 2005 and the number of graduates by
26.1 percent (National League for Nursing, 2005). In fact, 147,000 qualified
nursing school candidates were turned away in 2005, an 18 percent increase
over the previous year. It appears that the limiting factor in the growth of
the nursing workforce is the number of nursing programs and faculty.

Nevertheless, the shortages facing many hospitals today are acute and
extremely difficult to address on a day-to-day basis. These continuing short-

ages disrupt hospital operations, complicate attempts to deal with ED crowd-ing, and are detrimental to patient safety and quality of care. Until the nurs-ing school pipeline generates significant increases in the nursing workforce, the nursing shortage will continue to be a problem for hospitals and medical centers in all units. Indeed, the problem is expected to worsen before it gets better; as a result of the aging of the population, the demand for nursing services is expected to outpace the number of new nurses for some time. And robust research studies have shown a direct link between nurse staffing levels and patient outcomes (Aiken et al., 2002; Needleman et al., 2002).

EDs are particularly vulnerable to the nursing shortage. Because of the intensity of emergency care, EDs often have more vacant nursing positions than the hospital's average. Nationwide, it is estimated that 12 percent of RN positions for which hospitals are actively recruiting are in EDs. This makes the ED the third most common source of nursing position openings in hospitals (following general medical/surgical and critical care units). Among hospitals surveyed in New York City, 83 percent reported actively recruit-ing for nurses in their ED (Greater New York Hospital Association, 2004). A majority of nurses responding to a 2002 survey in New York State said there was "definitely" no shortage of jobs for nurses with their experience, training, and skills; however, there was "definitely" a shortage of qualified nurses with their experience, training, and skills. This trend was more pro-nounced among ED nurses than those working in other settings (New York State Education Department, 2003).

The impact of the nursing shortage on ED patient care has not been effectively evaluated; however, many speculate that the shortage has a negative impact on patient care for two reasons. First, as with other areas of the hospital, if the ED lacks appropriate nursing levels, patients will not receive the care or attention they need. For example, a triage nurse may be overwhelmed by the number of patients he or she has to evaluate and may miss an important sign of a severe illness or injury. Likewise, if a nurse in the ED must care for too many acutely ill and injured patients simultaneously while assessing newly arriving patients and monitoring admissions who are boarding in the ED, the potential for delayed care or medication errors is dramatically increased. Also, the nursing shortage adds to the problem of ED crowding by limiting the number of staffed inpatient beds available for emergency admissions.

Traditionally, hospitals have determined levels of nurse staffing in the ED using a productivity measure called hours per patient visit (HPPV). Under this system, the total number of paid nursing staff hours is divided by the total number of ED visits to generate a number of hours per patient visit. Obviously, the shortcoming of this method is that patients with vary-ing levels of severity of illness receive the same consideration with regard to nursing staff time (Robinson et al., 2004). More recently, labor unions, some nursing organizations, and the public have been advocating the use of mandatory nurse staffing ratios in an effort to promote patient safety and quality care (Hackenschmidt, 2004). In the ED, nurse staffing ratios tend to range from 1:4 for general ED patients to 1:1 for trauma patients (Robinson et al., 2004).

Hospitals have opposed mandatory nurse staffing ratios because of the nursing shortage, which makes meeting the ratios difficult; the potential increase in costs; and the increased risk of litigation if a hospital fails to comply with the ratios (Hackenschmidt, 2004). There are particular difficulties associated with maintaining nurse staffing ratios in the ED. The patient census may change rapidly, and the care requirements of patients change significantly during the course of their ED stay.

In 1999, California was the first state to introduce specific nurse-to-patient ratios in EDs, though the ratios were not instituted until 2004 (Hackenschmidt, 2004). The minimum staffing ratios used by the California Department of Health are one nurse to four general ED patients, one nurse to two critical care ED patients, and one nurse to one ED trauma patient. Triage nurses are not included in the ratios. The reaction to the staffing ratios in California among ED nurses is mixed. Some report feeling relieved about the improved staffing; others believe the law is too strict and does not allow for flexibility based on the unit and patient severity of illness. While individual patient care may improve as a result of mandatory ratios, wait times in the ED may increase if ED nurses may care for only a limited number of patients at a time (Hackenschmidt, 2004).

The ENA has spoken out against the use of HPPV and legislated nurse-to-patient staffing ratios, claiming that they are limited in scope and fail to consider the factors that affect the consumption of nursing resources. Indeed, there is a lack of scientific evidence to support the ratio numbers (Hackenschmidt, 2004). The ENA has in turn developed its own staffing guidelines based on six factors: patient census, patient severity of illness, patient length of stay, nursing time for nursing interventions and activities by severity of illness, skill mix for providing patient care based on nursing interventions that can be delegated to a non-RN, and an adjustment factor for the non–patient care time included in each full-time equivalent (FTE) position (Ray et al., 2003).

Despite the controversy over appropriate staffing levels, hospitals still struggle to fill vacant ED nursing positions. They have tried several strategies to compensate for the shortage of ED nurses, including recruiting nurses from foreign countries and using "float" or borrowed nurses from other units of the hospital when the ED is particularly busy. While recruitment from other countries, particularly Canada, has helped relieve the shortages, the use of float nurses is more problematic because those individuals are not familiar with the complexity of the ED or emergency nursing practice

(Schriver et al., 2003). Additionally, in many areas of the country, hospitals use mandatory overtime as a management tool to meet staffing requirements (Jacobsen et al., 2002). Mandatory overtime is a controversial practice, opposed by all of the major nursing organizations. While almost 20 states have considered banning mandatory overtime for nurses, only a handful have done so (Rogers et al., 2004).

Even offering voluntary overtime to nurses is not without controversy, however. Nurses often work longer than their scheduled time, and many shifts extend longer than 12 hours. Research has shown that the risk of medical errors increases significantly when nurses' shifts exceed 12 hours, when they work overtime, and when they work more than 40 hours per week (Rogers et al., 2004). In *Keeping Patients Safe: Transforming the Work Environment of Nurses*, the Institute of Medicine (IOM) recommended that voluntary overtime for nurses be limited (IOM, 2004a).

Physician Assistants

According to the American Association of Physician Assistants (AAPA), 4,508 physician assistants (PAs) (9.8 percent of all PAs) worked in EDs in 2003. PAs provide medical care to patients under the supervision of a licensed physician. They perform a number of functions, including conducting physical exams, diagnosing and treating illnesses, ordering and interpreting tests, counseling on preventive health care, and in most states, writing prescriptions (Allied Health Schools, 2005). PAs must be granted clinical privileges at the hospital in which they work.

Most PA programs can be completed through 2 years of training after college. The first year of training consists of coursework in the basic sciences, while the second gives students clinical experience in such areas as internal medicine, rural primary care, emergency medicine, surgery, pediatrics, neonatology, and occupational medicine. Some PAs pursue additional education in a specialty area, such as emergency medicine (Allied Health Schools, 2005). There are three PA educational programs in the United States offering specializations in emergency medicine, although PAs do not need to graduate from such a program to practice in EDs.

Racial and ethnic diversity is low among PAs practicing in EDs; 88 percent are non-Hispanic white. The majority are men. PAs in EDs generally tend to be older than other PAs, in direct contrast to the patterns found among other emergency care personnel (AAPA, 2005).

Pharmacists

The ED is a high-risk area that is prone to medical errors, including medication errors (Goldberg et al., 1996; Selbst et al., 1999; Schenkel, 2000;

Croskerry et al., 2004). In the 1970s, hospitals began integrating pharmacists into ED staff. Their roles generally involved improving medication billing and inventory control. Since that time, the role of pharmacists in the ED has grown to include clinical consultation, education of ED staff, and research (Thomasset and Faris, 2003). Clinical pharmacy specialists (CPSs) that work in EDs typically have a doctor of pharmacy degree and have completed a 1-year residency.

Substantial evidence indicates that including pharmacists on the care team can improve the quality and safety of patient care in both inpatient and outpatient settings (Bates et al., 1995; Leape et al., 1999; Kaushal et al., 2001; Kaushal and Bates, 2001). There are several reasons for including a CPS on the ED care team. The first is to ensure that patients' medication needs are met. With the growing number of drugs available and the increased complexity of drug selection, administration, and monitoring, there is some justification for having a doctorally trained pharmacist participate on the care team. Participation of a pharmacist on the care team is in line with guidelines of the Joint Commission on Accreditation of Healthcare Organizations (JCAHO) for promoting a multidisciplinary approach to patient care. Second, as noted, medication errors are a serious problem in EDs, and pharmacists may be able to lead system changes that can reduce or eliminate these errors. Finally, medication costs are rising, and pharmacists are in a good position to evaluate which medications are most cost-effective for patients and the hospital.

Still, the prevalence of pharmacists, particularly full-time pharmacists, in EDs remains limited. A 2001 survey of directors of pharmacy in hospitals with at least one accredited pharmacy residency program was conducted to ascertain the prevalence and characteristics of pharmaceutical services in EDs nationwide (Thomasset and Faris, 2003). Only 3 percent of respondents reported having a dedicated pharmacist in an ED satellite pharmacy; 14 percent reported having a dedicated pharmacist who provided services to ED patients. But the demand for pharmacists or pharmacy assistance may grow over the next few years as a result of JCAHO's 2005 National Patient Safety Goals and Requirements, which call for complete and accurate medication reconciliation across the continuum of care (JCAHO, 2005).

EMS Professionals

Increasingly, EMS professionals are supplementing their prehospital EMS practice by working in hospital EDs. Because of their relevant training and experience, they can serve as effective adjuncts to regular ED staff. According to a 2004 survey of EMS personnel conducted by the National Registry of EMTs, a considerable number of EMTs spend time working professionally in EDs—32.9 percent of EMT-Bs,[1] 34.9 percent of EMT-Is, and 29.8 percent of paramedics (NREMT, 2005). These figures represent a substantial increase over previous years. Anecdotal evidence suggests that this is a nationwide phenomenon that is prevalent in both rural and urban environments. There is substantial variation across states in how EMTs can be used in the ED, and some states (e.g., Kansas) have bridge courses that facilitate migration between EMT and RN credentials. This phenomenon may be explained in part by the substantial differences in pay and amenities between the two environments.

Psychologists, Social Workers, and Patient Advocates

A variety of patient care professionals play a critical and generally undervalued role in assisting patients with issues related to family, living arrangements, food and shelter, public and private insurance programs, mental health, and human dignity. The number of such practitioners in the ED is not well known. As the diversity of patients seen in the ED has increased, so, too, has the variety of their social and psychological needs. The importance of these providers has risen, by all accounts, at a much faster pace than their supply.

ENHANCING THE SUPPLY OF EMERGENCY CARE PROVIDERS

The ED workforce includes a broad cross section of the larger health care system—physicians in fields ranging from family medicine to neurosurgery, residents, nurses, pharmacists, and PAs—as well as those who specialize in emergency care, including emergency medicine physicians, emergency nurses, trauma surgeons, and certain medical and surgical specialists. There are substantial concerns about the long-term supply of emergency professionals in several of these categories.

Ensuring an adequate supply of highly trained professionals in every category is the goal. However, there are a number of challenges associated with enumerating the current ED workforce (e.g., how to count part-time workers, individuals who work in multiple EDs, different scopes of practice across states), and estimating the size of the ED workforce needed for the

---

[1]States commonly classify EMS field providers into four distinct levels. The first responder provides first aid and conducts basic assessments, usually in advance of the arrival of a higher-level EMT. The EMT-B (emergency medical technician-basic) is generally trained to provide basic, noninvasive prehospital care. The EMT-I (intermediate) performs some invasive procedures, such as delivery of intravenous fluids. The EMT-P (paramedic) is the most highly skilled EMS worker and is trained in advanced life support. Many states have additional categories, such as EMT-dispatch. There is wide variation across states in the scope of practice within each of these categories.

future is an even more challenging task. Bioterrorism preparedness, the aging of the population, changing morbidity patterns, potential reforms to the health care system, and technological advances are just some of the factors that will impact the size of the ED workforce needed in the future.

While the national supply of physicians and other medical specialists is critical, so is the distribution of the workforce. The most highly trained and specialized clinicians tend to cluster in metropolitan areas, while rural and frontier areas lack even basic medical coverage. This is not, of course, a problem that is restricted to emergency care. But the lack of qualified emergency care personnel in rural areas has a disproportionate impact on health because of the urgency involved: people can schedule elective visits and procedures at distant locations, but in an emergency, that may not be an option. Addressing the rural distribution of the emergency care workforce will require concerted efforts along many fronts, including training, incentives, and enhancement of the rural provider pipeline. For example, the frequently high debt burden of many emergency medicine residents and the limited opportunity to earn sufficient revenue to pay off educational debt in rural settings pose a significant barrier to rural practice, even for those who may prefer it. Enhanced rural training options combined with loan forgiveness programs is a possible approach for enhancing the rural emergency care workforce.

Developing effective strategies to ensure an adequate supply of trained ED professionals in the future requires an understanding of the needs of the nation 10 and 20 years into the future. The committee therefore recommends that **the Department of Health and Human Services, the Department of Transportation, and the Department of Homeland Security jointly undertake a detailed assessment of emergency and trauma workforce capacity, trends, and future needs, and develop strategies to meet these needs in the future (6.4).** This assessment should be conducted in the context of regionalized systems, which will require a different mix of skills than might otherwise be anticipated. Further, the assessment should consider optimal combinations of professional skills—including emergency and family physicians, NPs, PAs, pharmacists, hospitalists, trauma surgeons, on-call specialists, pediatric and geriatric specialists, social workers, psychologists, and EMS providers. Based on the findings of this assessment, targeted strategies should be considered to address long-term projected shortages, including subsidizing graduate and continuing education programs to increase the number of providers trained in those fields.

This assessment should also address such issues as the impact of graduate medical education allocations at medical centers. These allocations are usually capped, making it difficult for a newer specialty to increase the number of positions, which would require reducing positions in other, established departments. Also, even though emergency physicians are broadly trained (they are more "generalist" in their practice than any specialty other than family medicine), they are excluded from the definition of "primary care" because they do not generally provide continuity of care. Emergency physicians are thereby excluded from certain federal and state programs designed to promote the training of primary care physicians, although in some rural counties, primary care is provided predominantly through the ED.

The above discussion focuses only on emergency physicians, but concerns about the numbers of funded residency positions apply to virtually all specialties that provide emergency care. These concerns are especially important now that the physician workforce is projected to be inadequate for the nation's future needs.

BUILDING CORE COMPETENCIES

Core competencies are the critical skills, knowledge, abilities, and behaviors that a field or industry has agreed must be achieved if a person is to be accepted as competent at a particular level. The specialty of emergency medicine pioneered the concept of a core curriculum for training emergency medicine residents, and now has a detailed roadmap of the training and competencies required for the practice of emergency medicine. The core content eventually developed into a model of the clinical practice of emergency medicine that has served as the foundation for medical school training and residency curricula, certification exam specifications, continuing education objectives, and residency program review requirements (Hockberger et al., 2001). The model was revised in 2004 to incorporate the six core competencies promoted by ACGME: patient care, medical knowledge, practice-based learning and improvement, interpersonal skills, professionalism, and system-based practice (Chapman et al., 2004). The major professional organizations focused on emergency medicine, which include ACEP, SAEM, the Council of Emergency Medicine Residency Directors (CORD), ABEM, the Emergency Medicine Residents Association (EMRA), and the Residency Review Committee for Emergency Medicine (RRC-EM), ensure that the core content specific to the specialty is frequently updated.

As discussed earlier, however, a significant number of physicians practicing in EDs are not residency trained or board certified in emergency medicine (Moorhead et al., 2002). Their level of competency in emergency medicine is not well known. Only a small number of very limited studies have been conducted to compare the competencies of board-certified or residency-trained emergency physicians and those of other emergency physicians. Results of these studies suggest benefits of emergency medicine residency training in the performance of airway management and care of patients with acute myocardial infarction (Friedman et al., 1999; Jones et al., 2002; Weaver et al., 2004). Results of one study also indicate significantly fewer closed malpractice claims against emergency medicine residency–trained physicians relative to ED physicians without such training (Branney et al., 2000); however, there is a need for more robust research in this area.

Competencies in nursing are established and assessed in a similar manner. The ENA developed the Emergency Nursing Core Curriculum for nurses wishing to take the CEN exam. Those nurses with the CEN credential possess the basic competencies deemed appropriate by the ENA. However, most nurses working in EDs are not CENs, and their level of competency and training relevant to emergency care is not well known.

Furthermore, while specialties have established core competencies within their respective fields, there is no uniform standard of care for the multiple disciplines practicing within the ED. Although most EDs treat cardiac patients, not all hospitals require physicians and nurses to take the Advanced Cardiac Life Support course. Similarly, not all hospitals require ED nurses to take the Emergency Nursing Pediatric Course and the Trauma Nursing Core Course, and not all require ED physicians to take the Advanced Trauma Life Support Course. Yet while exposure to these courses may help improve the level of competency for some providers, particularly those with little formal training in emergency care, it does not ensure competency.

As a result of the variability in initial and continuing education received by ED providers, there is also variability in the emergency care received by the public. The committee believes the uncertainty about the quality and consistency of emergency care across the nation is unacceptable and that it is important to define clearly what qualifies as competent care and what does not. Therefore, the committee recommends that **the Department of Health and Human Services, in partnership with professional organizations, develop national standards for core competencies applicable to physicians, nurses, and other key emergency and trauma professionals, using a national, evidence-based, multidisciplinary process (6.5).** The core competencies developed should not simply represent one minimum level of competency that all ED providers must attain. If that were the case, the competencies would be a challenge for only the most resource-strapped hospitals. Instead, the core competencies should be tiered and reflect the categorization of the ED. EDs categorized at the highest levels should be subject to the most stringent competency requirements, while providers working in EDs with a lower categorization should be subject to less rigorous requirements. The competency standards should be developed to challenge hospitals, yet must be attainable. State regulatory agencies should monitor adherence to these standards.

These national standards should ensure that core competencies for all providers working in the ED are assessed in accordance with the level of ED in which they practice, regardless of board certification or CEN status. Research should be conducted to track patient outcomes as a means of monitoring the benefits of having such universal core competencies. Additionally, the efficacy of the core competencies should be periodically assessed and adjusted as necessary.

ADDRESSING THE ISSUE OF PROVIDER SAFETY

Working in an ED has the potential to be highly rewarding but is often very stressful, and at times dangerous. The work is complicated by limited access to patients' past medical history, the episodic nature of the care being provided, and the uncontrolled or unpredictable environments in which care must be provided (Cole et al., 1999). Physical threats to safety abound in the ED, ranging from a chance needle stick to the risk of assault, either physical or verbal, from patients who may be under psychological stress or the influence of intoxicants. Additionally, the psychological toll of working in a high-pressure environment, coupled with exposure to the pain and suffering of illness and injury, can result in tremendous stress on ED providers. This section reviews the day-to-day dangers that affect ED workers. The next chapter addresses provider safety in the context of disasters, including chemical and biological exposure.

Mental Stress

Numerous studies both in the United States and abroad have identified stress as a major concern for emergency care providers. Emergency physicians in 2002 spent an average of 55.7 hours per week on professional activities. This figure is slightly lower than the average number of hours spent on professional activities by all physicians (57.6); however, emergency physicians on average report more total patient visit hours (45.8 versus 43) and have more patient visits per week (118.4 versus 107.2) than other physicians (AMA, 2004). Furthermore, in contrast to most physicians, who follow an established panel of patients, most if not all ED physicians work with new patient encounters, which are often more demanding, time-consuming, and complex. Moreover, ED patients generally present with more acute conditions than are seen in a typical office practice. ED physicians also are prone to stress related to disruption of circadian rhythms because of the frequency and irregularity of night shifts, as well as stress related to the intensity and high levels of severity of illness among the patients they see, the unscheduled nature of emergency visits, the high medico-legal risk of missed diagnoses and complications of care, and the psychological drain of being second-guessed by consultants and admitting physicians. Emergency physicians must handle multiple patients at once and deal with a wide variety of social situations with little backup. As a result, emergency physicians who attempt to work a total number of hours similar to those of office-based practitioners are prone to burnout.

Nurses working in the ED also experience significant stress. Lambert and Lambert (2001) found a lack of job control, work overload, exposure to death and dying, and poor work relationships to be major sources of stress for nurses. A 2002 survey of registered nurses in New York State revealed that RNs working in EDs feel they are under great stress significantly more often relative to RNs working in other settings. Thirty-seven percent of ED RNs reported feeling under great stress "almost every day" (compared with 30 percent of other RNs), while only 10 percent said they felt great stress less than once a week (compared with 19 percent of other RNs), and none said that they "never" felt great stress (compared with 3 percent of other RNs) (New York State Education Department, 2003).

Violence

According to data from the Bureau of Labor Statistics for 1993, workers in the health care field experienced the highest incidence of assault injuries. One study found that 82 percent of nurses surveyed had been assaulted on the job, that 56 percent had been assaulted in the year prior to the survey, and that many assaults went unreported (Erickson and Williams-Evans, 2000). Several characteristics of the ED, the community it serves, and specific patients make the ED and its employees especially prone to such violence. Few steps have been taken to explore this issue and provide ED workers and patients the security they require. With the support of hospital administrators and in cooperation with local officials, security measures and specialized training can be instituted in EDs to enhance provider safety.

Workplace violence encompasses physical assaults and threats of assaults directed toward persons at work or on duty, and can encompass witnessing or being a victim of physical assaults, sexual assaults, nonverbal intimidation, and verbal threats (Flannery et al., 2000). Researchers have attempted to identify key risk factors associated with violence in the ED and the broader health care field in an effort to increase provider awareness and encourage the development of strong violence prevention programs. Those specific risk factors include staff shortages and long wait times, which can aggravate an already distraught patient or family member.

ED patients in poor mental health or those with substance-abuse problems may instigate violence in the ED. This threat has grown with the shift toward privatization and deinstitutionalization; the ED has seen an increase in visits from psychiatric patients (Flannery et al., 2000). High crime rates in larger urban communities can also translate into violent incidents in the ED; gang-related incidents are becoming more common, and weapons are increasingly being confiscated from patients and visitors upon entry into the ED (Ordog et al., 1995).

Safety measures to protect ED providers vary in cost and utilization. Many busy EDs are staffed with armed security personnel specially trained to handle disruptive or violent patients. Some EDs have metal detectors and controlled access to limit patients' ability to interfere with or threaten the care of others. Designated security phones or push buttons can provide direct links to local police departments. Additionally, assigning multiple staff members to violence-prone patients and ensuring two points of entry into an exam room can help protect providers.

Bloodborne and Airborne Pathogens

Health care delivery by nature poses unique threats to both patients and providers. Movement from one sick patient to another with the constant uncertainty of medical history or the presence of infectious disease makes the ED susceptible to a host of biological hazards, including bloodborne pathogens. Up to 800,000 injuries through the skin may occur annually in the United States, and these injuries account for approximately 82 percent of exposures to blood or other body fluids among health care workers (National Institute for Occupational Safety and Health, 2004). Although exposure to these occupational hazards and the prevalence of occupational injuries have increased for health care workers, the steady decline in rates of provider infection speaks to the value of nationwide protective measures. Over a 17-year period, the adoption of recommended universal precautions and the Occupational Safety and Health Administration's (OSHA) Bloodborne Pathogens Standard helped decrease the number of hepatitis B viral infections among health care workers from nearly 11,000 in 1983 to fewer than 400 in 1999 (CDC National Center for Infectious Disease, 2002). Yet while there is growing concern about the risk of exposure to airborne pathogens, including multidrug-resistant tuberculosis, severe acute respiratory syndrome (SARS), and emerging strains of influenza, most EDs have few negative pressure rooms to isolate staff and other patients from respiratory pathogens (Augustine et al., 2004).

The SARS outbreak in Toronto was triggered in part by a patient who sought care in a Toronto ED for fever and a cough. He stayed overnight in a crowded ED awaiting admission for what was thought at the time to be community-acquired pneumonia. Over the course of the night, he infected 2 nearby patients and several hospital staff members with SARS. Both this index case and the 2 patients he infected subsequently died from the disease, and a total of 31 patients and staff fell ill. Ironically, the same hospital where this incident occurred continues to board admitted patients in its ED (Cass, 2005).

Physical Stress

Nurses have the highest prevalence of back pain among health care workers and the highest incidence of workers' compensation claims for back injuries (Edlich et al., 2001). Estimates show that 12 percent of nurses leave the profession annually because of back injuries, and more than 52 percent report chronic back pain (Robinson et al., 2004). General back pain is often considered an inevitable consequence of nursing practice. Nurses spend much of their time standing. Additionally, they often work in physically awkward positions since they must maneuver around patient equipment; work in space that is often limited; and handle patients with unique sizes, shapes, or deformities. ED nurses also must lift heavy patients or equipment. National Institute for Occupational Safety and Health (NIOSH) guidelines state that the average provider must not lift more than 45 pounds; this translates to a need for more than three providers to be present when lifting the average patient (Edlich et al., 2001). However, time pressures and lack of sufficient resources may force a provider to administer care without adequate support. Specialized patient lifting techniques and machines can help prevent the common back injuries that many nurses experience. Several EDs have acquired lifting machinery to protect providers from injury and/or instituted guidelines for providers to assist each other in executing physically demanding or straining tasks.

It is imperative that EDs be as safe an environment as possible for emergency providers to deliver the highest level of care to patients. In fact, patient safety is positively impacted when a comfortable, supportive, and safe work setting is fostered.

INCREASING INTERPROFESSIONAL COLLABORATION

The concept of interprofessional collaboration gained strength in the late 1990s as attention to medical errors grew. Health services researchers and others interested in improving patient safety were energized by successes in the aviation industry, where teamwork training for the private and government aviation workforce led to reductions in errors and improved performance (Sprague, 1999). Research in the aviation industry indicated that effective teamwork does not arise spontaneously, but must be developed and practiced (Risser et al., 1999). The similarities between pilots and doctors—highly trained technically, accustomed to viewing themselves as bearers of ultimate authority and responsibility, independent yet increasingly dependent on others of varying skill levels—suggest that teamwork training may be influential in reducing errors in the medical field (Sprague, 1999).

Several organizations, including the IOM and the Institute for Healthcare Improvement (IHI), have embraced the concept of teamwork training for health professionals. In 2000, the IOM report *To Err Is Human: Building a Safer Health System* recommended that health care organizations establish team training programs for personnel in critical areas, including the ED (IOM, 2000). These recommendations are beginning to take hold. A November 2004 survey of members of ECRI's (formerly the Emergency Care Research Institute) Healthcare Risk Control System indicated that one-third of respondents provided teamwork training to employees, and nearly half that did not said they planned to do so in the next year (ECRI, 2005).

Teamwork training has considerable potential for improving the quality of care in EDs for several reasons. First, the ED parallels the environment in the aviation industry in many ways; high-stress, time pressure, and uncertainty abound in both (Small et al., 1999). Second, ED staff tend to have little or no formal training in teamwork skills, yet the delivery of emergency care requires rapid decision making and effective coordination of groups of caregivers, often from multiple disciplines, with vastly different training, professional missions, cultural identities, and feelings of empowerment. This unique environment joins together in real-time interaction such diverse providers as nurses, pharmacists, social workers, neurosurgeons, psychologists, and patients' attending physicians from the community. Patient outcomes can be undermined if caregivers do not work well together and coordinate their services appropriately (Risser et al., 1999). Third, teamwork failures in the ED are not uncommon. A review of closed malpractice claims from several EDs found that 43 percent of errors were due to problems with team coordination, and 79 percent of those errors could have been mitigated or prevented if there had been an effective team structure in the ED and ED personnel had received team behavior training. The researchers also concluded that better teamwork would have saved $3.50 per ED patient visit in legal costs (Risser et al., 1999; Shapiro et al., 2004). White and colleagues (2004) noted that communication issues were associated with 30 percent of the ED risk management files they studied and appeared to contribute directly to adverse medical outcomes in 20 percent of those cases.

Research on the impact of teamwork training in the ED is thin but promising. MedTeams, a Department of Defense project that introduced teamwork training to health care, developed an Emergency Team Coordination course—an 8-hour didactic course for physicians, nurses, technicians, and support personnel. An evaluation of the course revealed considerable success. EDs using it experienced a 67 percent increase in error-averting behavior and a 58 percent reduction in observable errors (Risser et al., 1999;

Shapiro et al., 2004). The research team also identified behaviors associated with teamwork failures, including failure to identify an established protocol for patient care and failure to cross-monitor the actions of other team members. They found as well that in most of the adverse events studied, some team member had a piece of information, observed an action, possessed a skill, or had a doubt or suspicion that, if acted upon, could have prevented or mitigated the error (Wears and Simon, 2000).

Key to teamwork training for ED providers is the use of simulations and promotion of interprofessional collaboration. Simulation training involves giving ED providers practice in performing tasks in lifelike circumstances using models or virtual reality, and includes feedback from observers, other team members, and video cameras to assist in the improvement of skills. Human simulators can give clinicians experience in dealing with high-risk, low-frequency events. For example, a pregnant human patient simulator can be used to train clinicians for emergency cesarean-section procedures. These simulators allow providers to learn from mistakes without harming an actual patient (ECRI, 2005). Moreover, the stress experienced by trainees when using a high-fidelity patient simulation model reproduces realistic patient encounters and reflects the difficulty associated with performing under stress (Vozenilek et al., 2004). The IOM report *To Err Is Human: Building a Safer Health System* recommended use of simulation training as a strategy to prevent medical errors (IOM, 2000).

Again, evidence of the effectiveness of simulation-based training is thin, but initial research indicates it has benefits. In one study, ED staff including nurses, physicians, emergency medicine residents, and technicians were randomly assigned to receive 8 hours of intensive training with a simulator in which three scenarios of increasing difficulty were presented following a didactic training session. Unlike a control group that received only the didactic training, the group that experienced the simulation training displayed an improvement in the quality of team behavior. Those who underwent the simulation training believed it was a useful educational method (Shapiro et al., 2004).

The use of simulation training is becoming more common. An example is the Advanced Cardiac Life Support course for third-year medical students at Brown University, which involves assigning students to multidisciplinary teams with nurses and technicians. The teams receive teamwork training while learning advanced cardiac life support using a high-fidelity simulation mannequin (Morchi, 2002). At Regions Hospital, emergency medicine residents spend 30 to 40 hours per year at a simulation center where, among other things, residents learn teamwork skills and develop their ED team leadership skills in realistically complex, challenging, and stressful emergency situations. The sessions are taped, and faculty and residents review and discuss the residents' performance (Patow, 2005).

Interprofessional collaboration is also a critical consideration in teamwork training, particularly in EDs where individuals from various medical disciplines must work together effectively (see Box 6-2). Differences in views often exist among health care professionals that can act as barriers to team performance (IOM, 2004a). Interprofessional collaboration in the ED may not develop naturally because of the high-pressure, high-stress environment, coupled with the strong personalities and egos of providers.

Interprofessional collaboration refers to an aggregation of attributes that include a shared understanding of goals and roles, effective communication, shared decision making, and conflict management. Evidence supports the effectiveness of interprofessional collaboration as a means of improving patient outcomes. There are several ways in which hospital leadership can nurture interprofessional collaboration through changes in organizational structure and processes. These strategies were endorsed by the IOM in the report *Keeping Patients Safe: Transforming the Work Environment of Nurses* (IOM, 2004a).

Most important in the present context is the need to enhance partnerships among the diverse professionals that function within the ED to solve the problems of crowding, diversion, communication, and coordination so as to provide better patient care. This collaboration goes beyond transforming the patient care work environment, but must take place in parallel with such changes. For example, the operations management solutions to crowding discussed in Chapter 4 cannot work without buy-in and collabo-

---

BOX 6-2
Example of Effective Collaboration in the ED

During an extremely busy shift in an ED whose entire staff had recently been trained in teamwork and collaboration, an emergency physician had just come from a resuscitation and was seeing a patient with an acute but non-life-threatening condition. During the history and physical exam, the patient told the physician twice about his severe allergy to a particular medication. The physician noted the allergy, and as he left the patient's room was pulled into another resuscitation. During a momentary break, the physician wrote orders on the patient's chart prescribing the medication to which he was allergic. An experienced nurse caught the mistake and showed no hesitation in bringing it to the physician's attention in a professional manner. Somewhat angry at himself for making the error, the physician was nonetheless very appreciative that the error had been caught and that the nurse had felt empowered to bring it to his attention.

ration among emergency physicians, admitting surgeons, and other critical specialists that make it possible to attempt changes in the status quo—in this case, changing long-established admitting and operating room (OR) blocking patterns. Likewise, unless emergency and trauma surgeons collaborate with on-call specialties, it will be difficult to fashion solutions to the on-call problems that plague hospitals and contribute substantially to crowding and boarding of patients.

Hospital leadership should model collaborative behaviors as a way to persuade other ED staff to adopt the same behaviors. Moreover, hospital leadership should support the ongoing acquisition and maintenance of staff members' clinical knowledge and skills. Research indicates that individual clinical competence is an essential precursor to collaborative practice. ED work and workspaces should be designed to facilitate collaboration. Workspaces should encourage physical proximity among ED personnel who work together, and staffing patterns should ensure that personnel have the time to participate in collaborative activities. Hospital leadership should encourage mechanisms for interprofessional practice. Structured interprofessional forums, such as patient rounds or regularly scheduled interprofessional meetings, are effective in improving patient care. Sharing of patient records and documents also promotes interprofessional collaboration.

Finally, human resource policies should be designed to support collaboration. Hostile behaviors, such as verbal abuse, should be identified and addressed. Managers should set practice expectations for staff, endorsing cooperation and communication with others while displaying regard for their dignity; shouting, foul language, and rudeness must be restricted. Performance evaluations might include measures of the extent to which staff are viewed as collaborators by staff from other disciplines.

ADDRESSING THE SHORTAGE OF
RURAL EMERGENCY CARE PROVIDERS

The workforce in rural EDs has mirrored many of the challenges of overall recruitment and retention of health care providers in rural areas. A recent IOM study, *Quality Through Collaboration: The Future of Rural Health*, described the special problems of rural health care and the unique challenges of providing high-quality medical services in rural areas, particularly core health services such as emergency care. The report highlighted the urgent shortages of medical personnel in rural areas, the critical need to address these shortages, and the complex challenges associated with strengthening the rural workforce (IOM, 2004b). Although 21 percent of Americans live in rural areas, only slightly more than 12 percent of emergency physicians, regardless of training or certification status, practice in these settings (Moorhead et al., 2002). Thus a pattern of population-based maldistribution exists, and in fact has worsened since 1997, when 15 percent of emergency physicians practiced in rural areas (Moorhead et al., 1998; Williams et al., 2001). This change may reflect the rapid growth in urban areas with rising numbers of emergency medicine residency training programs rather than a sharp decline in rural communities. Nevertheless, this maldistribution is a problem that must be addressed.

The specialty of emergency medicine has focused on strategies for increasing the number of emergency medicine specialists in rural areas, but workforce issues in rural EDs may never be resolved by such efforts alone. The difficulties of recruitment and retention in rural EDs are due to a variety of causes, but are generally assignable to either work-related factors or personal and community characteristics (Pan et al., 1996). There exists a strong correlation between where a physician is raised and the community in which he or she later chooses to practice (Williams et al., 2001). Additionally, the location of residency training is a major factor in the choice of practice location for emergency medicine residency graduates regardless of previous geographic ties (Steele et al., 1998). Rural hospitals that have residency training programs are more successful in recruiting and retaining physicians when they complete their residency (Connor et al., 1994; Cutchin, 1997). The fact that the majority of emergency medicine residency programs are located in urban areas suggests that residency graduates will likely continue to choose to practice in those areas. Graduates also are faced with lower levels of compensation in rural than in urban areas (Bullock et al., 1999). The high debt burden of many emergency medicine residents, coupled with the limited opportunity to earn sufficient income to pay off educational debt in rural settings, is a significant barrier to rural practice. Increased workload in rural areas is another barrier: rural emergency medicine physicians spend 35 percent more time in on-call backup relative to the average for all emergency physicians (Moorhead et al., 2002). Given the fewer resources and consultants typical of rural settings (Sklar et al., 2002), the lack of physicians trained in emergency medicine in these settings is not surprising.

One strategy for increasing the emergency care workforce in rural areas would be to increase the number of emergency medicine residency programs in these areas. However, ACGME program requirements enforced by the Residency Review Committee (RRC) make it virtually impossible to gain certification for a "rural" residency program unless it is situated in a large referral hospital. The RRC is equally reluctant to recognize satellite sites at rural hospitals if they are geographically remote from the program's base hospital, regardless of distance. Changes in such ACGME requirements might increase rural emergency medicine training during residency and ultimately benefit the rural emergency medicine workforce and the quality of care provided in rural settings. Another approach would be to develop programs that would cover the costs of medical education in return for future assignment to a rural area, based on the National Health Service Corps or Public Health Service Commissioned Corps model but specifically targeting emergency medicine.

To compensate for manpower shortages, rural EDs have resorted to alternative methods and providers in an effort to maintain minimum levels of staffing. This strategy is evident if one examines the physician characteristics in rural EDs. In one survey of random hospitals across the United States, rural EDs, comprising 25 percent of all EDs, reported an average of 4.74 physicians per institution, 40 percent fewer than the average for all locales (Moorhead et al., 2002). Numbers of FTEs, defined as those working 40 clinical hours per week, were also significantly lower in rural EDs; there were 3.42 FTEs per rural ED—35 percent fewer than average. Rural EDs were noted to have the highest percentage of osteopathic physicians (14 percent) and non-U.S.-trained physicians (14 percent). It is significant that 67 percent of rural emergency medicine physicians are neither residency trained nor board certified in emergency medicine. Of the 33 percent of physicians with emergency medicine credentials, fewer than half are both emergency medicine residency trained and board certified. Only 12 percent of rural respondents in the survey reported requiring any emergency medicine credentials for ED hiring. In summary, rural EDs have lower levels of staffing, and when they are staffed by physicians, these physicians are much less likely to be emergency medicine specialists and more likely to be trained in family practice or other primary care specialties.

Although ideally all EDs would be staffed by residency-trained, board-certified emergency physicians, this is highly unlikely to occur in the near to mid term, if ever. Therefore, alternative staffing models must be developed. Clinicians other than physicians—such as PAs, NPs, CNMs, and CNSs—are often used in the staffing of rural EDs (Moorhead et al., 2002). With national efforts to lower costs and the demonstrated success of using nonphysician clinicians in certain prescribed roles, their use in the staffing of rural EDs may increase (Blunt, 1998). At the same time, it should be noted that rural EDs experience problems with recruitment and retention of all clinicians, not just physicians, and for similar reasons (Bullock et al., 1999).

Rural ED providers exhibit wide variability in their skill levels and the competence with which they provide emergency care. Care often falls short of established guidelines. In a study of acute stroke care in nonurban EDs, patients were found to have been treated in ways discordant with AHA recommendations. Hypertension was often treated too aggressively, and inappropriate medications were sometimes used. Additionally, it was suggested that nonmotor symptoms of stroke were less likely to be recognized or were treated with less urgency than motor symptoms of stroke (Burgin et al., 2001). Although these data are far from conclusive, results of such studies may explain in part the stigma of decreased competence attributed to rural emergency physicians (Leap, 2000). Yet the reality is that rural emergency physicians are often called upon to care single-handedly for critically ill and injured patients in a challenging setting typically lacking in manpower, equipment, and access to consultants. The deficit of rural health care providers has complicated the roles these providers must fill. It is typical for rural primary care physicians' practices to entail management of patients in EDs, outpatient clinics, inpatient wards, and ICUs, as well as additional duties related to health care administration. Additionally, the low patient census in a rural ED may contribute to the difficulty experienced by physicians and midlevel providers in maintaining a high level of proficiency in emergency medicine.

Furthermore, certain specialists who provide on-call emergency and trauma services are even scarcer in rural areas. Substantial near-term increases in the capacity to provide advanced emergency and trauma care in rural settings are unlikely. This situation makes effective regional solutions to the transport of patients to definitive emergency and trauma care essential. But effective transport requires effective stabilization, critical care management, and in some cases surgical intervention. The proposed subspecialty in emergency surgery described earlier in this chapter has particular applicability to rural settings, where there are unlikely to be other specialists with the skills to adequately address certain serious emergencies.

All patients, regardless of setting, deserve prompt access to high-quality emergency care. Initiatives to improve the quality of emergency care in rural areas have recognized the need to develop strategies for enhancing the knowledge and training and expanding the size of the rural emergency care workforce. Given current workforce shortages in emergency care and economic conditions in the health system, rural EDs are unlikely to have residency-trained, board-certified emergency physicians on a round-the-clock basis. Approaches recommended to address this situation include increased collaboration between emergency medicine and primary care specialties (such as family practice physicians who provide emergency medical care in rural areas) and increased links between academic medical centers and rural hospitals (Williams et al., 2001). Emergency physicians and family practitioners in Minnesota, for example, have developed a course for training teams of health care providers in comprehensive advanced life support that can serve as a model for collaborative training in rural emergency medicine (Carter et al., 2001).

The committee supports these efforts, and recommends that **states link rural hospitals with academic health centers to enhance opportunities for professional consultation, telemedicine, patient referral and transport, and continuing professional education (6.6).**

SUMMARY OF RECOMMENDATIONS

6.1: Hospitals, physician organizations, and public health agencies should collaborate to regionalize critical specialty care on-call services.

6.2: Congress should appoint a commission to examine the impact of medical malpractice lawsuits on the declining availability of providers in high-risk emergency and trauma care specialties, and to recommend appropriate state and federal actions to mitigate the adverse impact of these lawsuits and ensure quality of care.

6.3: The American Board of Medical Specialties and its constituent boards should extend eligibility for certification in critical care medicine to all acute care and primary care physicians who complete an accredited critical care fellowship program.

6.4: The Department of Health and Human Services, the Department of Transportation, and the Department of Homeland Security should jointly undertake a detailed assessment of emergency and trauma workforce capacity, trends, and future needs, and develop strategies to meet these needs in the future.

6.5: The Department of Health and Human Services, in partnership with professional organizations, should develop national standards for core competencies applicable to physicians, nurses, and other key emergency and trauma professionals, using a national, evidence-based, multidisciplinary process.

6.6: States should link rural hospitals with academic health centers to enhance opportunities for professional consultation, telemedicine, patient referral and transport, and continuing professional education.

REFERENCES

AAPA (American Association of Physician Assistants). 2005. *2005 AAPA Physician Assistant Census Report*. [Online]. Available: http://www.aapa.org/research/05census-intro.html [accessed June 16, 2006].

ABPS (American Board of Physician Specialties). 2005. *Eligibility Requirements*. [Online]. Available: http://www.abpsga.org/certification/emergency/eligibility.html [accessed August 10, 2005].

ACEP (American College of Emergency Physicians). 2004. *Two-Thirds of Emergency Department Directors Report On-Call Specialty Coverage Problems*. [Online]. Available: http://www.acep.org/1,34081,0.html [accessed September 28, 2004].

ACEP. 2006. *The National Report Card on the State of Emergency Medicine: Evaluating the Environment of Emergency Care Systems State by State.* Dallas, TX: ACEP.

ACEP Research Committee. 2005. *Report on Emergency Medicine Research.* Washington, DC: ACEP.

Aiken LH, Clarke SP, Sloane DM. 2002. Hospital staffing, organization, and quality of care: Cross-national findings. *International Journal for Quality in Health Care* 14(1):5–13.

All Nursing Schools. 2005. *Entry Level Nursing Programs.* [Online]. Available: http://www.allnursingschools.com/faqs/programs.php [accessed February 15, 2005].

Allied Health Schools. 2005. *Become a Physician Assistant (PA): Physician Assistant Training and Careers.* [Online]. Available: http://www.allalliedhealthschools.com/faqs/physician_assistant.php [accessed August 9, 2005].

AMA (American Medical Association). 2003. *Physician Socioeconomic Statistics.* Chicago, IL: AMA.

AMA. 2004. *Physician Characteristics and Distribution in the U.S.: 2004 Edition.* Chicago, IL: AMA.

Augustine J, Kellermann A, Koplan J. 2004. America's emergency care system and severe acute respiratory syndrome: Are we ready? *Annals of Emergency Medicine* 43(1):23–26.

Bates DW, Boyle DL, Vander Vliet MB, Schneider J, Leape L. 1995. Relationship between medication errors and adverse drug events. *Journal of General Internal Medicine* 10(4):199–205.

Berenson RA, Kuo S, May JH. 2003. Medical malpractice liability crisis meets markets: Stress in unexpected places. *Issue Brief (Center for Studying Health System Change)* (68):1–7.

Blunt E. 1998. Role and productivity of nurse practitioners in one urban emergency department. *Journal of Emergency Nursing* 24(3):234–239.

Branney SW, Pons PT, Markovchick VJ, Thomasson GO. 2000. Malpractice occurrence in emergency medicine: Does residency training make a difference? *The Journal of Emergency Medicine* 19(2):99–105.

Brewster LR, Felland LE. 2004. Emergency department diversions: Hospital and community strategies alleviate the crisis. *Issue Brief (Center for Studying Health System Change)* (78):1–4.

Bullock K, Rodney WM, Gerard T, Hahn R. 1999. Advanced practice family physicians as the foundation for rural emergency medicine services (part I). *Texas Journal of Rural Health* 17(1):19–29.

Burgin WS, Staub L, Chan W, Wein TH, Felberg RA, Grotta JC, Demchuk AM, Hickenbottom SL, Morgenstern LB. 2001. Acute stroke care in non-urban emergency departments. *Neurology* 57(11):2006–2012.

Byrne RW, Bagan B. 2004. Academic center ERs bear brunt of Chicago-area transfers. *American Association of Neurological Surgeons Bulletin* 13(4):14–15.

California Healthcare Association. 2003. *On-Call Physician ED Backup Survey.* Sacramento, CA: California Healthcare Association.

Carter DL, Ruiz E, Lappe K. 2001. Comprehensive advanced life support. A course for rural emergency care teams. *Minnesota Medicine* 84(11):38–41.

Cass D. 2005. Once upon a time in the emergency department: A cautionary tale. *Annals of Emergency Medicine* 46(6):541–543.

CDC (Centers for Disease Control and Prevention) National Center for Infectious Disease. 2002. *National Notifiable Diseases Surveillance System (NNDSS).* Unpublished.

Center for Health Workforce Studies. 2000. *2000 Survey of Nurse Practitioners Licensed in New York State.* Rensselaer, NY: Center for Health Workforce Studies, School of Public Health, SUNY Albany.

Chapman D, Hayden S, Sanders A, Binder L, Chinnis A, Corrigan K, LaDuca T, Dyne P, Perina D, Smith-Coggins R, Sulton L, Swing S. 2004. Integrating the accreditation council for graduate medical education core competencies into the model of the clinical practice of emergency medicine. *Annals of Emergency Medicine* 43(6):756–769.

Church A. 2003. Critical care and emergency medicine. *Critical Care Clinician* 19(2): 271–278.

Cole FL, Ramirez E, Luna-Gonzales H. 1999. *Scope of Practice for the Nurse Practitioner in the Emergency Setting*. Des Plaines, IL: Emergency Nurses Association.

Cole FL, Kuensting LL, Maclean S, Abel C, Mickanin J, Bruske P, Wilson ME, Rehwaldt M. 2002. Advance practice nurses in emergency care settings: A demographic profile. *Journal of Emergency Nursing* 28(5):414–419.

Committee on Trauma, ACS (American College of Surgeons). 1998. *Resources for Optimal Care of the Injured Patient: 1999*. Chicago, IL: ACS.

The Committee to Develop the Reorganized Specialty of Trauma, Surgical Critical Care and Emergency Surgery. 2005. Acute care surgery: Trauma, critical care, and emergency surgery. *The Journal of Trauma* 58(3):614–616.

Connor RA, Hillson SD, Kralewski JE. 1994. Association between rural hospitals' residencies and recruitment and retention of physicians. *Academic Medicine* 69(6):483–488.

Couldwell WT, Gottfried ON, Weiss MH, Popp AJ. 2003. Too many? Too few. New study reveals current trends in U.S. neurosurgical workforce. *AANS Bulletin* 7–9.

Croskerry P, Shapiro M, Campbell S, LeBlanc C, Sinclair D, Wren P, Marcoux M. 2004. Profiles in patient safety: Medication errors in the emergency department. *Academic Emergency Medicine* 11(3):289–299.

Cutchin MP. 1997. Community and self: Concepts for rural physician integration and retention. *Social Science & Medicine* 44(11):1661–1674.

Danzl D, Munger B. 2000. *History of Academic Emergency Medicine. Emergency Medicine: An Academic Career Guide* (2nd edition). Lansing, MI: Society for Academic Emergency Medicine and Emergency Medicine Residents Association.

DHHS (U.S. Department of Health and Human Services). 2000. *National Sample Survey of Registered Nurses*. Rockville, MD: Health Resources and Services Administration, Bureau of Health Professions, National Center for Health Workforce Analysis.

DHHS. 2002. *Projected Supply, Demand, and Shortages of Registered Nurses, 2000–2020*. Rockville, MD: Health Resources and Services Administration, Bureau of Health Professions, National Center for Health Workforce Analysis.

Dresnick S. 1997. The future of the private practice of emergency medicine. *Annals of Emergency Medicine* 30(6):754–756.

ECRI. 2005, March 25. Teamwork takes hold to improve patient safety. *The Risk Management Reporter*.

Edlich RF, Woodard CR, Haines MJ. 2001. Disabling back injuries in nursing personnel. *Journal of Emergency Nursing* 27(2):150–155.

ENA (Emergency Nurses Association). 2005a. *ENA History*. [Online]. Available: http://www.ena.org/about/history/ [accessed February 9, 2005].

ENA. 2005b. *History of the Certification Examination for Emergency Nurses*. [Online]. Available: http://www.ena.org/bcen/about/History.asp [accessed February 9, 2005].

Encinosa WE, Hellinger FJ. 2005. Have state caps on malpractice awards increased the supply of physicians? *Health Affairs (Millwood, VA) Suppl. Web Exclusives* W5-250–W5-258.

Erickson L, Williams-Evans SA. 2000. Attitudes of emergency nurses regarding patient assaults. *Journal of Emergency Nursing* 26(3):210–215.

Flannery RB Jr, Fisher W, Walker A, Kolodziej K, Spillane MJ. 2000. Assaults on staff by psychiatric patients in community residences. *Psychiatric Services* 51(1):111–113.

Friedman L, Vilke GM, Chan TC, Hayden SR, Guss DA, Krishel SJ, Rosen P. 1999. Emergency department airway management before and after an emergency medicine residency. *Journal of Emergency Medicine* 17(3):427–431.

GAO (U.S. Government Accountability Office). 2003a. *Hospital Emergency Departments: Crowded Conditions Vary among Hospitals and Communities* (GAO-03-460). Washington, DC: GAO.

GAO. 2003b. *Medical Malpractice: Implications of Rising Premiums on Access to Health Care* (GAO-03-836). Washington, DC: GAO.

Glabman M. 2005. Specialist shortage shakes emergency rooms; more hospitals forced to pay for specialist care. *The Physician Executive* 6–11.

Goldberg RM, Mabee J, Chan L, Wong S. 1996. Drug-drug and drug-disease interactions in the ED: Analysis of a high-risk population. *American Journal of Emergency Medicine* 14(5):447–450.

Greater New York Hospital Association. 2004. *Survey of Nurse Staffing in GNYHA Member Hospitals, 2003.* New York: Greater New York Hospital Association.

Green L, Melnick GA, Nawathe A. 2005. *On-Call Physicians at California Emergency Departments: Problems and Potential Solutions.* Oakland, CA: California Healthcare Foundation.

Hackenschmidt A. 2004. Living with nurse staffing ratios: Early experiences. *Journal of Emergency Nursing* 30(4):377–379.

Hellinger FJ, Encinosa WE. 2005. *Impact of State Laws Limiting Malpractice Awards on Geographic Distribution of Physicians.* Rockville, MD: Department of Health and Human Services, Agency for Healthcare Research and Quality.

Hockberger RS, Binder LS, Graber MA, Hoffman GL, Perina DG, Schneider SM, Sklar DP, Strauss RW, Viravec DR, Koenig WJ, Augustine JJ, Burdick WP, Henderson WV, Lawrence LL, Levy DB, McCall J, Parnell MA, Shoji KT, American College of Emergency Physicians Core Content Task Force II. 2001. The model of the clinical practice of emergency medicine. *Annals of Emergency Medicine* 37(6):745–770.

Holliman CJ, Wuerz RC, Chapman DM, Hirshberg AJ. 1997. Workforce projections for emergency medicine: How many emergency physicians does the United States need? *Academic Emergency Medicine* 4(7):725–730.

Hurley RE, Pham HH, Claxton G. 2005. A widening rift in access and quality: Growing evidence of economic disparities. *Health Affairs* Web Exclusive.

IOM (Institute of Medicine). 2000. *To Err Is Human: Building a Safer Health System.* Washington, DC: National Academy Press.

IOM. 2004a. *Keeping Patients Safe: Transforming the Work Environment of Nurses.* Washington, DC: The National Academies Press.

IOM. 2004b. *Quality Through Collaboration: The Future of Rural Health.* Washington, DC: The National Academies Press.

Jacobsen C, Holson D, Farley J, Charles J, Suel P. 2002. Surviving the perfect storm: Staff perceptions of mandatory overtime. *JONA's Healthcare Law, Ethics and Regulation* 4(3):57–66.

JCAHO (Joint Commission for the Accreditation of Healthcare Organizations). 2005. *2005 Hospitals' National Patient Safety Goals.* [Online]. Available: http://www.jcaho.org/accredited+organizations/patient+safety/05+npsg/05_npsg_hap.htm [accessed August 9, 2005].

Jones JH, Weaver CS, Rusyniak DE, Brizendine EJ, McGrath RB. 2002. Impact of emergency medicine faculty and an airway protocol on airway management. *Academic Emergency Medicine* 9(12):1452–1456.

Kaiser Commission on Medicaid and the Uninsured. 2003. *Medicaid Benefits.* [Online]. Available: http://www.kff.org/medicaid/benefits/index.cfm [accessed August 20, 2004].

Kane CK. 2003. *Physician Marketplace Report: The Impact of EMTALA on Physician Practices*. Chicago, IL: American Medical Association, Center for Health Policy Research.

Kaushal R, Bates DW, Landrigan C, McKenna KJ, Clapp MD, Federico F, Goldmann DA. 2001. Medication errors and adverse drug events in pediatric inpatients. *Journal of the American Medical Association* 285(16):2114–2120.

Kaushal R, Bates D. 2001. The clinical pharmacist's role in preventing adverse drug events. In: *Making Health Care Safer: A Critical Analysis of Patient Safety Practices* (Evidence Report/Technology Assessment, No. 43). Rockville, MD: Agency for Healthcare Research and Quality.

Keim S, Chisholm C. 2000. Moonlighting and emergency medicine: Raising the standard. *Academic Emergency Medicine* 7(8):927–928.

Kellermann AL. 1995. Moonlighting. *Annals of Emergency Medicine* 26(1):83–84.

Lambert VA, Lambert CE. 2001. Literature review of role stress/strain on nurses: An international perspective. *Nursing & Health Sciences* 3(3):161–172.

Leap E. 2000. The stigma of being a rural EP. *EM News*. P. 12.

Leape L, Cullen D, Dempsey Clapp M, Burdick E, Demonaco H, Ives Errickson J, Bates D. 1999. Pharmacist participation on physician rounds and adverse drug events in the intensive care unit. *Journal of the American Medical Association* 281(3):267–270.

The Leapfrog Group. 2004. *ICU Physician Staffing Factsheet*. Washington, DC: The Leapfrog Group.

Li J, Tabor R, Martinez M. 2000. Survey of moonlighting practices and work requirements of emergency medicine residents. *American Journal of Emergency Medicine* 18(2):147–151.

Macasaet A, Zun A. 2005. *The On-Call Physician*. [Online]. Available: http://www.Emedicine.com [accessed February 10, 2006].

MacKenzie EJ, Rivara FP, Jurkovich GJ, Nathens AB, Frey KP, Egleston BL, Salkever DS, Scharfstein DO. 2006. A national evaluation of the effect of trauma-center care on mortality. *New England Journal of Medicine* 354(4):366–378.

Maguire P. 2001, November. Wanted: Doctors willing to take ER call. *ACP-ASIM Observer*.

Marx J. 2005. *Education*. [Online]. Available: http://www.carolinas.org/education/meded/emergency/emergency_chairman.cfm [accessed February 8, 2005].

Matsa D. 2005. *Does Malpractice Liability Keep the Doctor Away? Evidence from Tort Reform Damage Caps*. Boston, MA: MIT.

Mays GP, Bodenheimer T, Felland LE, McKenzie KL, Regopoulos LE. 2005. *Uninsured Patients, Malpractice Insurance Woes Stress Miami Health Care Market*. Washington, DC: Center for Studying Health System Change.

McCaig LF, Burt CW. 2005. *National Hospital Ambulatory Medical Care Survey: 2003 Emergency Department Summary*. Hyattsville, MD: National Center for Health Statistics.

McNamara R. 2006. *Emergency Medicine and the Physician Practice Management Industry: History, Overview, and Current Problems*. [Online]. Available: http://www.aaem.org/corporatepractice/history.shtml [accessed March 1, 2006].

Moorhead JC, Gallery ME, Mannle T, Chaney WC, Conrad LC, Dalsey WC, Herman S, Hockberger RS, McDonald SC, Packard DC, Rapp MT, Rorrie CC Jr, Schafermeyer RW, Schulman R, Whitehead DC, Hirschkorn C, Hogan P. 1998. A study of the workforce in emergency medicine. *Annals of Emergency Medicine* 31(5):595–607.

Moorhead JC, Gallery ME, Hirshkorn C, Barnaby DP, Barsan WG, Conrad LC, Dalsey WC, Fried M, Herman SH, Hogan P, Mannle TE, Packard DC, Perina DG, Pollack CV Jr, Rapp MT, Rorrie CC Jr, Schafermeyer RW. 2002. A study of the workforce in emergency medicine: 1999. *Annals of Emergency Medicine* 40(1):3–15.

Morchi R. 2002. High-fidelity medical simulation and teamwork training to enhance medical student performance in cardiac resuscitation [Abstract]. *Academic Emergency Medicine* 9(10):1055.

National Institute for Occupational Safety and Health. 2004. *Worker Health Chartbook, 2004*. Cincinnati, OH: Department of Health and Human Services.

National League for Nursing. 2005. *Despite Encouraging Trends Suggested by the NLN's Comprehensive Survey of All Nursing Programs, Large Number of Qualified Applications Continue to be Turned Down*. [Online]. Available: http://www.nln.org/newsreleases/nedsdec05.pdf [accessed February 17, 2006].

Needleman J, Buerhaus P, Mattke S, Stewart M, Zelevinsky K. 2002. Nurse-staffing levels and the quality of care in hospitals. *New England Journal of Nursing* 346(22):1715–1722.

New York State Education Department. 2003. *Registered Nurses in New York State, 2002, Survey Data*. Albany, NY: NY State Education Department.

NHT (Nurses for a Healthier Tomorrow). 2006. *Emergency Nurse*. [Online]. Available: http://www.nursesource.org/emergency.html [accessed February 1, 2006].

NREMT (National Registry of EMTs). 2005. *National EMS Practice Analysis*. Columbus, OH: NREMT.

O'Malley AS, Gerland AM, Pham HH, Berenson RA. 2005. *Rising Pressure: Hospital Emergency Departments: Barometers of the Health Care System*. Washington, DC: The Center for Studying Health System Change.

Ordog GJ, Wasserberger J, Ordog C, Ackroyd G, Atluri S. 1995. Weapon carriage among major trauma victims in the emergency department. *Academic Emergency Medicine* 2(2):109–113; discussion 114.

Osborn TM, Scalea TM. 2002. A call for critical care training of emergency physicians. *Annals of Emergency Medicine* 39(5):562–563.

Pan S, Geller JM, Muus KJ, Hart LG. 1996. Predicting the degree of rurality of physician assistant practice location. *Hospital & Health Services Administration* 41(1):105–119.

Patow CA. 2005, March/April. Advancing medical education and patient safety through simulation learning. *Patient Safety & Quality Healthcare*.

Perception Solutions, Inc. 2004. *AANS-CNS Neurological Survey—Emergency and Trauma Services: Analysis & Result Reporting*. Aurora, IL: Perception Solutions, Inc.

Pham HH, Devers KJ, Kuo S, Berenson R. 2005. Health care market trends and the evolution of hospitalist use and roles. *Journal of General Internal Medicine* 20(2):101–107.

Plantz SH, Kreplick LW, Panacek EA, Mehta T, Adler J, McNamara RM. 1998. A national survey of board-certified emergency physicians: Quality of care and practice structure issues. *American Journal of Emergency Nursing* 16(1):1–4.

Pronovost P, Wu AW, Dorman T, Morlock L. 2002. Building safety into ICU care. *Journal of Critical Care* 17(2):78–85.

Pronovost PJ, Jenckes MW, Dorman T, Garrett E, Breslow MJ, Rosenfeld BA, Lipsett PA, Bass E. 1999. Organizational characteristics of intensive care units related to outcomes of abdominal aortic surgery. *Journal of the American Medical Association* 281(14):1310–1317.

Ray C, Jagim M, Agnew J, McKay J, Sheehy S. 2003. ENA's new guidelines for determining emergency department nurse staffing. *Journal of Emergency Nursing* 29(3):245–253.

Risser DT, Rice MM, Salisbury ML, Simon R, Jay GD, Berns SD. 1999. The potential for improved teamwork to reduce medical errors in the emergency department. The MedTeams Research Consortium. *Annals of Emergency Medicine* 34(3):373–383.

Robinson KS, Jagim MM, Ray CE. 2004. *Nursing Workforce Issues and Trends Affecting U.S. Emergency Departments*. Falls Church, VA: KAR Associates.

Rogers AE, Hwang W-T, Scott LD, Aiken LH, Dinges DF. 2004. The working hours of hospital staff nurses and patient safety. *Health Affairs* 23(4):202–212.

Rosen P. 1995. *History of Emergency Medicine*. New York: Josiah Macy, Jr. Foundation. Pp. 59–79.

Russell T. 2004. Understanding the latest changes in EMTALA: Our country's emergency care safety net. *ACS Cross Country* (February). [Online]. Available: www.facs.org/ahp/feb04crosscountry.html 89 [accessed June 22, 2006].

Salsberg E. 2005. *Physician Workforce Issues and Trends: Implications for Surgical Specialties.* Presentation at the meeting of the ACS Meeting on Workforce Issues, Chicago, IL.

Scaletta T. 2003. *Performing without a Net.* [Online]. Available: http://www.aaem.org/commonsense/rules5.shtml [accessed January 26, 2005].

Scheck A. 2004. Payments to specialists are rescuing on-call panels. *Emergency Medicine News* 26(10):1, 28–29.

Schenkel S. 2000. Promoting patient safety and preventing medical error in emergency departments. *Academic Emergency Medicine* 7(11):1204–1222.

Schriver J, Talmadge R, Chuong R, Hedges J. 2003. Emergency nursing: Historical, current, and future roles. *Academic Emergency Medicine* 10(7):798–804.

Selbst SM, Fein JA, Osterhoudt K, Ho W. 1999. Medication errors in a pediatric emergency department. *Pediatric Emergency Care* 15(1):1–4.

Shapiro MJ, Morey JC, Small SD, Langford V, Kaylor CJ, Jagminas L, Suner S, Salisbury ML, Simon R, Jay GD. 2004. Simulation based teamwork training for emergency department staff: Does it improve clinical team performance when added to an existing didactic teamwork curriculum? *Quality and Safety in Healthcare* 13(6):417–421.

Sklar D, Spencer D, Alcock J, Cameron S, Saiz M. 2002. Demographic analysis and needs assessment of rural emergency departments in New Mexico (DANARED–NM). *Annals of Emergency Medicine* 39(4):456–457; author reply 457.

Small SD, Wuerz RC, Simon R, Shapiro N, Conn A, Setnik G. 1999. Demonstration of high-fidelity simulation team training for emergency medicine. *Academic Emergency Medicine* 6(4):312–323.

Society of Hospital Medicine. 2006. *FAQ's.* [Online]. Available: http://www.hospitalmedicine.org/AM/Template.cfm?Section=FAQs&Template=/FAQ/FAQListAll.cfm [accessed February 1, 2006].

Sprague L. 1999. *Reducing Medical Error: Can You Be As Safe in a Hospital As You Are in a Jet?* Washington, DC: National Health Policy Forum.

Steele MT, Schwab RA, McNamara RM, Watson WA. 1998. Emergency medicine resident choice of practice location. *Annals of Emergency Medicine* 31(3):351–357.

Taheri PA, Butz DA. 2004. *Specialist On-Call Coverage of Palm Beach County Emergency Departments.* Palm Beach County, FL: Palm Beach County Medical Society Services.

Thomasset KB, Faris R. 2003. Survey of pharmacy services provision in the emergency department. *American Journal of Health-System Pharmacy* 60(15):1561–1564.

Thorpe K. 2004. The medical malpractice "crisis": Recent trends and the impact of state tort reforms. *Health Affairs Web Exclusive* W4–20.

Valadka A. 2004. RE: The ER, who is answering call? *American Association of Neurological Surgeons* 13(4):6–12.

Vozenilek J, Huff JS, Reznek M, Gordon JA. 2004. See one, do one, teach one: Advanced technology in medical education. *Academic Emergency Medicine* 11(11):1149–1154.

Wachter R. 2004. The hospitalist movement: Ten issues to consider. *Hospital Practice* 2.

Wears RL, Simon R. 2000. Testimony of Robert L. Wears and Robert Simon. Panel 2: Broad-based Systems Approaches. Written Statement: Creating Complementary Roles for Behavioral Solutions and Technology Applications to Patient Safety. National Summit on Medical Errors and Patient Safety Research.

Weaver CS, Avery SJ, Brizendine EJ, McGrath RB. 2004. Impact of emergency medicine faculty on door to thrombolytic time. *The Journal of Emergency Medicine* 26(3):279–283.

Whaley S. 2002, July 10. Opinion offers hope for trauma center. *The Las Vegas Review Journal.* P. 18.

White AA, Wright SW, Blanco R, Lemonds B, Sisco J, Bledsoe S, Irwin C, Isenhour J, Pichert JW. 2004. Cause-and-effect analysis of risk management files to assess patient care in the emergency department. *Academic Emergency Medicine* 11(10):1035–1041.

Williams J, Ehrlich P, Prescott J. 2001. Emergency medical care in rural America. *Annals of Emergency Medicine* 38(3):323–327.

Yoo GJ, Dawson-Rose C, Chang YJ, Aquino J. 2001. *Factors Impacting the Availability of Emergency On-Call Coverage in California: Report to the California State University Faculty Fellows Program.* [Online]. Available: http://www.csus.edu/calst/Government_ Affairs/reports/Emergency_Room_On-Call_Coverage.pdf [accessed June 23, 2005].

7

Disaster Preparedness

The day before September 11, 2001, the cover story of *U.S. News and World Report* described an emergency care system in critical condition as a result of demand far in excess of its capacity (Shute and Marcus, 2001; see Figure 7-1). While the article focused on the day-to-day problems of diversion and boarding, the events of the following day brought home a frightening realization to many. If we cannot take care of our emergency patients on a normal day, how will we manage a large-scale disaster? Federal, state, and local government entities have since realized the importance of hospitals, particularly emergency departments (EDs), in planning for such events, and significant progress has been made on integrating inpatient resources into planning for disasters (Schur, 2004). More than 4 years after September 11, however, Hurricane Katrina revealed how far we have to go in this regard. While Katrina was unusual in its size and scope, the capacity of the emergency care system to respond effectively even to smaller disasters is still in question (GAO, 2003a).

Disaster response involves many different community resources—from police and fire to medical providers, structural and environmental engineers, and transportation and housing experts. The hospital plays a small but crucial role in this larger picture. It is the epicenter of medical care delivered to those who are injured. Running a hospital is an enormously complex task under the best of circumstances; preparing a hospital for a disaster is infinitely more complicated. Planning for disasters involves a range of difficult questions: For what types of disaster events should hospitals prepare? Should every hospital prepare for disasters, or should medical response be regionalized? When does "busy" rise to the level of disaster, who makes that

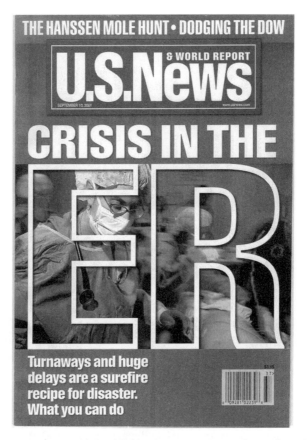

FIGURE 7-1 *U.S. News and World Report*, cover story on September 10, 2001.
SOURCE: Reprinted from Shute and Marcus, 2001, with permission.

decision, and how does a large, complex organization shift from routine to disaster mode? How does a hospital protect itself and its staff from chemical or biological agents when patients are contaminated?

This chapter examines these and other questions, and considers the current level of hospital disaster preparedness. It also explores the special problems associated with rural hospitals, and presents the committee's recommendations for enhancing hospital preparedness.

DEFINING DISASTER

The term "disaster" denotes a low-probability but high-impact event that causes a large number of individuals to become ill or injured. The International Federation of Red Cross and Red Crescent Societies defines a disaster as an event that causes more than 10 deaths, affects more than 100 people, or leads to an appeal for assistance by those affected (Bravata et al., 2004b). This report expands that definition in the context of hospital-based emergency and trauma care to include any event that creates a significant, short-term spike in the demand for emergency care services that requires extraordinary measures to address adequately.

Disasters can range from large multiple-vehicle crashes to massive events such as the North Ridge earthquake, Hurricane Katrina, and the terrorist attacks of September 11. Disasters can be natural, such as earthquakes, floods, and disease outbreaks; or they can be man-made, such as transportation incidents, terrorist bombings, and biological or chemical attacks. The federal government has grouped terrorist threats into five categories—chemical, biological, radiological, nuclear, and explosive (CBRNE)—which are also useful for classifying general threats (see Box 7-1).

Each type of threat presents different challenges to hospitals, which must able to respond to each in some capacity. Given finite resources, however, hospitals must attempt to focus their resources on the most likely and potentially serious scenarios. Bombings are the most common form of terrorist attack (Frykberg, 2004). They often result in the worst forms of both blunt and penetrating trauma in addition to burns, as shown by recent experience; examples include the train and subway attacks in Madrid (Gutierrez de Ceballos et al., 2004) and London, Oklahoma City bombing (Teague, 2004), and the Atlanta Centennial Olympics bombing (Feliciano et al., 1998). Worldwide, there were more than 500 terrorist bombings between 2001 and 2003, resulting in 4,600 deaths (U.S. Department of State, 2005a,b,c). Over the past 25 years, few acts of global terrorism have involved the use of chemical or biological agents. In contrast, explosives and/or firearms have been used to commit countless acts of terrorism in Israel, Egypt, Kenya, Argentina, Colombia, Bali, Yemen, Russia, the United Kingdom, Germany, France, Italy, and many other countries. The possibility of bioterrorism or a nuclear attack is also real, however, and the impact of such incidents on public health would be catastrophic.

To some degree, each region must prioritize its response preparedness according to the likelihood of the different types of events it could face. Thus New York City should probably spend more resources than Topeka, Kansas, on preparation for biological or nuclear attack; Topeka, on the other hand, should focus more of its preparedness efforts on tornados. The scope of various types of disasters is illustrated by selected recent events, which are summarized in Table 7-1.

The federal government has promoted the idea of preparing for "all hazards." But federal disaster planning has paid much more attention to biological and chemical threats than to explosive attacks by terrorists or,

BOX 7-1
Classification of Terrorist Threats

The federal government groups terrorist threats into five categories—chemical, biological, radiological, nuclear, and explosive—commonly referred to as CBRNE. Each type of threat has unique characteristics and medical impacts:

- **Chemical.** A chemical emergency occurs when a hazardous chemical has been released, and the release has the potential to harm people's health. In the United States, 60,000 chemical spills, leaks, and explosions involving more than 300 deaths occur each year (Geiger, 2001; Kaji and Waeckerle, 2003). Many hazardous chemicals are used in industry (for example, chlorine, ammonia, and benzene). Chemical releases can be unintentional, as in the case of an industrial incident, or intentional, as in the case of a terrorist attack. Examples are nerve agents, such as sarin; mustard gas; and choking agents, such as phosgene. Others are found in nature (for example, poisonous plants).
- **Biological.** This category includes bioterrorism agents, such as anthrax, smallpox, botulism, and plague. In the nonterrorism context, it can include outbreaks of infectious disease with a high risk of transmission and serious health effects, such as severe acute respiratory syndrome (SARS) and avian influenza.
- **Radiological.** Widescale exposure to radiation could result from a dirty bomb, in which radioactive material is dispersed through an explosive device, or by a compromise of the containment of nuclear power stations or nuclear storage facilities.
- **Nuclear.** Resulting from the detonation of a nuclear device, this type of incident can result in a wide range of injuries, including explosive, radiological, and burns.
- **Explosive.** Explosive injuries can include blunt and shock wave–induced trauma, as well as burns, hearing loss, and injuries from shrapnel and the secondary collapse of structures.

until Hurricane Katrina, to natural disasters (Arkin, 2005). Of the 15 National Planning Scenarios introduced by the Department of Homeland Security (DHS) to guide disaster preparation efforts, only two involve natural disasters and only one an attack using explosives (see Box 7-2). Following Hurricane Katrina, however, DHS altered the selection process for its Urban Area Security Initiatives grants to ensure that the program would place as much weight on cities under threat from natural disasters as those likely to be terrorism targets (Jordan, 2006).

Because of the unpredictability of demand for emergency services, hospitals face fluctuations in utilization on an hourly, daily, and weekly basis. With many hospitals already operating at or near full capacity (as detailed in Chapter 2), temporary surges can exacerbate chronic ED crowding, boarding, and ambulance diversion. While these surges in demand can severely stretch the resources of a hospital's staff and diminish the quality and safety of patient care, hospitals generally maintain their normal standard of care through these surges. In a disaster situation, however, hospitals may need to shift to a sufficiency-of-care mode, in which the focus is on saving as many lives as possible rather than ensuring that each patient receives the usual standard of care (AHRQ, 2005). In the most extreme cases—for example, a full-blown influenza pandemic such as that experienced worldwide in 1918—this could mean assigning the most severely ill or injured patients to "expectant care," a strategy that withholds treatment for those who have

TABLE 7-1 Recent Disaster Events (United States and Worldwide)

Type	Examples	Locations	No. of Deaths
Natural	Hurricane (Katrina)	New Orleans/Louisiana/ Mississippi/Alabama (2005)	1,326
	Avian influenza	6 countries (2005–2006)	118 (as of October 20, 2005)
	Earthquake	Kashmir (2005)	73,000 (69,000 injured)
	Tsunami	12 countries (2004)	212,611
	SARS	25 countries (2002–2003)	774
	Earthquake	Northridge, California (1994)	57 (5,000+ injured)
Man-made	Subway bombing	London (2005) Madrid (2004)	52 (700 injured) 191 (2,000 injured)
	Nightclub fire	Rhode Island (2003)	100 (200+ injured)
	Nightclub bombing	Bali (2002)	202
	Anthrax	Washington, D.C. (2001)	5 (13 injured)
	Terrorist attacks of September 11	New York and Washington, D.C. (2001)	2,752
	Embassy bombings	Nairobi and Tanzania (1998)	224 (4,000+ injured)
	Release of sarin gas	Tokyo, Japan (1995)	12 (5,000 injured)

SOURCES (in order listed): Associated Press, 2006a; BBC News, 2006b; Times Foundation, 2005; CNN.com, 2005a; IOM, 2004; Insurance Information Network of California, 2006; CNN.com, 2005b; Gutierrez de Ceballos et al., 2004; Associated Press, 2006b; BBC News, 2006a; CNN.com, 2002; Hirschkorn, 2003; Rand Corporation, 2004; Accountability Review Boards on the Embassy Bombings in Nairobi and Dar es Salaam, 1999; BBC News, 2005.

BOX 7-2
Department of Homeland Security's
15 National Planning Scenarios

1. Nuclear Detonation: 10-Kiloton Improvised Nuclear Device
2. Biological Attack: Aerosol Anthrax
3. Biological Disease Outbreak: Pandemic Influenza
4. Biological Attack: Plague
5. Chemical Attack: Blister Agent
6. Chemical Attack: Toxic Industrial Chemical
7. Chemical Attack: Nerve Agent
8. Chemical Attack: Chlorine Tank Explosion
9. Natural Disaster: Major Earthquake
10. Natural Disaster: Major Hurricane
11. Radiological Attack: Radiological Dispersal Device
12. Explosives Attack: Bombing Using Improvised Explosive Devices
13. Biological Attack: Food Contamination
14. Biological Attack: Foreign Animal Disease (Foot and Mouth Disease)
15. Cyber Attack

SOURCE: DHS, 2005b.

---

very little chance of survival to focus resources on saving the largest possible number of lives.

A hospital's decision to switch from routine to disaster mode has enormous implications. When to make that decision and what actions to take as a result are complex. A number of initiatives are exploring these questions. For example, within the Department of Health and Human Services (DHHS), the Centers for Disease Control and Prevention's (CDC) National Center for Injury Prevention and Control, Division of Injury Response, is developing a consensus report describing the detailed actions to be taken by hospital and trauma center departments and personnel in the event of an explosive mass casualty event (CDC National Center for Injury Control and Prevention, 2006). The Agency for Healthcare Research and Quality (AHRQ) has sponsored research, convened expert panels, and published guidance for hospitals and communities on preparing for biological and other terrorist events. The Health Resources and Services Administration's (HRSA) Bioterrorism Hospital Preparedness Program specifically targets hospital preparedness, with a focus on the development and implementation of regional plans to improve the capacity of hospitals to respond to bioterrorist attacks.

CRITICAL HOSPITAL ROLES IN DISASTERS

Evaluations of ED disaster preparedness consistently yield the same finding: EDs are better prepared than they used to be, but still fall short of where they should be (Schur et al., 2004). A survey conducted by CDC in 2003 gives a comprehensive picture of hospital preparedness in the years following September 11 (Niska and Burt, 2005). Hospitals vary widely in the degree to which they have prepared for the range of possible threats. At the time of the survey, almost all hospitals (97.3 percent) had plans for responding to natural disasters because holding natural disaster drills is a requirement for accreditation by the Joint Commission for Accreditation of Healthcare Organizations (JCAHO). More than 80 percent of hospitals had plans for chemical (85.5 percent) and biological (84.8 percent) threats, and more than 70 percent had plans for nuclear and radiological (77.2 percent) and explosive (76.9 percent) threats.

The remainder of this section reviews the current status of and recommended actions for enhancing hospital preparedness across five critical hospital roles during disasters: maintaining surge capacity, carrying out planning and coordination with the wider health and public safety communities, conducting training and disaster drills, protecting the hospital and its staff, and performing surveillance.

Surge Capacity

Hospitals in most large population centers are operating at or near full capacity. In many cities, hospitals and trauma centers have problems dealing with a multiple-car highway crash, much less the volume of patients likely to result from a large-scale disaster. During emergencies, hospitals can do a number of things to free up capacity and extend their resources, but there are serious physical limitations on this expansion of their capabilities. Surveys indicate that the numbers of available beds, ventilators, isolation rooms, and pharmaceuticals may be insufficient to care for victims of a large-scale disaster (Kaji and Lewis, 2004). The Rhode Island nightclub fire (discussed further below) demonstrated that even medium-sized incidents can overwhelm local hospital capacities (Hick et al., 2004). The frequent ambulance diversions and ED boarding discussed earlier in this report also signal limitations on hospital surge capacity.

The issue of capacity is an immediate problem because many hospitals and their EDs are already maximizing their existing capacity after years of capacity shedding designed to reduce costs. According to the American

Hospital Association (AHA), 60 percent of hospitals were operating at or over capacity in 2001 (The Lewin Group, 2002). Many hospitals have already opened up additional beds in an effort to alleviate overcrowding, but continue to face nursing shortages and staffing issues in supporting the existing beds (Derlet and Richards, 2000; Asplin and Knopp, 2001).

The limiting factor in the ability to respond to a disaster will vary by hospital and by type of disaster. An important limiting factor is the availability of specialists who can treat the types of cases resulting from a disaster event. For an event involving a rare biological or chemical agent, there may be limited expertise in the community. For more common types of events, such as blast injuries, the limitation will likely be an inadequate supply of surgical specialists (including neurosurgeons, orthopedic surgeons, and burn surgeons) to treat the volume of cases requiring their specialized services. While other staff, such as emergency physicians, critical care specialists, and nurses, are important, they are less likely to represent a major constraint on the ability to treat additional patients. One way in which hospitals can alleviate staff shortages is to use emergency medical services (EMS) personnel as physician extenders. In many disaster scenarios, the prehospital component is over in 1–2 hours, making a large number of EMS personnel available just as hospital activity is peaking.

Physical space is an important consideration, but probably not the most critical factor. Hospitals can add to available capacity on short notice by halting elective admissions and discharging noncritical patients. In addition, they can sometimes use ED hallways, inpatient hallways, and nonclinical areas to house victims in an emergency. According to the CDC survey, however, only 61 percent of hospitals had developed plans for the use of nonclinical space in such cases (Niska and Burt, 2005). In some instances, particularly a more circumscribed disaster, hospitals can make room for patients by transferring existing inpatients to more distant facilities. But the CDC study revealed that only 46 percent of hospitals had agreements with other hospitals to accept patients in the case of a disaster (Niska and Burt, 2005).

Intensive care unit (ICU) beds are much more difficult to empty on short notice than other beds and are probably the key limiting factor in terms of physical capacity, as they often are in day-to-day crowding (GAO, 2003a). Another physical limitation is the number of negative pressure rooms needed to prevent the spread of airborne pathogens. Limitations in available equipment, such as mechanical ventilators and decontamination showers, are also important. The committee concludes that the lack of adequate hospital surge capacity is a serious and neglected element of current disaster preparedness efforts.

Planning and Coordination

When a disaster occurs, the normal operating assumptions about patients, responses, and treatments often must be jettisoned. Depending on the type of event, some of the nonroutine things that can happen include the following (Ackermann et al., 1998; Auf der Heide, 2006):

• Victims who are less injured and mobile (the so-called "walking wounded") will often self-transport to the nearest hospitals, quickly overwhelming those facilities.
• Casualties are likely to bypass on-site triage, first aid, and decontamination stations.
• EMS responders will often self-dispatch. Providers from other jurisdictions may appear at the scene and transport patients, sometimes without coordination or communication with local officials.
• In some cases, local facilities are not aware of the event until or just before patients start arriving. Hospitals may receive no advance notice of the extent of the event or the numbers and types of patients they can expect.
• There may be little or no communication among regional hospitals, incident commanders, public safety, and EMS responders to coordinate the response regionwide.

Consider the regional response needed after the Rhode Island nightclub fire in February 2003. During a concert, a fire broke out on the stage in the small venue and quickly spread throughout the nightclub before many patrons could escape. The fire consumed the building in 3 minutes, and 96 people were killed. It took 160 firefighters from 15 communities to put out the flames; 65 ambulances also responded (Gutman et al., 2003; Ginaitt, 2005).

The first patients began to arrive at local hospitals minutes after the fire broke out. Most hospitals received notification from EMS before patients began to arrive, but several others said they received no notification, or there was limited or incorrect information regarding the number of patients to expect. A total of 273 victims sought care at hospitals. The closest hospital to the nightclub (3 miles away), Rhode Island's second largest, is a 359-bed acute care hospital that handles 58,000 ED visits per year. It received 82 patients, 25 percent of whom were admitted and 25 percent of whom were transferred to other hospitals. A level I trauma center located 12 miles away from the nightclub received 68 patients; approximately 63 percent were admitted (Gutman et al., 2003). A number of other Rhode Island hospitals, as well as Massachusetts General, University of Massachusetts Medical Center, and Shriners Hospital for Children, also received patients. It was only the second time that Shriners had opened its doors to adult patients (Ginaitt, 2005).

However, there was limited communication between hospitals and no means for hospital coordination and prioritization of helicopter transfers of patients to burn centers. As a result, 10 transfers by helicopter occurred from four different hospitals within the first few hours. All air medical resources available in New England were used that evening (Gutman et al., 2003). The amount of regional resources needed to respond to this medium-sized emergency incident is striking. It demonstrates the need for hospitals to coordinate planning with each other as well as other responders, including prehospital providers and air medical personnel. This often means working and planning with groups across state lines to decide on and implement the surge capacity, workforce training, protective equipment, and surveillance and communications systems appropriate for the region.

Coordination among Local, Regional, State, and Federal Entities

The underlying philosophy of disaster management is that every event is handled at the lowest possible geographic, organizational, and jurisdictional level (DHS, 2004). When a disaster event becomes larger than can be handled adequately by local response capabilities, the state usually gets involved, enabling the allocation of statewide resources to the affected area. The state government has ultimate responsibility for the health and well-being of its citizens, and can allocate funding and statewide emergency resources, utilize National Guard troops, and draw on state supplies of drugs and vaccines. When an event becomes too big to be handled at the state and local levels, it may be declared an "incident of national significance." In this case, the command structure shifts to the federal response outlined by the National Incident Management System (NIMS) through DHS, opening the way for federal resources, including federal stockpiles, disaster management assistance teams (DMATs), and federal dollars, to be deployed to support operations.

Most agree that for disaster response to be effective, incident control must be clear, communications good, and providers at the local level involved in the process. In the event of a disaster, local emergency providers must respond as additional resources are mobilized at state or federal levels. The medical care component of most disasters is usually over after a few hours, so even if these additional resources can be assembled, they may arrive too late to be of much help (Waeckerle, 1991). Further, only regional and local planning can adequately anticipate and address local utilization patterns that will impact the execution of disaster plans. Therefore, all hospitals must be prepared to receive patients suffering from any type of illness, injury, or exposure.

To respond effectively, hospitals must interface with incident command at multiple levels and be prepared to deal with transitions between levels, for example, when incident command shifts from the local to the state or federal level. Each hospital should be familiar with the local office of emergency preparedness and know how hospitals are represented at the emergency operations center during an event, whether through the hospital association, the health department, the EMS system, or some other mechanism. Using an existing program, such as the Hospital Emergency Incident Command System (HEICS), can aid hospitals in internal preparedness and coordination with the rest of the system. HEICS is a standardized approach to disaster management—essentially an internal hospital application of NIMS—that was developed and has been used nationwide for a decade.

Regionalization

Current federal preparedness funding has been geared toward preparing all hospitals to respond at some level to all hazards. Because the range of possible threats is so broad, the feasibility of meaningfully preparing all hospitals is unrealistic. Regionalization of certain aspects of preparedness may facilitate a more timely and effective response (Bravata et al., 2004a). The benefits of regionalizing disaster response include consolidation of inventories of drugs and vaccines; surveillance to identify outbreaks of disease; efficiency of concentrating certain types of medical response at fewer hospitals; and improved communications, command, and control associated with regionwide events (GAO, 2003a). Regionalization is also likely to benefit triage, medical care, outbreak investigations, security management, emergency management, and training.

Regional trauma systems are critical to planning for the care of severely injured patients during a disaster. While 47 states have developed or are developing a statewide trauma system plan and 38 states now designate trauma systems, there is wide variation across states in the level of development of these systems and in the degree of coordination with disaster planning. In one example of a regional approach to disaster planning, Connecticut developed a statewide system for hospital preparedness for bioterrorism that was built on the trauma system (Jacobs et al., 2003). The Connecticut Department of Public Health contracted with two level I trauma centers, which were designated as regional centers of excellence for bioterrorism preparedness. The existing trauma system and communications network provide the basic infrastructure for the system, which links to the Metropolitan Medical Response System centered in Hartford. The two centers of excellence serve to coordinate all aspects of medical disaster response activities within their regions, including surveillance, training, planning, facilities, equipment, and supplies. This model is based on the realization that resources are too scarce for a haphazard approach—disaster funding should be targeted to those regions and hospitals where it will do the most good for the community in the event of a disaster. Ideally, all assets required for a community or a state to mount an effective response should be developed within the regional context described in Chapter 3.

Federal funding for the development of such approaches is currently limited. The establishment of the Division of Trauma and EMS within DHHS in 1990 helped jump start the development of trauma systems through state grants. But this program was eliminated in 1995, leaving a gap in federal leadership until the creation of the Trauma/EMS Systems program within HRSA's Division of Healthcare Preparedness in 2001. This program was also recently defunded. While the program operated on a relative shoestring—approximately $3.5 million in fiscal years 2002 to 2005—it provided critical national leadership for planning, infrastructure development, standards development, and coordination with other federal agencies.

Communications

Good communications among the many community services involved in disaster response are essential to an effective response—to ensuring that patients will be directed to the most appropriate facilities, that hospitals will not be overwhelmed with patients, that hospitals will be alerted sufficiently in advance of the arrival of patients to be able to mount the appropriate response, and that resources will be allocated effectively throughout the community. Unfortunately, communication is a significant weakness of the current system, reflecting the existing fragmentation of emergency care. According to the 2003 CDC survey, surprisingly few hospitals had provisions in their bioterrorism response plans for contacting outside entities such as EMS (72 percent), fire departments (66 percent), or other hospitals (51 percent). Hospital collaboration in mass casualty drills with outside organizations followed a similar pattern—only 71 percent collaborated with EMS, 67 percent with fire departments, and 46 percent with other hospitals (Niska and Burt, 2005).

In addition to coordinated communications, investments should be made in enhanced communications equipment. Hospitals should have reliable and redundant digital and voice communications with the regional and state public safety, emergency management, and public health agencies. The loss of hospital communications capabilities during Hurricane Katrina turned out to be a major obstacle to coordinating the evacuation and care of victims. Hospitals should have some satellite telecommunications capability in preparation for a catastrophic event.

Veterans Health Administration

With hospitals, nursing homes, ambulatory care clinics, and counseling clinics in many communities across the country, the Veterans Health Administration (VHA) is well positioned to enhance regional response, particularly since its hospitals are required by law to maintain excess capacity. The VHA currently deploys personnel to all presidentially declared disasters, including Hurricane Andrew, the Northridge earthquake, and the September 11 terrorist attacks. VHA staff also support such events as the Super Bowl, presidential inaugurations, and papal visits. An Emergency Management Academy is being developed to train and equip VHA staff with emergency management skills. In addition, the VHA procures, stores, and maintains pharmaceutical stockpiles for incidents involving weapons of mass destruction (WMD) (Emergency Management Strategic Healthcare Group et al., 2005). The committee recognizes the importance of the VHA in emergency planning and response, and recommends that **the Department of Homeland Security, the Department of Health and Human Services, the Department of Transportation, and the states collaborate with the Veterans Health Administration (VHA) to integrate the VHA into civilian disaster planning and management (7.1).**

Training and Disaster Drills

The unique aspects of disaster response require specialized training, both in the clinical management of disaster victims and in institutional procedures that may be quite different from those under normal operating conditions (HRSA, 2002; Treat et al., 2001; GAO, 2003a,b; Rivera and Char, 2004). There are strong indications that training is inadequate in both areas.

Hospital Training and Drills

Results of the 2003 CDC survey indicate that progress has been made since September 11 in training hospital staff to deal with emergencies, but deficiencies remain. Training in response to terrorism-related threats varied widely among staff: 92 percent of hospitals trained their nursing staffs in at least one type of threat, while residents and interns received training at only 49 percent of hospitals (Niska and Burt, 2005) (see Figure 7-2). This nevertheless represents an improvement over training prior to September 11. Treat and colleagues (2001), for example, found that fewer than 25 percent of hospitals in and around Washington, D.C., had staff trained in WMD before September 11 (Treat et al., 2001). The CDC survey revealed that staff at most hospitals (89 percent) had received training since September 11 in the

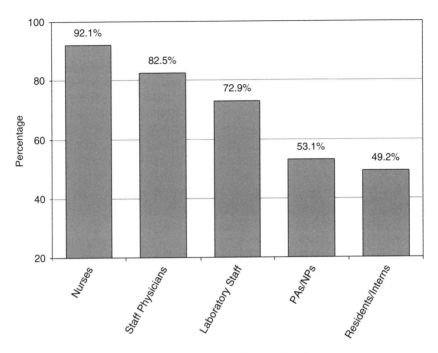

FIGURE 7-2 Percentage of hospitals with staff trained in disaster response.
NOTE: NP = nurse practitioner; PA = physician assistant.
SOURCE: Niska and Burt, 2005.

diagnosis and treatment of exposure to biological agents—most frequently smallpox and anthrax. And three-quarters of hospitals had trained staff in implementing an incident command system.

According to the CDC survey, nearly 90 percent of hospitals (88.4 percent) had conducted a mass casualty drill. The most common scenario was a general disaster response, with far fewer hospitals addressing other types of threats—chemical (44.7 percent), biological (37.5 percent), explosive or incendiary (21.3 percent), nuclear or radiological (15.4 percent), and severe epidemic (7.1 percent).

JCAHO requires hospitals to have an emergency management plan and to evaluate the plan by conducting practice drills, but this effort focuses mainly on logistical aspects rather than personnel training. Some hospitals have developed their own curriculum or training guides for staff (Zavotsky, 2000; Phillips and Lavin, 2004). Researchers have aided these efforts by outlining key recommendations for training components (Waeckerle et al., 2001; Greenberg et al., 2003), developing ideas for future training approaches (Terndrup et al., 2005), and suggesting best practices based on provider feedback (Alexander et al., 2005). States can overcome the lack of standardized disaster training guidelines and other barriers by expanding and supporting continuing education and facility preparedness requirements.

Introducing on-the-job training for ED personnel is difficult for a number of reasons, however. Many hospitals report inadequate funding to cover the attendance costs (e.g., time off, tuition, travel) of training (ACEP Nuclear, Biological and Chemical Task Force, 2001). At the University of Pittsburgh Medical Center, a disaster drill in the ED costs $3,000 per hour in staff salaries alone (AHRQ, 2004). Also, the ED may experience personnel shortages during training unless coverage is provided for the staff being trained. Additionally, the failure of hospital administrators or ED personnel to recognize the importance of training can result in a lack of support (ACEP Nuclear, Biological and Chemical Task Force, 2001).

HRSA's National Bioterrorism Hospital Preparedness Program (HRSA, 2006) (discussed in more detail below) provides grants to states to improve hospital preparedness. Guidance to grantees in the initial year of the program (HRSA, 2002) made training a secondary priority, and in the following year it was made optional. However, all grantees noted that they were providing training for bioterrorism and other public health emergencies. The most frequently addressed subject was worker safety, followed by psychosocial issues for both patients and providers. Other topics addressed included responding to CBRNE events, incident command, risk communication, and treatment of special populations (AHRQ, 2004). The grantees used a variety of different methods for training, including face-to-face training, distance learning, field exercises and drills, and distribution of written materials.

Professional Training Curricula

Training currently provided to physicians in medical school and continuing education programs does not uniformly address the threat of disasters, types of WMD agents, and procedures for handling mass casualty incidents and events. WMD-related training is only a small component of emergency medicine residency programs, but, as mentioned earlier, approximately 38 percent of practicing emergency physicians are neither residency trained nor board certified in emergency medicine and are therefore not exposed to that curriculum. Barriers to training include an already full medical school and residency curriculum and a lack of instructor expertise, equipment, and advocates to lobby for the inclusion of disaster preparedness training (Waeckerle et al., 2001; ACEP Nuclear, Biological and Chemical Task Force, 2001). But opportunities for training in CBRNE agents exist at various levels; medical schools can incorporate instruction on these agents into current coursework (e.g., toxicology, epidemiology) and clerkships, residency programs can dedicate time to these agents in both the ED and planned educational experiences, and states can require a certain amount of continuing education on these agents for relicensure (Waeckerle et al., 2001).

Disaster training is also currently not a core component of the nursing curriculum. WMD topics and agents have been added to the Emergency Nurses Association (ENA) Emergency Nurses Core Curriculum; however, only a small percentage of ED nurses receive this training. Additionally, disaster response is not included on the emergency nursing certification exam. Opportunities exist for integrating WMD agents and disaster response techniques into the nursing curriculum. Additional steps might include incorporating articles on disaster response and associated topics in professional nursing journals and introducing related questions into the certified emergency nurse (CEN) board exam (Waeckerle et al., 2001).

The lack of standardized training for ED workers is recognized, and there have been several efforts to improve their competencies. For example, the American Medical Association (AMA) developed courses for physicians and other health professionals in disaster preparedness, including courses in basic disaster life support (BDLS) and advanced disaster life support (ADLS) (AMA, 2003). Additionally, the federal Office of Emergency Preparedness (formerly in DHHS, now in DHS) contracted with the American College of Emergency Physicians (ACEP) to identify the core content of a national program for training prehospital emergency personnel and emergency physicians and nurses to detect and respond to nuclear, biological, and chemical agents. Phase 2 of the contract, which has not yet been funded, would assist with the implementation of that curriculum (ACEP, 2005).

Serious clinical and operational deficiencies, fragmentation, and lack of standardization exist across a broad spectrum of key professional personnel (nurses, physicians, ancillary care providers, administrators, and public health officials) in both individual training and coordination of a team response. The committee believes a concerted effort to integrate disaster preparedness and education into established professional curricula, continuing education, and certification programs is the most reasonable solution to these shortcomings at this point in time. Therefore, to address the need for competency in disaster medicine across disciplines, the committee recommends that **all institutions responsible for the training, continuing education, and credentialing and certification of professionals involved in emergency care (including medicine, nursing, emergency medical services, allied health, public health, and hospital administration) incorporate disaster preparedness training into their curricula and competency criteria (7.2).**

Protecting the Hospital and Staff

Protecting the Hospital

The hospital represents a critical asset in the event of a disaster, but it is also a vulnerable one. Hospitals can fall victim to the disaster event itself, as occurred in the cases of Katrina and other recent hurricanes. Obviously, each hospital must have procedures in place to maintain essential services when necessary and transport patients to alternative facilities. In addition, when a hospital shuts down, its staff, vehicles, equipment, and supplies may still be useful. Regional disaster planning should include plans to distribute these assets as needed by the community.

Hospitals can be targeted by terrorism directly or indirectly, and there has been little preparation for or even discussion of that possibility. Hospitals should plan for direct attacks and establish plans for limiting access, securing perimeters, protecting water and power supplies, and sheltering staff. A particular vulnerability, because of the information intensity of the hospital environment, is the hospital's exposure to cyber attack. Such an attack could have a profound impact on clinical operations, communications, telemetry, records, and many other critical functions.

Hospitals are also vulnerable to an influx of disaster victims. Large numbers of victims descending on a hospital can be overwhelming and diminish its effectiveness in dealing with casualties. Patients suspected of exposure to chemical or biological agents can completely shut down a facility if they are not decontaminated properly before entering (the same applies to vehicles as well). Every hospital must have adequate decontamination showers and procedures for dealing with contaminated patients because experience has taught that many victims "self-evacuate" from the scene of a disaster, bypassing on-scene triage and decontamination (Auf der Heide, 2006). In extreme cases, the hospital must be prepared to lock down to prevent the entry of contaminated patients who would otherwise disable the facility—an action antithetical to the open way in which hospitals typically operate.

Protecting Staff

The risk of chemical or biological exposure of hospital staff occurs when exposed patients are not properly decontaminated before arriving at the ED or as ED personnel are in the process of decontaminating victims. The risk of secondary contamination is present if the substance is toxic and likely to be carried on a victim's clothing, skin, or hair in sufficient quantities to threaten rescuers or health care providers (Horton et al., 2005). There may also be a risk if victims of chemical contamination exhale the fumes they have inhaled in breathing space shared with others.

The sarin attacks in Tokyo and the severe acute respiratory syndrome (SARS) epidemic in China and Toronto are examples of exposure of emergency care providers. The SARS epidemic (see Box 7-3) demonstrated the difficulties associated with containing even a small outbreak—particularly when health professionals themselves are inadequately protected and become both victims and spreaders of disease (Donovan, 2003; Augustine et al., 2004). One of the most important tools in such an event is the availability of negative pressure rooms that prevent the spread of airborne pathogens throughout the ED or inpatient ward. The potential for a major outbreak of avian influenza further highlights the need for this capacity. Unfortunately, the number of such rooms is minimal and is often restricted to a handful of tertiary hospitals in major population centers. The committee believes the lack of an adequate supply of negative pressure rooms is a critical vulnerability of the current system and that the existing capacity of this resource could be quickly overwhelmed by either a terrorist event or a major outbreak of avian influenza or some or other airborne disease, posing an extreme danger to hospital workers and patients. It may be hoped that future ED and hospital bed construction will include designs that allow any patient room to be converted to a negative pressure room.

While an adequate number of negative pressure rooms is essential for control of airborne infections, it is only part of the solution. There must also be substantial training in disease recognition and in decontamination and containment procedures. In addition, it is necessary to learn from SARS and similar experiences and to develop techniques and approaches that add to our understanding of the management of disease outbreaks. One possible containment strategy is to use cohort staffing techniques similar to those employed in neonatal intensive care. In this approach, groups of providers are linked with groups of patients for the episode of care to prevent spread to other patients and providers.

During the sarin event in Tokyo, the failure of hospital providers to wear personal protective equipment (see the discussion below), coupled with a decision to contain the still-clothed contaminated patients in a poorly ventilated hospital chapel, contributed to hospital workers' secondary sarin exposure (Hick et al., 2004; see Box 7-4). This incident raises an important issue with regard to disasters involving exposures, alluded to above: most ambulatory patients are unlikely to wait for hazardous materials teams to deploy and set up decontamination equipment; instead, victims self-refer to the nearest emergency room (Hick et al., 2004; Horton et al., 2005).

Personal Protective Equipment

The use of personal protective equipment by hospital workers is complicated by the fact that different types of such equipment are needed for

BOX 7-3
The SARS Outbreak and Its Implications

The 2003 outbreak of severe acute respiratory syndrome (SARS) speaks volumes about the global health care community's deficiencies in recognizing, controlling, and communicating information about potential infectious diseases. The rapid spread of SARS in early 2003 caught the world off guard and challenged the global public health infrastructure. A clinical syndrome characterized by fever, lower respiratory symptoms, and radiographic evidence of pneumonia (CDC, 2005), SARS is caused by a coronavirus originally transmitted from an animal source. Case control studies suggest that China's Guangdong Province was the initial focus of infection and transmission (IOM, 2004). Between November 16, 2002, and February 10, 2003, the disease quietly spread throughout provinces in China, as well as neighboring countries, before being officially recognized. Striking mainly adults aged 18–64, the disease was quickly spread by infected travelers and "superspreaders"—people who may infect many others because they have high levels of contact, go undiagnosed for a long period, and may have secondary conditions that aid the spread of disease. Nosocomial transmission made health care providers, patients, and family members of both groups especially susceptible.

Deficiencies in both global and local public health infrastructures were apparent at every stage of the epidemic. The virus went unreported from China for 3 months, and later warnings and alerts were slow to be released. Most warnings about symptoms were unrecognized, and guidelines for the use of isolation or personal protective equipment were ignored (Donovan, 2003).

The SARS outbreak in Toronto was triggered in part by a patient who sought care in a Toronto ED for fever and a cough. He spent the night in a crowded ED awaiting admission for what was thought at the time to be community-acquired pneumonia. Over the course of the night, he infected 2 nearby patients and several hospital staff members with SARS. Both this index case and the 2 patients he infected subsequently died from the disease, and a total of 31 patients and staff fell ill. Ironically, the same hospital where this incident occurred continues to board admitted patients in its ED (Cass, 2005).

But health care workers clearly suffered the most. The aggressive respiratory care provided actually helped spread SARS, while insufficient availability of isolation rooms and personal protective equipment helped boost the case fatality rate for the disease to 10–15 percent (Augustine et al., 2004). Based on data as of December 2003, there were 8,094 total suspected SARS cases, 774 of whom died (WHO, 2005).

BOX 7-4
The Tokyo Subway Attack

At approximately 7:45 AM on March 20, 1995, five men, all members of a religious cult, boarded five separate subway trains in Tokyo. Witnesses reported that one of the men boarded a train wearing a sanitary mask and after taking a seat, opened his briefcase and removed a box wrapped in newspaper. The man put the box at his feet and leisurely read the newspaper until the next stop, when he exited the train, leaving the package behind. This man and the four others each released one or more containers of sarin, a lethal, colorless gas. Riders on the subway were immediately affected. Subway stations evacuated all passengers, many choking, vomiting, and blinded by the chemical. More than 4,000 victims of the attack sought treatment at hospitals; most were self-transported. Lacking initial knowledge of the sarin attack and proper personal protective equipment, hospital workers became victims when they were exposed to the nerve agent on the clothing of patients. Twenty-three percent of the hospital house staff (100 health care workers) showed signs of sarin poisoning (Pangi, 2002).

various types of exposures. Biological and chemical agents require different types of respiratory and dermal protection (Arnold and Lavonas, 2004). Proper selection of personal protective equipment is particularly challenging when the identity of the contaminating agent is unknown. Additionally, such equipment is often restrictive and cumbersome, making triage and patient care more difficult (Suner et al., 2004; Horton et al., 2005).

Until recently, hospitals had little guidance to follow regarding the specific personal protective equipment that should be available (Hick et al., 2004; OSHA, 2005). JCAHO requires each institution with an ED to have a plan for treating at least one contaminated patient (Arnold and Lavonas, 2004). In January 2005, the Occupational Safety and Health Administration (OSHA) compiled a set of best practices that specifies the personal protective equipment hospitals can use to protect first receivers assisting victims contaminated with unknown substances. This equipment includes a powered air purifying respirator, a chemical-resistant protective garment, head covering if it is not already included in the respirator, double-layer protective gloves, and chemical-protective boots. However, this recommendation assumes that hospitals will make a conscientious effort to limit the secondary exposure of health care workers (e.g., that hospitals will have protocols in place for removing the clothing of and properly decontaminating victims). Additionally, OSHA recommended that hospitals assess specific local hazards and augment its recommendations accordingly (OSHA, 2005). The committee believes that protection of emergency care and other hospital personnel is a critical deficiency of the current system.

Surveillance

EDs are well positioned to collect and analyze, in collaboration with state and local health departments, data on injury incidence, disease trends, and potential bioterrorism threats in the community (Garrison et al., 1994). The role of EDs in surveillance has been demonstrated by the National Electronic Injury Surveillance System (NEISS), operated by the U.S. Consumer Product Safety Commission. The commission uses data from the NEISS to monitor consumer product–related injuries under its regulatory jurisdiction and recommend changes in policy regarding those products. For example, NEISS helped the commission identify an outbreak of injuries from all-terrain vehicles, which ultimately led to direct intervention by the federal government to restrict access to such vehicles (Garrison et al., 1994). ED surveillance data have played a crucial role in our current understanding of nonfatal injuries, leading to physical safety improvements (better-designed highways) and public safety legislation (changes to speed limits).

To address the threat of bioterrorism and disease outbreaks, hospital EDs can learn to recognize the diagnostic clues that may indicate an unusual infectious disease outbreak so public health authorities can respond quickly (GAO, 2003c). During the SARS outbreak in 2003, hospitals played an important role in identifying infected individuals. ED staff routinely used questionnaires to screen patients for fever, cough, and travel to a country with active SARS. But this screening of patients for SARS symptoms was reactive—EDs were performing it because SARS had become a problem in Toronto, and there was a real possibility of its spreading to cities in the United States. The greater challenge is preparing ED staff and their public health partners to identify an initial outbreak.

Surveillance systems vary considerably from region to region, and according to a recent Government Accountability Office (GAO) report, there are serious gaps in our ability to detect an outbreak. The majority of surveillance systems in existence today are manual ones that rely heavily on ED personnel to communicate information to public health personnel. There are two types of manual surveillance systems: active and passive. With active systems, hospital staff are responsible for reporting incidents and conveying data on illnesses to public health officials, for example, through phone calls or faxes (GAO, 2003c; McHugh et al., 2004). An example of an active system is that operating in Santa Clara County, California. ED nurses make note of every patient who has a chief complaint compatible with one of six syndromes: flu-like symptoms, fever with mental status changes, fever with skin rash, diarrhea with dehydration, visual or swallowing difficulties/ slurred speech or dry mouth, and acute respiratory distress syndrome. The information is then faxed to the local health department at the end of each nursing shift (Henning, 2003). Because of underreporting by hospitals and the time lag between the diagnosis and the health department's receipt of information, active systems are not effective in identifying a rapidly spreading outbreak at its earliest stage (GAO, 2003c). Other regions use passive systems, in which information is automatically collected in the course of patient care, and either automatically reported or "mined" by public health workers to solicit information from hospitals (GAO, 2003c; Schur, 2004). Passive systems tend to provide more complete reporting of surveillance data than a system that is fully dependent on voluntary reporting (GAO, 2003c).

In an effort to improve disease surveillance capabilities, some hospitals use electronic surveillance systems to passively collect surveillance data and automatically transfer the data from the ED to health departments. Electronic systems are beneficial in that they allow more timely transmission of data, but are inappropriate for local health departments that do not have adequate resources to manage, analyze, and interpret large influxes of data (Bravata et al., 2004b). CDC funds three ongoing electronic surveillance system networks that collect data from a sample of hospitals. One of these is EMERGency ID NET, which collects data from 11 academically affiliated EDs that cumulatively account for approximately 1 percent of all ED visits (Talan et al., 1998; Barthell et al., 2002). The data are collected during evaluation of patients with specific clinical syndromes; entered into the program's software within 1 day of a patient visit; and electronically stored, transferred, and analyzed at a central receiving site. With these data, research on emerging infectious disease can be conducted (Talan et al., 1998). But data from systems such as EMERGency ID NET may be limited in that the systems collect data only on certain types of patients, collecting all the data is difficult and time-consuming, distribution to individuals assigned to analyze the data may be delayed, and findings may have little relevance for local efforts (Barthell et al., 2002). This type of system is too slow to trigger rapid response by public health officials.

Some surveillance systems, whether manual or electronic, capture syndromics. Syndromic surveillance is surveillance for disease syndromes (signs and symptoms), rather than for specific clinical or laboratory-defined diseases (Henning, 2003). It is a relatively new concept in public health surveillance. The problem with nonsyndromic systems is that outbreaks of disease may be difficult to diagnose, and delays in diagnosis can result in a larger number of casualties and a more prolonged outbreak. Syndromic surveillance may improve early detection of an outbreak (Henning, 2003). The key is to have systems that can help staff recognize index cases (i.e., the first one to three patients), as well as clusters of cases presenting to different hospitals in an area.

The most sophisticated of surveillance systems are real-time syndromic surveillance systems. Several large cities (New York, Chicago, Boston, Seattle) began operating such systems, beginning largely in 1999, with special funding from CDC (Henning, 2003). An example is Insight, a computer-based clinical information system at the Washington Hospital Center (WHC) in Washington, D.C., designed to record and track patient data, including geographic and demographic information. The software proved useful during the 2001 anthrax attacks, when it enabled WHC to send complete, real-time data to CDC while other hospitals were sending limited information with a lag of one or more days. The success of Insight attracted considerable grant funding for its expansion; WHC earmarked $7 million for Insight to link it to federal and regional agencies and integrate it with other hospital systems (Kanter and Heskett, 2002).

Although most public health officials are quickly embracing surveillance systems, particularly syndromic systems, more research is needed on their effectiveness. Bravata and colleagues (2004b) recently undertook a review of surveillance systems to evaluate their utility for detecting illnesses and syndromes related to bioterrorism. Researchers reviewed 115 systems (at EDs and other locations), including 9 syndromic surveillance systems. The authors found that few surveillance systems have been comprehensively evaluated; therefore, information is lacking on the ability of such systems to facilitate decision making by clinicians and public health officials (Bravata et al., 2004b).

CHALLENGES IN RURAL AREAS

The focus of emergency preparedness has been on urban areas in part because of the perceived increased risk of terrorism in these areas. However, there is a danger associated with neglecting rural areas. Indeed, one might argue that rural areas may be even more vulnerable to a terrorist attack. Many nuclear power facilities, hydroelectric dams, uranium and plutonium storage facilities, and agricultural chemical facilities, as well as all U.S. Air Force missile launch facilities, are located in rural areas and are potential targets for attack. Additionally, if individuals with infectious diseases, such as smallpox, enter the country through Canadian or Mexican borders, rural providers may be the first to identify the threat (ORHP, 2002). Although fewer individuals may be harmed by an incident in a rural area as compared with an urban area, mass disasters are relative, depending on the size of the local population and hospital capacity. The demand for health and hospital care by 200 people could overwhelm a 20-bed facility (AHA, 2001).

The emergency preparedness challenges EDs face are exacerbated in rural areas because rural hospitals often lack the resources and staff needed to respond swiftly to a catastrophic event (ORHP, 2002). In fact, results of several studies indicate that urban areas are generally further along in bioterrorism preparedness planning than rural areas because they have more experience in dealing with public health emergencies and more resources upon which to draw (Schur et al., 2004). Rural facilities tend to be limited in medical supplies, life-sustaining equipment (such as ventilators), and auxiliary power sources (Gursky, 2004). Additionally, rural hospitals have even more limited surge capacity than hospitals in urban areas; 500 rural hospitals are Critical Access Hospitals, which are limited to 15 beds (ORHP, 2002). Rural hospitals also tend to lack decontamination facilities. In a 2001 study of hospitals in Federal Emergency Management Agency (FEMA) region III, none of the 22 rural hospitals had decontamination stations that could process 10 to 15 patients at a time; 4 of those hospitals had no decontamination plans in place (Treat et al., 2001). Some rural hospitals rely on local EMS personnel to perform decontamination; however, this is concerning because past experience has shown that the vast majority of disaster victims seek care in emergency rooms without accessing EMS (Treat et al., 2001). Moreover, communications systems in rural EDs tend to be unreliable and interrupted by terrain and weather (Gursky, 2004).

Staffing is another crucial problem for rural hospitals. Although the American Hospital Association (AHA) and other groups recommend that rural hospitals develop a reserve staff (retired health workers, persons in training), existing shortages make it difficult to do so. Additionally, some hospital personnel, particularly nurses, work part-time in nearby urban areas and may not be available in the event of a crisis. Training of staff in emergency preparedness is often complicated by the fact that training meetings are frequently held in urban areas that may be quite far away from rural hospitals. One day of training may require 2 or 3 days away from the hospital to accommodate travel time (Schur et al., 2004). Additionally, rural hospitals that rely heavily on contract staff may be reluctant to invest in training opportunities for those individuals since they may not continue working at that hospital in the long term.

Rural hospitals may not have access to the same federal funding for bioterrorism as urban hospitals. This may be particularly problematic because many rural hospitals are older and more isolated, making preparedness measures more expensive (Schur et al., 2004). Rural hospitals have not benefited from Metropolitan Medical Response System (MMRS) funding since that funding is targeted to metropolitan areas. On the other hand, rural hospitals have access to other funding streams not available to urban hospitals; in 2003, DHHS allocated $45 million in federal grants for rural and frontier hospitals (Gursky, 2004).

FEDERAL FUNDING FOR HOSPITAL PREPAREDNESS

Total federal preparedness funding has increased substantially in the 5 years since September 11, 2001. Emergency preparedness funding in DHHS, for example, rose from $237 million in fiscal year 2000 to $9.6 billion in fiscal year 2006 (Broder, 2006). But while the vast majority of terrorist events worldwide have involved conventional explosives and nonbiological agents, federal spending on preparedness has focused heavily on bioterrorism at the expense of other priorities (DePalma et al., 2005). Furthermore, the proportion of these dollars allocated to hospitals for infrastructure, technology, equipment, and training enhancements has been very limited.

Federal preparedness funding has been made available indirectly to hospitals primarily through two programs: MMRS and the Bioterrorism Hospital Preparedness Program. A review of each of these programs indicates that the amount provided to hospitals specifically for improving preparedness efforts has been small (IOM, 2002).

MMRS was created in 1996 to enhance and coordinate local and regional response capabilities for highly populated areas that could be targeted by a terrorist attack using WMD. A total of 124 jurisdictions receive funding under the program. The organizing principles and resources of the program are also applicable to large-scale incidents, such as hazardous material incidents, natural disasters, and disease outbreaks. MMRS was funded at $50 million for both fiscal years 2003 and 2004, and was reduced to $30 million in both fiscal years 2005 and 2006. Each of the 124 jurisdictions will receive $232,030 for fiscal year 2006. Hospitals are aided indirectly through this program by participation in preparedness planning. However, hospitals initially did not participate in the program; it took several years before they were integrated into MMRS planning (DHS, 2005a). MMRS was transferred from DHHS to DHS in 2003 and now resides in the Office of Grants and Training (GAO, 2003b).

The Bioterrorism Hospital Preparedness Program is targeted more specifically to hospital preparedness. The primary focus of the program is on developing and implementing regional plans to improve the capacity of hospitals to respond to bioterrorist attacks. The program made its initial awards in 2002, and the funding is distributed through cooperative agreements with states and selected municipalities, which have considerable flexibility in determining how the funding is allocated across hospitals. The cooperative agreements consist of two phases. In phase I, states are required to develop a needs assessment for a comprehensive bioterrorism preparedness program for hospitals and other health care entities and to begin the initial implementation of the plan. In phase II, states are required to submit more detailed implementation plans, including how they are going to address a series of critical benchmarks outlined by HRSA (GAO, 2003a). Funding for this program grew from $125 million in 2002 to $498 million in fiscal year 2003 and $515 million in fiscal year 2004 (Gursky, 2004), but fell to $491 million in fiscal year 2005 (HRSA, 2006). The amount going directly to hospitals varied greatly by state, and in many cases hospitals received only a limited amount of the funding. According to one study, the "typical" award to hospitals was approximately $5,000–10,000, though some hospitals received funding in the range of $50,000–100,000 (McHugh et al., 2004). The funding under the program has generally not been sufficient to purchase the equipment needed for one critical care room or to retrofit an airborne infection isolation room in one hospital (Hick et al., 2004).

In addition, CDC funds 52 Centers for Public Health Preparedness (CPHPs). CPHPs are academic institutions that provide a focal point for planning, training, and collaboration between health departments and other community partners in preparing for public health crises.

The allocation of preparedness funding across states has been controversial. The 2005 appropriations bill allocated "hospital preparedness" funding to states on a per hospital bed basis, rather than on the basis of the likelihood of disaster. Critics argue that this apportionment is essentially "pork" rather than an attempt to allocate preparedness dollars rationally according to need. States facing limited risk can receive substantial funding under this approach, while cities such as Washington, D.C., which face a much greater risk, receive a lesser share (ER One, 2005).

Trauma systems also represent a critical component of disaster response. Federal support for the development of these systems and their coordination with other regional disaster planning efforts does not appear to reflect recognition of this fact. Federal funding for state trauma system development and planning has been inconsistent; it was recently dealt a blow with the defunding of the Trauma/EMS Systems program for fiscal year 2006.

States and communities should play an important role in determining how they will prepare for emergencies. To the extent that they are supported in this effort through federal preparedness grants, the critical role and vulnerabilities of hospitals must be more widely acknowledged, and the particular needs of hospitals and hospital personnel must be taken explicitly into account. Therefore, the committee recommends that **Congress significantly increase total preparedness funding in fiscal year 2007 for hospital emergency preparedness in the following areas: strengthening and sustaining trauma care systems; enhancing emergency department, trauma center, and inpatient surge capacity; improving emergency medical services' response to explosives; designing evidence-based training programs; enhancing the availability of decontamination showers, standby intensive care unit capacity, negative pressure rooms, and appropriate personal protective equipment; and conducting international collaborative research on the civilian consequences of conventional weapons terrorism.**

SUMMARY OF RECOMMENDATIONS

7.1: The Department of Homeland Security, the Department of Health and Human Services, the Department of Transportation, and the states should collaborate with the Veterans Health Administration (VHA) to integrate the VHA into civilian disaster planning and management.

7.2: All institutions responsible for the training, continuing education, and credentialing and certification of professionals involved in emergency care (including medicine, nursing, emergency medical services, allied health, public health, and hospital administration) should incorporate disaster preparedness training into their curricula and competency criteria.

7.3: Congress should significantly increase total preparedness funding in fiscal year 2007 for hospital emergency preparedness in the following areas: strengthening and sustaining trauma care systems; enhancing emergency department, trauma center, and inpatient surge capacity; improving emergency medical services' response to explosives; designing evidence-based training programs; enhancing the availability of decontamination showers, standby intensive care unit capacity, negative pressure rooms, and appropriate personal protective equipment; and conducting international collaborative research on the civilian consequences of conventional weapons terrorism.

REFERENCES

Accountability Review Boards on the Embassy Bombings in Nairobi and Dar es Salaam. 1999. Report of the Accountability Review Boards on the Embassy Bombings in Nairobi and Dar es Salaam on August 7, 1998. Washington, DC.

ACEP Nuclear, Biological and Chemical Task Force (American College of Emergency Physicians Nuclear, Biological and Chemical Task Force). 2001. *Developing Objectives, Content, and Competencies for the Training of Emergency Medical Technicians, Emergency Physicians, and Emergency Nurses to Care for Casualties Resulting from Nuclear, Biological, or Chemical (NBC) Incidents.* Dallas, TX: Department of Health and Human Services, ACEP.

ACEP. 2005. *Nuclear, Biological, and Chemical Terrorism.* [Online]. Available: http://www.acep.org/webportal/PatientsConsumers/HealthSubjectsByTopic/NuclearBiologicaland-ChemicalTerrorism/default.htm [accessed July 7, 2005].

Ackermann RJ, Kemle KA, Vogel RL, Griffin RC Jr. 1998. Emergency department use by nursing home residents. *Annals of Emergency Medicine* 31(6):749–757.

AHA (American Hospital Association). 2001. *Public Health System's Capacity to Respond to Bioterrorism.* Committee on Government Reform: Subcommittee on Technology and Procurement Policy. Chicago, IL: AHA.

AHRQ (Agency for Healthcare Research and Quality). 2004. *Optimizing Surge Capacity: Hospital Assessment and Planning. Bioterrorism and Health System Preparedness* (Issue Brief No. 3, AHRQ Publication No. 04-P008). Rockville, MD: AHRQ. [Online]. Available: http://www.ahrq.gov/news/ulp/btbriefs/btbrief3.htm [accessed: May 20, 2006].

AHRQ. 2005. *Bioterrorism and Other Public Health Emergencies: Altered Standards of Care in Mass Casualty Events.* Rockville, MD: AHRQ.

Alexander AJ, Bandiera GW, Mazurik LA. 2005. A multiple disaster training exercise for emergency medicine residents: Opportunity knocks. *Academic Emergency Medicine* 12(5):404–409.

AMA (American Medical Association). 2003. *AMA Announces New Emergency and Disaster Preparedness Coursework for Physicians and Other Health Care Professionals.* [Online]. Available: http://www.ama-assn.org/ama/pub/article/print/1616-7771.html [accessed December 9, 2003].

Arkin WM. 2005. *Michael Brown Was Set Up: It's All in the Numbers.* [Online]. Available: http://blogs.washingtonpost.com/earlywarning/2005/09/michael_brown_w.html [accessed November 1, 2005].

Arnold JL, Lavonas E. 2004. *CBRNE: Personal Protective Equipment.* [Online]. Available: http://www.emedicine.com/emerg/topic894.htm [accessed May 20, 2006].

Asplin BR, Knopp RK. 2001. A room with a view: On-call specialist panels and other health policy challenges in the emergency department. *Annals of Emergency Medicine* 37(5):500–503.

Associated Press. 2006a. *Four Bodies Found Since Dec. 21; Katrina Death Toll Now 1,326.* [Online]. Available: http://www.katc.com/global/story.asp?s=4317545&ClientType= Printable [accessed May 1, 2006].

Associated Press. 2006b. *Band Ex-Manager Sentenced to Four Years in R.I. Club Fire Case.* [Online]. Available: http://www.usatoday.com/news/nation/2006-05-09-fire-hearing_ x.htm [accessed May 11, 2006].

Auf der Heide E. 2006. The importance of evidence-based disaster planning. *Annals of Emergency Medicine* 47(1):34–49.

Augustine J, Kellermann A, Koplan J. 2004. America's emergency care system and severe acute respiratory syndrome: Are we ready? *Annals of Emergency Medicine* 43(1):23–26.

Barthell EN, Cordell WH, Moorhead JC, Handler J, Feied C, Smith MS, Cochrane DG, Felton CW, Collins MA. 2002. The frontlines of medicine project: A proposal for the standardized communication of emergency department data for public health uses including syndromic surveillance for biological and chemical terrorism. *Annals of Emergency Medicine* 39(4):422–429.

BBC News. 2005. *Sarin Attack Remembered in Tokyo.* [Online]. Available: http://news.bbc. co.uk/2/hi/asia-pacific/4365417.stm [accessed May 1, 2006].

BBC News. 2006a. *Bali Death Toll Set at 202.* [Online]. Available: http://news.bbc.co.uk/1/hi/ in_depth/asia_pacific/2002/bali/default.stm [accessed May 1, 2006].

BBC News. 2006b. *Q&A: Bird Flu.* [Online]. Available: http://news.bbc.co.uk/2/hi/ health/3422839.stm [accessed May 1, 2006].

Bravata DM, McDonald K, Owens DK. 2004a. *Regionalization of Bioterrorism Preparedness and Response.* Rockville, MD: Agency for Healthcare Research and Quality.

Bravata DM, McDonald KM, Smith WM, Rydzak C, Szeto H, Buckeridge DL, Haberland C, Owens DK. 2004b. Systematic review: Surveillance systems for early detection of bioterrorism-related diseases. *Annals of Internal Medicine* 140(11):910–922.

Broder DS. 2006, July 16. Unprepared for the attacks: Preparing for flu pandemic. *The Washington Post.* P. A11.

Cass D. 2005. Once upon a time in the emergency department: A cautionary tale. *Annals of Emergency Medicine* 46(6):541–543.

CDC (Centers for Disease Control and Prevention) National Center for Injury Control and Prevention. 2006. *Presentation at the meeting of the Surge Capacity Expert Meeting.* Atlanta, GA: CDC.

CDC. 2005. *Severe Acute Respiratory Syndrome (SARS).* [Online]. Available: http://www.cdc. gov/ncidod/sars/ [accessed October 15, 2005].

CNN.com. 2002. *Anthrax Terror Remains a Mystery.* [Online]. Available: http://archives.cnn. com/2002/US/03/26/anthrax.investigation/ [accessed March 14, 2006].

CNN.com. 2005a. *Tsunami Deaths Soar Past 212,000.* [Online]. Available: http://www.cnn. com/2005/WORLD/asiapcf/01/19/asia.tsunami/ [accessed May 1, 2005].

CNN.com. 2005b. *Four Sought in Attempted Attacks: Police Say Man Shot and Killed in Underground Not One of Four.* [Online]. Available: http://www.cnn.com/2005/WORLD/ europe/07/22/london.tube/index.html [accessed May 1, 2006].

DePalma RG, Burris DG, Champion HR, Hodgson MJ. 2005. Blast injuries. *New England Journal of Medicine* 352(13):1335–1342.

Derlet RW, Richards JR. 2000. Overcrowding in the nation's emergency departments: Complex causes and disturbing effects. *Annals of Emergency Medicine* 35(1):63–68.

DHS (U.S. Department of Homeland Security). 2004. *National Response Plan.* Washington, DC: DHS.

DHS. 2005a. *Metropolitan Medical Response System (MMRS): The First Decade (1995–2005).* Washington, DC: DHS.

DHS. 2005b. *National Planning Scenarios: Created for Use in National, Federal, State, and Local Homeland Security Preparedness Activities.* Washington, DC: DHS.

Donovan K. 2003, April 19. How world let virus spread. *Toronto Star.* P. A.01.

Emergency Management Strategic Healthcare Group, Veterans Health Administration, Department of Veterans Affairs. 2005. *Overview of EMSHG and the 4th Mission.* [Online]. Available: http://www1.va.gov/emshg/docs/EMSHGOverview.ppt#256,1,Overview of EMSHG and the 4th Mission [accessed March 1, 2005].

ER One. 2005, December 13. *The Washington Post.* P. A26.

Feliciano DV, Anderson GV Jr, Rozycki GS, Ingram WL, Ansley JP, Namias N, Salomone JP, Cantwell JD. 1998. Management of casualties from the bombing at the centennial Olympics. *American Journal of Surgery* 176(6):538–543.

Frykberg ERMF. 2004. Principles of mass casualty management following terrorist disasters. *Annals of Surgery* 239(3):319–321.

GAO (U.S. Government Accountability Office). 2003a. *Hospital Emergency Departments: Crowded Conditions Vary Among Hospitals and Communities.* Washington, DC: GAO.

GAO. 2003b. *Hospital Preparedness: Most Urban Hospitals Have Emergency Plans but Lack Certain Capacities for Bioterrorism Response.* Washington, DC: GAO.

GAO. 2003c. *Infectious Diseases: Gaps Remain in Surveillance Capabilities of State and Local Agencies* (GAO-03-1176T). Washington, DC: GAO.

Garrison H, Runyan C, Tintinalli J, Barber C, Bordley W, Hargarten S, Pollock D, Weiss H. 1994. Emergency department surveillance: An examination of issues and a proposal for a national strategy. *Annals of Emergency Medicine* 24(5):849–856.

Geiger J. 2001. Terrorism, biological weapons, and bonanzas: Assessing the real threat to public health. *American Journal of Public Health* 91(5):708–709.

Ginaitt PT. 2005. *Statewide Emergency Preparedness in Rhode Island: Lessons Learned "The Station" Nightclub Fire.* Presentation, Rhode Island Hospital Association. [Online]. Available: http://www.emlrc.org/pdfs/disaster2005presentations/RhodeIslandStationClubFire-LessonsLearned.pdf [accessed May 20, 2006].

Greenberg MI, Hendrickson RG, CIMERC, Drexel University Emergency Department Terrorism Preparedness Consensus, Panel. 2003. Report of the Cimerc/Drexel University Emergency Department Terrorism Preparedness Consensus Panel. *Academic Emergency Medicine* 10(7):783–788.

Gursky, E. 2004. *Hometown Hospitals: The Weakest Link? Bioterrorism Readiness in America's Rural Hospitals.* Washington, DC: National Defense University, Center for Technology and National Security Policy.

Gutierrez de Ceballos JP, Turegano-Fuentes F, Perez-Diaz D, Sanz-Sanchez M, Martin-Llorente C, Guerrero-Sanz JE. 2004. 11 March 2004: The terrorist bomb explosions in Madrid, Spain—an analysis of the logistics, injuries sustained and clinical management of casualties treated at the closest hospital. *Critical Care* 8.

Gutman D, Biffl WL, Suner S, Cioffi WG. 2003. The station nightclub fire and disaster preparedness in Rhode Island. *Medicine and Health, Rhode Island* 86(11):344–346.

Henning KJ. 2003. *Syndromic Surveillance. Microbial Threats to Health: Emergence, Detection, and Response.* Washington, DC: National Academy Press.

Hick JL, Hanfling D, Burstein JL, DeAtley C, Barbisch D, Bogdan GM, Cantrill S. 2004. Health care facility and community strategies for patient care surge capacity. *Annals of Emergency Medicine* 44(3):253–261.

Hirschkorn P. 2003. *New York Reduces 9/11 Death Toll by 40.* [Online]. Available: http://www.cnn.com/2003/US/Northeast/10/29/wtc.deaths/ [accessed May 1, 2006].

Horton DK, Burgess P, Rossiter S, Kaye WE. 2005. Secondary contamination of emergency department personnel from o-chlorobenzylidene malononitrile exposure, 2002. *Annals of Emergency Medicine* 45(6):655–658.

HRSA (Health Resources and Services Administration). *A 2002 National Assessment of State Trauma System Development, Emergency Medical Services Resources, and Disaster Readiness for Mass Casualty Events.* Rockville, MD: HRSA.

HRSA. 2006. *National Bioterrorism Hospital Preparedness Program.* [Online]. Available: http://www.hrsa.gov/bioterrorism/ [accessed April 16, 2006].

IOM (Institute of Medicine). 2002. *Preparing for Terrorism: Tools for Evaluating the Metropolitan Medical Response System.* Washington, DC: The National Academies Press.

IOM. 2004. *Learning from SARS: Preparing for the Next Disease Outbreak. Workshop Summary.* Washington, DC: The National Academies Press.

Insurance Information Network of California. 2006. *Earthquakes.* [Online]. Available: http://iinc.org/pdf/EQ%20Kit%20final.updated.pdf [accessed May 1, 2006].

Jacobs LM, Burns KJ, Gross RI. 2003. Terrorism: A public health threat with a trauma system response. *The Journal of Trauma, Injury, Infection, and Critical Care* 55:1014–1021.

Jordan LJ. 2006, January 2. Homeland security to re-prioritize grants. *Washington Dateline.*

Kaji AH, Waeckerle JF. 2003. Disaster medicine and the emergency medicine resident. *Annals of Emergency Medicine* 41(6):865–870.

Kaji AH, Lewis R. 2004. Hospital disaster preparedness in Los Angeles County, California. *Annals of Emergency Medicine* 44(4).

Kanter RM, Heskett M. 2002. *Washington Hospital Center (B): The Power of Insight.* Boston, MA: Harvard Business School.

The Lewin Group. 2002. *Emergency Department Overload: A Growing Crisis, the Results of the AHA Survey of Emergency Department (ED) and Hospital Capacity.* Washington, DC: American Hospital Association.

McHugh M, Staiti AB, Felland LE. 2004. How prepared are Americans for public health emergencies? Twelve communities weigh in. *Health Affairs (Millwood, VA)* 23(3):201–209.

Niska RW, Burt CW. 2005. Bioterrorism and mass casualty preparedness in hospitals: United States, 2003. *Advance Data* (364):1–14.

ORHP (Office of Rural Health Policy). 2002. *Rural Communities and Emergency Preparedness.* Rockville, MD: ORHP.

OSHA (Occupational Safety and Health Administration). 2005. *OSHA Best Practices for Hospital-Based First Receivers of Victims from Mass Casualty Incidents Involving the Release of Hazardous Substances.* Washington, DC: OSHA.

Pangi R. 2002. *Consequence Management in the 1995 Sarin Attacks on the Japanese Subway System* (BCSIA Discussion Paper 2002–4, ESDP Discussion Paper ESDP-2002–01).Boston, MA: Harvard University, John F. Kennedy School of Government.

Phillips S, Lavin R. 2004. Readiness and response to public health emergencies: Help needed now from professional nursing associations. *Journal of Professional Nursing* 20(5):279–280.

Rand Corporation. 2004. *RAND Study Shows Compensation for 9/11 Terror Attacks Tops $38 Billion; Businesses Receive Biggest Share.* [Online]. Available: http://www.rand.org/news/press.04/11.08b.html [accessed May 1, 2006].

Rivera A, Char D. 2004. Emergency department disaster preparedness: Identifying the barriers. *Annals of Emergency Medicine* 44(4).

Schur C. 2004. *Understanding the Role of the Rural Hospital Emergency Department in Responding to Bioterrorist Attacks and Other Emergencies: A Review of the Literature and Guide to the Issues.* Bethesda, MD: NORC Walsh Center for Rural Health Analysis.

Schur CL, Berk ML, Mueller CD. 2004. *Perspectives of Rural Hospitals on Bioterrorism Preparedness Planning* (W Series, No. 4). Bethesda, MD: NORC Walsh Center for Rural Health Analysis.

Shute N, Marcus MB. 2001. Crisis in the ER. Turning away patients. Long delays. A surefire recipe for disaster. *U.S. News & World Report* 131(9):54–61.

Suner S, Williams K, Shapiro MM, Kobayashi L, Woolard R, Sullivan F. 2004. Effect of personal protective equipment (PPE) on rapid patient assessment and treatment during a simulated chemical weapons of mass destruction (WMD) attack. *Academic Emergency Medicine* 11(5):605.

Talan D, Moran G, Mower W, Newdow M, Ong S, Slutsker L, Jarvis W, Conn L, Pinner R. 1998. EMERGEncy ID NET: An emergency department-based emerging infections sentinel network. *Annals of Emergency Medicine* 32(6):703–711.

Teague DC. 2004. Mass casualties in the Oklahoma City bombing. *Clinical Orthopaedics & Related Research* (422):77–81.

Terndrup T, Nafziger S, Weissman N, Casebeer L, Pryor E. 2005. Online bioterrorism continuing medical education: Development and preliminary testing. *Academic Emergency Medicine* 12(1):45–50.

Times Foundation. 2005. *Kashmir Earthquake: A Situation Report.* India: The Times Group.

Treat KN, Williams JM, Furbee PM, Manley WG, Russell FK, Stamper CD Jr. 2001. Hospital preparedness for weapons of mass destruction incidents: An initial assessment. *Annals of Emergency Medicine* 38(5):562–565.

U.S. Department of State. 2005a. *Patterns of Global Terrorism 2001.* [Online]. Available: http://www.state.gov/documents/organization/10319.pdf [accessed November 1, 2005].

U.S. Department of State. 2005b. *Patterns of Global Terrorism 2002.* [Online]. Available: http://www.state.gov/documents/organization/20177.pdf [accessed November 1, 2005].

U.S. Department of State. 2005c. *Patterns of Global Terrorism 2003.* [Online]. Available: http://www.state.gov/documents/organization/31912.pdf [accessed November 1, 2005].

Waeckerle JF. 1991. Disaster planning and response. *New England Journal of Medicine* 324(12):815–821.

Waeckerle JF, Seamans S, Whiteside M, Pons PT, White S, Burstein JL, Murray R, Task Force of Health Care and Emergency Services Professionals on Preparedness for Nuclear BaC Incidents. 2001. Executive summary: Developing objectives, content, and competencies for the training of emergency medical technicians, emergency physicians, and emergency nurses to care for casualties resulting from nuclear, biological, or chemical incidents. *Annals of Emergency Medicine* 37(6): 587–601.

WHO (World Health Organization). 2005. *Summary of Probable SARS Cases with Onset of Illness from 1 November 2002 to 31 July 2003.* [Online]. Available: http://www.who. int/csr/sars/country/table2004_04_21/en/index.html [accessed November 10, 2005].

Zavotsky KE. 2000. Developing an ED training program: How to "grow your own" ED nurses. *Journal of Emergency Nursing* 26(5):504–506.

8

Enhancing the
Emergency Care Research Base

Emergency care is a broad field of inquiry involving many disciplines and cross-cutting themes. Unlike many other areas of medical research, which tend to be defined by organ systems or types of conditions, emergency care is uniquely defined by the urgency and location of treatment. The emergency care research field has spawned multiple branches, generally defined by specialty or research discipline, that have developed distinct but overlapping identities. The field also extends into disciplines well outside the traditional scope of medical research. Each branch includes basic science, clinical research, and health services research activities.

The fact that emergency care research defies easy description has been proven to be one of the principal challenges facing the field as it seeks its niche in the medical research and funding establishment. Figure 8-1 is an attempt to depict the scope of the field and necessarily is an oversimplification; the lines demarcating the three branches tend to suggest stronger distinctions than actually exist.

The first branch, emergency medicine research, is defined by time and place. It addresses principally conditions and interventions common to pre-hospital emergency medical services (EMS) and hospital emergency department (ED) settings, and its focus is on the acute management of patients. The research is conducted by emergency physicians, often in collaboration with specialists in other fields, such as pediatrics or cardiology. Emergency care research also extends significantly into prevention.

Trauma research is a parallel field of study that is also defined by time and place. It deals principally with the acute management of patients with traumatic injuries. Like emergency medicine research, it is concerned with

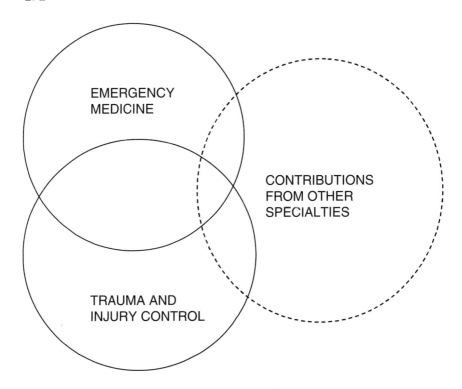

FIGURE 8-1 The scope of emergency care research.

the care of these patients in the prehospital and hospital settings; however, it reaches further into the inpatient setting, particularly the intensive care unit (ICU) and surgical departments, and deals with critical care and the operative management of trauma patients. In addition to trauma surgeons, the research involves specialists in critical care and anesthesiology, as well as collaborators in organ and disease specialties such as neurology and orthopedics. A significant focus of trauma research is service delivery and the effectiveness of trauma care systems.

The injury control field can be thought of as an arm of trauma research that has developed a distinct or rather several distinct areas of focus. It is concerned principally with the prevention of injury, but also overlaps significantly with the acute management of injury and has an additional focus on long-term rehabilitation following traumatic injury. It is one of the most interdisciplinary fields in all of medicine, involving the collaboration of trauma surgeons, numerous medical specialties, engineers, behavioral scientists, and epidemiologists, to name but a few.

The third branch represents many other specialties—disease-, organ system-, and population-based—that lack a direct link to the emergency care setting but either independently or through collaboration with emergency medicine researchers make research contributions that impact emergency care. A significant amount of the research effort in both emergency and trauma care involves translation of findings from these fields into practice in emergency care settings. There has also been substantial research in emergency care that has flowed back to the specialties.

Finally, nursing research is a growing field that spans all three branches. Its principal focus is the clinical management of patients in all settings.

This chapter describes the development and current status of emergency medicine and trauma and injury research, the branches most germane to the present study, with reference to the other specialties as appropriate. The focus is on hospital-based, adult emergency care research; pediatric and prehospital EMS research are addressed in the two companion reports in the *Future of Emergency Care* series. The chapter also examines barriers to emergency care research and presents the committee's recommendations for enhancing the emergency care research enterprise.

EMERGENCY MEDICINE RESEARCH

Emergency care research is vital to the health of Americans. It addresses the care of patients in their most vulnerable moments—when injury or sudden illness strikes. While most Americans have a need for emergency care only rarely, they count on it to be there when needed. Nearly 114 million visits were made to EDs in 2003, and traumatic injury is the leading cause of death among nonelderly adults. In contrast to the vast majority of patient encounters in medicine, the quality and speed of the care that is provided in the relatively brief emergency care encounter can mean the difference between life and death or a prolonged period of disability.

Although emergency medicine and trauma surgery are relatively young specialties, researchers have made important contributions to both basic science and clinical practice that have dramatically improved emergency care and resulted in significant advances in general medicine. Examples include assessment and management of cardiac arrest, including the development and refinement of guidelines for cardiopulmonary resuscitation (CPR) and the pharmacology of resuscitation; understanding and treatment of hemorrhagic shock; electrocardiogram (EKG) analysis of ventricular fibrillation; toxicology and detoxification; injury prevention and control; and uses of diagnostic methods and treatment protocols.

Emergency Care Research Infrastructure and Funding

Because emergency medicine and trauma surgery are young fields, they are not strongly represented in the political infrastructure of the National Institutes of Health (NIH), its various institutes, and its study sections. As a result, scant resources are allocated to advance the science of emergency care, and few training grants are offered to develop researchers who want to focus their work in the field.

A conference held in 1994 highlighted the need to strengthen the academic structure and funding for emergency care research (Josiah Macy, Jr. Foundation, 1995). The report resulting from that conference recommended that academic departments in emergency medicine be increased in number and enhanced, and that the specialty develop a research agenda and a strategic plan for its implementation. In response, the specialty took a number of actions to enhance academic departments and develop the capacity and funding of research in emergency care. In 2003, the American College of Emergency Physicians' (ACEP) Research Committee reported on progress in emergency medicine research (Pollack et al., 2003). Their findings include the following:

• Academic departments in emergency medicine more than doubled between 1991 and 2001, growing from 18 to 48 percent of medical schools. These increases occurred disproportionately among higher-ranked medical schools. At the time of the study, 63 percent of medical schools had either an academic department or a residency program in the field, and 44 percent had both.
• Postresidency fellowships in the field increased from 18 in 1988 to 74 in 2002, although only 12 percent of available fellowships had a primary focus on research.
• By 1999, 54 investigators had been named as principal investigators (PIs) on grants from NIH, the Centers for Disease Control and Prevention (CDC), the Agency for Healthcare Research and Quality (AHRQ), and others. In 2001 there were 40 active grants with emergency-trained PIs, but there are no data on the number of applications rejected.
• The Emergency Medicine Foundation, a small specialty-supported foundation administered by ACEP, has provided development awards to 89 investigators at 53 academic institutions. However, more than 50 percent of those awards have gone to 12 individuals at 7 institutions.

A 2005 report of the ACEP Research Committee noted that emergency medicine residency programs had grown rapidly, from 1 such program in 1970 to 81 in 1990 to 132 in 2005. Currently there are 3,909 emergency medicine residents. The number of federally funded emergency medicine investigators has also increased rapidly but remains low—only 87 in 2005

(ACEP Research Committee, 2005). Just 0.05 percent of NIH training grants awarded to medical schools goes to departments of emergency medicine—an average of only $51.66 per graduating resident. In contrast, other medical specialties have much higher levels of support; for example, internal medicine receives approximately $5,000 per graduating resident per year (see Table 8-1).

While the pace and quality of emergency care–related research have improved steadily over the last two decades, further progress is limited by several factors. These include (1) a limited number of adequately trained laboratory, clinical, and health services investigators; (2) poorly defined professional research tracks (Stern, 2001; Lewis, 2004); (3) limited inter-disciplinary collaboration and multi-institutional research networks; and (4) funding streams that are poorly geared to the nature of emergency care investigations (ACEP Research Committee, 2005).

Research Training Support

Research training grants and fellowships related to emergency care are funded by a number of sources, including institutions, foundations, and federal agencies. Postgraduate fellowships can be categorized into those that

TABLE 8-1 NIH Funding to Medical School Departments for Training Grants in 2003

Field	No. of Awards	Dollar Amounts	Percentage of Total	Active Residents/ Fellows	NIH Training Grant Dollars per Resident
Overall	1,281	370,186,331	100.00		
Internal Medicine	354	107,209,870	29.00	21,351	5,021.30
Pathology	78	28,289,147	7.64	2,257	12,533.96
Psychiatry	78	18,176,767	4.91	4,522	4,019.63
Pediatrics	81	17,547,387	4.74	7,773	2,257.48
Surgery	41	8,302,760	2.24	7,623	1,089.17
Neurology	24	5,654,160	1.53	1,339	4,222.67
Ophthalmology	16	3,346,324	0.90	1,260	2,655.81
Anesthesiology	10	2,640,197	0.71	4,719	559.48
Obstetrics/Gynecology	13	2,324,220	0.63	4,681	496.52
Dermatology	13	2,183,009	0.59	994	2,196.19
Otolaryngology	11	1,989,202	0.54	1,071	1,857.33
Urology	9	1,138,828	0.31	1,038	1,097.14
Neurosurgery	2	599,544	0.16	775	773.61
Orthopedics	4	390,055	0.11	3,024	128.99
Emergency Medicine	**1**	**198,012**	**0.05**	**3,909**	**50.66**
Family Medicine	0	0	0.00	9,529	0.00

SOURCE: ACEP Research Committee, 2005.

are primarily clinical but include a research component (e.g., EMS, pediatric emergency medicine, toxicology) and those that are dedicated to research training. The former category is often funded by institutional resources. Frequently, patient care provides the financial support for the fellowship, limiting the amount of "protected time" trainees have to develop their research careers. It is generally accepted, however, that unless a research training program includes 2 years of dedicated research training (e.g., greater than 80 percent research time), it is unlikely to result in long-term success in today's research climate (NIH, 2003). Thus postgraduate fellowship programs that are supported by clinical activity are unlikely to be an effective means of improving the nation's research capacity in emergency care.

A substantial number of institutions offer dedicated postgraduate research fellowships, which may be funded using institutional resources, may be contingent on the individual applicant's securing extramural funding, or may be funded by extramural support to the institution through an Institutional (T32) Grant. Currently, there is only one emergency care–related institutional training program supported by the T32 mechanism, and its focus is pediatric emergency medicine. No Institutional or Career Development (K12) Grant has ever been awarded directly to an academic department of emergency medicine (ACEP Research Committee, 2005), although some departments may have submitted grant applications under the name of the academic medical center hospital rather than the medical school.

The primary foundation-based supporters of emergency care research training are the Emergency Medicine Foundation (EMF), affiliated with ACEP, and the Society for Academic Emergency Medicine (SAEM). Both entities fund individual research fellowships for trainees who have completed residency training in emergency medicine, or in the case of SAEM, in pediatrics with the intent to pursue pediatric emergency medicine fellowship training. Currently, the EMF fellowship grants supply only a single year of training, although 2-year fellowships may be added. The SAEM individual research training grants provide 2 years of training. SAEM also funds an institutional training grant, through which 2 years of support is provided to the institution with the intent that the institution will then recruit an appropriate trainee. This funding mechanism was explicitly modeled after the T32 mechanism.

A handful of emergency care research trainees have secured individual NIH F32 National Research Service Award (NRSA) fellowship funding. Further, a notable number of emergency care researchers have obtained support for career development and educational activities through the K08 and K23 mechanisms (ACEP Research Committee, 2005).

As detailed in the 2005 ACEP report (ACEP Research Committee, 2005), a substantial proportion of all emergency medicine trainees intend to pursue an academic career, yet paradoxically, the support devoted to emergency care research and research training is very low, especially compared with other medical specialties. While existing foundation support has modestly increased the number of well-trained emergency care investigators, substantial growth in the total available research training support will be required to expand the emergency care research capability nationwide.

Many have noted a concerning lack of young investigators, both in industry-sponsored clinical trials and among the ranks of federally supported clinical investigators. Sung and colleagues (2003, p. 1282) reported that "8 percent of principal investigators conducting industry-sponsored clinical trials are younger than forty years," and "less than 4 percent of competing research grants awarded by the National Institutes of Health (NIH) in 2001 were awarded to investigators aged thirty-five years or younger" (see also Zisson, 2001; Goldman and Marshall, 2002). By contrast, investigators in emergency care specialties, including emergency medicine, pediatric emergency medicine, and EMS, are characterized by their relative youth. Physician-scientists in these fields are generally recently trained, and with the receipt of additional clinical research training may be well positioned to initiate productive, long-term clinical research careers. In its 2005 report, ACEP called for the development of 100 new investigators within 10 years through the NIH Mentored Career Development Award Program (K12) at an estimated cost of $50 million over 10 years. Sung and colleagues (2003, p. 1283) recommended that, as part of a strategy to increase the number of well-trained clinical investigators, academic health centers and research sponsors, including federal sponsors, "increase opportunities for training in all areas of clinical research, including health services and outcomes research, clinical trials, and research synthesis, and develop a mechanism for collecting longitudinal data on training program outcomes."

Similarly, many have noted the lack of a sufficient pool of well-trained laboratory and patient-oriented investigators in emergency care. Nevertheless, emergency medicine investigators have made important contributions in laboratory investigations of shock, ischemia–reperfusion, cellular injury, early biomarkers for cardiac ischemia, cerebral resuscitation, and neuroprotection. For many years, medical training in the specialties of emergency medicine, pediatric emergency medicine, and trauma surgery were heavily focused on the development of clinical skills, with little formal training in research methodology. As noted by Stern (2001), formal fellowship training is now a well-recognized requirement for those embarking on a successful long-term research-based academic career. To address the shortage of training for new investigators in emergency medicine, the committee recommends that **academic medical centers support emergency and trauma care research by providing research time and adequate facilities for promising emergency care and trauma investigators, and by strongly considering the establishment of autonomous departments of emergency medicine (8.1).**

Research Funding

A 1994 review of nonmilitary research articles published in three emergency medicine journals revealed that the majority of articles did not list a source of funding. This is in contrast to other specialties, in which the majority of published research was funded. The literature review also found that funded studies published in the emergency medicine literature were less likely to be federally supported and more likely to be supported by industrial sources relative to studies published in the literature of other specialties (Wright and Wrenn, 1994). Although these results may be dated, federal funding, and in particular NIH funding, remains difficult for emergency medicine researchers to obtain (Morris and Manning, 2004). The limited amount of funding available for emergency care research extends across a wide range of institutes, programs, and sponsors, although NIH remains the key sponsor.

As noted earlier, because of the cross-cutting nature of emergency care, the field overlaps with many other medical disciplines. This makes it difficult to establish a unique funding home for emergency care within NIH and other research sponsors that tend to have a traditional orientation based on diseases or body parts. On the other hand, the cross-cutting nature of emergency care exposes it to many opportunities for collaboration with other research specialties and disciplines, and collaborating with established researchers in other fields may be a good way for emergency care investigators to obtain or expand their research funding.

National Institutes of Health   NIH includes 20 institutes, seven centers, and four program offices contained within the Office of the Director (OD). NIH is the largest single source of support for biomedical research in the world, with a budget of over $27 billion in 2004 (IOM, 2004). All institutes but only some of the centers (e.g., the Center on Scientific Review [CSR]) provide research funding, while several other centers provide general support. All institutes and four of the centers receive individual congressional appropriations. The NIH institutes are organized into five categories, some by disease (e.g., the National Institute of Neurological Disorders and Stroke [NINDS]), some by organ system (e.g., the National Heart, Lung and Blood Institute [NHLBI]), some by stage of life (e.g., the National Institute of Child Health and Human Development [NICHD]), some by scientific discipline (e.g., the National Human Genome Research Institute [NHGRI]), and some by profession or technology (e.g., the National Institute of Nursing Research [NINR] and the National Institute of Biomedical Imaging and Bioengineering [NIBIB]) (IOM, 2003). None of the current institutes or centers is defined either by the site of care or the timing or urgency of care—defining characteristics of emergency care research. Perhaps for this reason, NIH does not have an institute or center focused specifically on emergency services. Thus, many important emergency care clinical questions extend beyond the domains of single NIH institutes or centers. While both a 2003 Institute of Medicine (IOM) report (IOM, 2003) and the NIH Roadmap Initiative (Zerhouni, 2003) emphasized the importance of stimulating and funding trans-NIH research, and emergency care research questions naturally span the domains of multiple institutes and centers, the lack of attention to emergency care has not been effectively addressed. In fact, the term "emergency care" does not appear in the NIH Roadmap.

Other federal agencies   Many other federal agencies provide small amounts of research funding in emergency care. AHRQ, for example, like NIH, does not have a dedicated funding stream for research on emergency services. However, it does have a long track record of funding grants in emergency care, such as a study on the effects of cost sharing on use of the ED, evaluation of technologies for identifying acute cardiac ischemia in EDs, and measurement of ED crowding (AHRQ, 2004).

The Health Resources and Services Administration (HRSA), through its Emergency Medical Services for Children (EMS-C) Program, sponsors the Pediatric Emergency Care Applied Research Network (PECARN), the first federally funded multi-institutional network for research in pediatric emergency medicine. The EMS-C Program also sponsors the National EMS Data Analysis Resource Center (NEDARC), which was established in 1995 to help states collect and analyze data on pediatric EMS systems and to populate the pediatric trauma registry. The HRSA Trauma-EMS Systems Program and the Office of Rural Health Policy also support research efforts in emergency care.

CDC's National Center for Injury Prevention and Control (NCIPC) sponsors investigations in injury prevention and control and recently developed an Acute Care Research Agenda for the Future. NCIPC/CDC and the Consumer Product Safety Commission cosponsor the National Electronic Injury Surveillance System (NEISS), a longitudinal database with information from 100 hospital EDs on consumer product–related injuries, and since 2000 on all injuries. NCIPC also sponsors the Data Elements for Emergency Department Systems (DEEDS) project, a national effort to develop uniform specifications for data entered in ED patient records.

The Office of EMS in the National Highway Traffic Safety Administration (NHTSA) plays a lead role in coordinating activities related to EMS system development and research. Together with HRSA, NHTSA sponsored the development of the National Emergency Medical Services Research Agenda (NHTSA, 2001). The Office currently funds two key research initiatives: the Emergency Medical Services Outcomes Project, a study to develop metrics for use in EMS-related outcomes research, and the Emergency Medical Services Cost Analysis Project, a study to develop metrics for assessing the costs and benefits of EMS. NHTSA and HRSA cosponsor the National EMS Information System (NEMSIS), a national database on EMS systems and outcomes that is operated by the National Association of State EMS Directors. NHTSA's Office of Human-Centered Research sponsors the Crash Injury Research and Engineering Network (CIREN), a network of level I trauma centers that collect and share detailed research data on automobile crashes, injuries, and outcomes.

Although not research funding per se, funds are being provided by NHTSA's Office of EMS for the National EMS Scope of Practice Model project, a joint initiative of the National Association of State EMS Directors and the National Council of State EMS Training Coordinators. The Longitudinal Emergency Medical Technician Attribute and Demographics Study (LEADS) is a NHTSA-funded project of the National Registry of Emergency Medical Technicians. An annual LEADS survey collects information on the EMS workforce.

The Centers for Medicare and Medicaid Services (CMS), the Department of Homeland Security, and the Department of Veterans' Affairs also provide small amounts of funding related to emergency care research.

Private Funders

SAEM and EMF both provide investigator training grants, as described earlier. EMF awarded 18 grants in 2004–2005 totaling almost $500,000 (Pollack and Cairns, 1999; ACEP, 2005). The Robert Wood Johnson Foundation funded the Urgent Matters project, which provided grants to 10 hospitals and their communities for evaluating approaches to reducing crowding and improving patient flow. A small number of emergency medicine researchers received research training through The Robert Wood Johnson Clinical Scholars program. The National Emergency Medicine Association also provides research grants in trauma and emergency care.

Future Directions in Emergency Care Research

Pressing gaps remain in our understanding of emergency care in all three research areas: basic science, clinical research, and health services research. There have been several recent attempts to identify research priorities and key opportunities in emergency care (Aghababian et al., 1996; Maio et al., 1999; Seidel et al., 1999; Becker et al., 2002). The EMS Research Agenda for the Future project (Sayre et al., 2005) identified priority issues for targeted research efforts, including asthma, acute cardiac ischemia, circulatory shock, major injury, pain, acute stroke, and traumatic brain injury, as well as education and system design issues. Critical research questions identified by these groups cut across basic science, clinical research, and health services research. Some fertile topics for research in each area are described below.

Basic Science

Because emergency medicine is defined by time and place, rather than body part or disease process, research in the field is often mischaracterized as being strictly translational in nature. But emergency medicine requires both basic discoveries and translation of those discoveries to the clinical setting. Basic research projects involving emergency medicine investigators focus on the following:

- Characterization of the molecular events that cause delayed neuronal death after brain ischemia and other studies on neuronal injury (multiple NINDS grants).
- The pathophysiology of carbon monoxide poisoning and mechanisms for the benefit of hyperbaric oxygen therapy (multiple NIH grants).
- Understanding of the events that occur following ischemia–reperfusion injury from cardiac arrest, using animal models, cardiomyocyte cell culture models, and methods for inducing hypothermia for treatment of patients following cardiac arrest (NIH).
- The pathophysiology of acute lung injury and acute respiratory failure (NHLBI).
- Means of minimizing the risk of secondary ischemic brain injury during limited resuscitation from hemorrhagic shock and traumatic brain injury (Department of Defense [DoD]).
- Identification of effective neuroprotective agents to limit tissue loss and enhance recovery following acute traumatic brain injury or stroke (NINDS, CDC).
- Pathophysiology and treatment of traumatic spinal cord injury (NIH).
- Hypothermia and gene expression following cardiac arrest (NIH).
- Pathophysiological processes that contribute to the destruction of articular cartilage in a variety of disorders, including an evaluation of immunoprobes for lubricin from human synovial fluid (NIH).
- Understanding of the human genomic and proteomic response to injury and injury recovery.

Clinical Research

Because of the wide range of patients, diseases, and interventions seen by physicians in emergency practice, these practitioners have a unique window on the state of treatment options available, including their shortcomings.

Thus emergency physicians have both the motivation and opportunity for focused efforts aimed at translating research into better modes of treatment. As a result, clinical research represents the most active area of emergency care research. Examples include the following:

- The efficacy, safety, and dosages of medications for infants, children, adolescents, adults, and the elderly.
- Definition of an effective and practical diagnostic and risk-stratification strategy for patients with possible pulmonary embolism (Kline and Wells, 2003; Brown et al., 2005; Courtney and Kline, 2005; Kline et al., 2004, 2005).
- Development of evidenced-based protocols for common pediatric conditions (e.g., fever).
- Evaluation of the pharmacokinetics and efficacy of promising clinical therapies for treatment of acute traumatic brain injury (Wright et al., 2005).
- Development and testing of new therapies and strategies for resuscitation of the multiply injured trauma patient (Bickell et al., 1992; Coimbra et al., 1997; Angle et al., 1998; Sloan et al., 1999a; Cooper, 2004).
- Evidence-based criteria for determining which patients with community-acquired pneumonia require hospitalization (current national guidelines are based largely on a risk stratification model created from data that did not include manipulation of the decision to admit (Fine et al., 1997).
- Definition and testing of strategies for determining which patients with possible acute coronary syndromes require hospitalization and for those who do, definition of the appropriate level of care.
- Identification and testing of new strategies for the prevention of secondary brain injury after both traumatic and ischemic insults (The Hypothermia after Cardiac Arrest Study Group, 1921; Stern et al., 2000; Neumar, 2000; Bernard et al., 2002; Nolan et al., 2003; Abella et al., 2004).
- Use of blood substitutes by paramedics.
- Evaluation of simplified methods of CPR instruction (Kellermann et al., 1989; Eisenberg et al., 1995; Todd et al., 1998, 1999).
- Assessment of the potentially deleterious effects of hyperventilation on successful resuscitation following cardiac arrest (Auf der Heide et al., 2004).

Health Services Research

Emergency medicine by definition requires timely and efficient approaches to the delivery of services. The impact of the organization and mode of delivery has long been recognized as having a major impact on the quality of care and outcomes—first codified in Crowley's "golden hour" and Pantridge's cardiac care in the field, and reinforced through military and civilian experience. But the organization and delivery of services is perhaps the weakest link in the emergency care evidence base. Even accepted doctrine, such as the value of paramedics in the field, has recently been overturned. This, then, represents a formative and essential area for research. Some of the key research questions in service delivery include the following:

- The impact of bottlenecks in different hospital units (e.g., ICU, telemetry) on ED crowding and patient flow.
- The effectiveness of queuing theory in smoothing patient volume to alleviate crowding, boarding, and diversion.
- The effect of timeliness of out-of-hospital response, stratified by etiology and/or severity of injury.
- Identification of which components of trauma systems impact outcomes and cost-effectiveness.
- The causes of and solutions for missed diagnoses in the ED.
- Validation of the use of prehospital 12-lead electrocardiography to direct patients with acute ST-elevation myocardial infarction (STEMI) to interventional cardiac centers.
- The impact of medical direction in EMS systems.
- Use of prehospital electrocardiography to identify and directly transport patients to a cardiac catheterization laboratory for percutaneous coronary intervention.
- The impact of prearrival information from dispatchers about the condition of patients with respect to both arrival at the hospital and long-term outcome.
- Evaluation of safe alternatives to endotracheal intubation for securing the airway in prehospital and ED settings.
- The feasibility and cost-effectiveness of implementing point-of-care HIV testing of high-risk patients in the ED.
- Development of a practical testing technology for evaluating mild traumatic brain injury and other causes of cognitive impairment in prehospital, sports, and ED settings.
- Use of computers to screen ED patients for a variety of health risk behaviors, including intimate partner violence, depression, substance abuse, and suicide.

This and the above lists of basic science and translational research are not meant to be all-inclusive or even representative of current research challenges or priorities, but merely to suggest the breadth of important research questions in need of attention.

Multicenter Research Collaborations

Many of the important successes in emergency care research have been based on the establishment of large-scale multicenter research collaborations. Such collaborations enable researchers to assemble sufficiently large datasets to establish robust research findings.

There are a number of examples of successful studies by multicenter research collaborations. The National Emergency X-Radiography Utilization Study (NEXUS), for example, has investigated the use of cervical spine radiography in patients suffering blunt trauma (Hoffman et al., 1998, 2000). The Multicenter Airway Research Collaboration (MARC)/Emergency Medicine Network (EMNet) is studying respiratory disease management strategies in the ED (EMNet, 2005). The EMERGEncy ID Net collaboration provides important information on the characteristics and management of infectious diseases in the ED (Cydulka et al., 2003; Kim et al., 2004), as well as sentinel detection of emerging infectious diseases (Talan et al., 1998, 1999, 2003; Moran et al., 2000). The Resuscitation Outcomes Consortium network, sponsored by NIH and DoD, is addressing prehospital-based trauma and cardiac arrest resuscitation in North America. A number of emergency medicine departments are participating in or heading programs related to this endeavor. The Inflammation and the Host-Response to Injury study is a National Institute of General Medical Sciences (NIGMS) Glue Grant[1] that has joined clinical level I trauma centers, genomic centers, and proteomic high-throughput centers in a multi-institutional, multidisciplinary attempt to explore the genomic, proteomic, and phenotypic host response to the stress of severe injury (Calvano et al., 2005). Finally, PECARN, sponsored by HRSA's EMS-C program, focuses on prevention and management of acute illnesses and injuries in children through four research nodes (PECARN, 2003, 2005). The publication records of these collaborative efforts, as well as the impact of those publications on clinical care, illustrate the power of such research collaborations to address pressing clinical questions, as well as the ability of the emergency care research community to organize and conduct large-scale clinical research endeavors.

TRAUMA AND INJURY CONTROL RESEARCH

It is difficult to characterize the field of trauma and injury control research. For one thing, the field has expanded dramatically in scope from its early focus on treatment of injuries. It has become increasingly interdisciplinary and now includes investigators from a broad range of fields, such as

---

[1]Glue Grants are NIH research initiatives that bring together multidisciplinary teams of researchers from different centers to solve a research problem.

engineering, epidemiology, behavioral sciences, biomechanics, criminology, molecular biology, and human factors research.

While trauma and injury are, by and large, identical or at least overlapping, the terms do suggest some differences in focus, type of investigator, and setting. Historically, trauma research was focused clinically on treatment of injury and was strongly influenced by advances in trauma treatment gleaned from battlefield experiences. Injury research can be viewed as a newer endeavor, and one that has branched out in new directions. But even here the distinctions are nuanced rather than clear cut. The modern fields of trauma and injury research began to take shape in the 1960s as a result of the increasing number of highway deaths. The National Academy of Sciences/National Research Council (NAS/NRC) report *Accidental Death and Disability* (NAS and NRC, 1966) was followed by a burst of regulatory activity, including passage of the Highway Safety Act; establishment of NHTSA, the Occupational Safety and Health Administration, and the Consumer Product Safety Commission; and the founding of the American Trauma Society. These events collectively signaled a new national commitment to reducing death and disability due to injury.

The new field of injury science was based on the recognition that patterns of injury could be determined with the epidemiological tools of public health. William Haddon, a public health physician, set forth a scientific paradigm for analyzing injury based on the interaction between human and environmental factors (Haddon, 1968). The 1985 NRC/IOM report *Injury in America* (NRC and IOM, 1985) presented the idea of injury prevention and control as a separate discipline. It proposed the establishment of an injury center at CDC, which led to passage of the Injury Control Act of 1990. As a result of this legislation, the Division of Injury Epidemiology and Control was elevated to NCIPC. NCIPC's focus on nonoccupational injuries was designed to complement a new center at NIH focused on occupational injuries—the National Institute on Occupational Safety and Health (NIOSH). While establishing a science base in injury prevention and surveillance, the development of these centers represented a divergence from trauma research, which remained more focused on treatment and service delivery.

The Trauma Field

The U.S. military experience during the Korean and Vietnam wars provided evidence that an organized health system with medical capabilities could improve chances of survival from trauma (GAO, 1991). Physicians returning from the war tried to apply the advances made and lessons learned during the war to civilian life. Through the availability of helicopters, the time required to evacuate the wounded from the battlefield was cut dramatically, resulting in decreased mortality rates. Other advances during the period include the availability of whole blood, well-organized medical teams, well-equipped forward hospitals, and more effective management of medical resources.

Along with advances made during the Korean and Vietnam wars, several medical and technology advances during this period coincided with the development of trauma centers. In 1956, Drs. Elan and Safar developed mouth-to-mouth resuscitation. In 1959, researchers at Johns Hopkins developed the first portable defibrillator and perfected CPR; the first out-of-hospital defibrillation occurred in 1969. These advances provided a means to stabilize victims, thereby making it possible for more critically ill patients to arrive at the hospital for care. During this period, prehospital EMS became more sophisticated, while at the same time trauma centers and systems were developed and formalized.

The American College of Surgeons Committee on Trauma (ACS COT) has also made significant contributions and played a major leadership role in the development of trauma centers. In 1976 ACS COT first published *Optimal Hospital Resources for Care of the Seriously Injured* (ACS COT, 1976). This document, updated most recently in 1999, identified the key characteristics for the categorization of hospitals as trauma centers. In 1987 ACS COT initiated an external review process for trauma centers. ACS COT also recently published *Consultation for Trauma Systems*, which provides guidelines for evaluating trauma system development (ACS, 1987).

In 1981 a seminal article, "Regionalization of Trauma Care," outlined the key elements of the modern trauma system (Trunkey, 1981). The Major Trauma Outcome Study was undertaken in 1982 to improve scoring systems for trauma centers, establish national outcome data, and provide objective evaluations of quality assurance and outcomes for trauma care; by 1989, data on 170,000 patients from more than 150 institutions had been recorded (IOM, 1999). In addition, in 1986 ACEP published *Guidelines for Trauma Care Systems*, addressing prehospital care (ACEP, 1986).

A significant body of research has focused on the effectiveness of trauma systems. In 1998 the Skamania Conference was convened to review the medical evidence on trauma systems.[2] The conference called for renewed federal funding for trauma system development and the drafting of a visionary document on the subject.

Trauma research has also focused on injury scales/scoring systems, leading to a succession of refinements to the precision and usefulness of these scales (e.g., the Abbreviated Injury Scale, the Injury Severity Score, the Anatomic Profile, the New Injury Severity Score, the Glasgow Coma Scale,

---

[2]A September 1999 supplemental issue of the *Journal of Trauma* was devoted to the Skamania Conference. See *Journal of Trauma*, v. 47, No. 3 (supplement).

and the Revised Trauma Score). These scales are important for standardizing the measurement of injury and have multiple applications, including triage, diagnosis, and research.

Injury Control

The injury control field is focused less on treatment and more on surveillance and prevention. It links researchers in public health, medicine, and engineering and includes many disciplines. Systematic collection of injury data through such databases as NEISS, the National Trauma Data Bank, the Fatality Analysis Reporting System (FARS), and state trauma registries is critical to gathering sufficient observations to permit meaningful research. Most states have trauma registries, but the data elements are variable and generally not linked with one another. The American College of Surgeons (ACS) established the National Trauma Data Bank (NTDB) as a voluntary repository of trauma records. In 2005 the NTDB contained almost 1.5 million records from 565 trauma centers in 45 states, U.S. territories, and the District of Columbia. It represents 70 percent of level I and 53 percent of level II trauma centers (ACS, 2005).

Injury research has led to a wide range of prevention successes. By far the most important of these successes have occurred in prevention and control of motor vehicle crash injuries. Others include childproof containers; mandated use of smoke alarms; laws requiring motorcycle and bicycle helmets, sports pads, and mouth guards; and safe refrigerator disposal to prevent suffocation. Successes related to motor vehicles range from seatbelts, airbags, and child safety restraint systems to graduated driver's license programs and improvements in highway design. An important current initiative is CIREN, whose mission is "to improve the prevention, treatment and rehabilitation of motor vehicle crash injuries to reduce deaths, disabilities, and human and economic costs" (NHTSA and CIREN Center Staffs, 2003, p. 1). CIREN researchers have had a significant impact in improving safety research, automobile safety, and emergency medical care.

Much of this research is concerned with the field of injury biomechanics—the study of physical and physiological responses to both penetrating and nonpenetrating impacts. Examples of the disciplines involved in this branch of study are robotics, physical therapy, orthopedics, physical and sports medicine, prosthetics, orthotics, and tissue engineering.

One area that has been highly underresearched relative to the magnitude of its impact is primary and secondary prevention of falls. Falls are a significant problem among toddlers and the elderly and are now the most common cause of traumatic brain injuries among the latter. With the aging of the population, this problem will only grow in importance over time (Wadman et al., 2003).

The injury field has focused largely on unintentional injuries but has begun to address intentional injuries—for example, those caused by firearms and suicide. Whereas the trauma field has long been interested in gunshot injuries from a treatment perspective, the injury field has looked at such injuries from the prevention perspective. Although widely accepted today, this new area of focus led to substantial debate about priorities in the field. Prevention of suicide and violence extends into the realms of behavioral science, sociology, and even economics. Indeed, the scope of injury research now encompasses many disciplines—epidemiology, behavioral sciences, biomedical science, biomechanics, criminology, sociology, engineering, law, molecular biology, and others.

Research Infrastructure and Funding

The majority of support for trauma and injury research comes from NIH and CDC, with limited support being provided by NHTSA, HRSA, AHRQ, DoD, and others.

National Institutes of Health

By far the most important source of funding for trauma research is NIH. The 1966 report *Accidental Death and Disability* recommended that NIH establish an Institute for Trauma. While this recommendation was never implemented, trauma research at NIH has grown. NIH convened a task force to study the needs and gaps in trauma research and produced the *Report of the Task Force on Trauma Research* (NIH, 1994). This report recommended doubling funding for trauma research centers, but sufficient funding was never appropriated to carry out this recommendation. Relevant areas of trauma and injury research funding are spread across multiple NIH institutes and centers—for example, NIGMS Research Centers in Trauma, Burn, and Perioperative Injury; the National Heart Attack Alert Program within NHLBI; and NINDS, which includes a Program on Trauma, Regeneration and Pain focused almost exclusively on neurotrauma. Finally, NICHD has a National Center for Medical Rehabilitation Research, which includes both injury-related and non-injury-related rehabilitation.

Total NIH support for research on trauma and injury is very limited in relation to the importance of both in terms of mortality, disability, and costs. The costs of trauma approach 10 percent of health care spending, and injury is the number one killer of nonelderly adults (IOM, 1999). Traumatic injury has surpassed heart disease as the most expensive category of medical treatment, resulting in $71.6 billion dollars in expenditures per year (AHRQ, 2006). In 1998, injury was the third-leading cause of death in terms of years of potential life lost (YPLL), yet NIH injury research was collectively funded at a level of less than $200 million. In terms of YPLL, trauma received only $.10, compared with $3.51 for HIV/AIDS and $1.65 for cancer (IOM, 1999).

Just as important, with research spread across programs, there is little opportunity for coordination or the development of comprehensive research centers. The 1999 IOM report *Reducing the Burden of Injury: Advancing Prevention and Treatment* stated that "NIH lacks a focal point and a mechanism for coordinating disparate injury research projects and programs" (IOM, 1999, p. 229). The report recommended expanding the program within NIGMS and elevating the Trauma and Burn Program to a division. In addition, there is scant support for the development of investigators in the field.

Centers for Disease Control and Prevention

As noted earlier, the NRC/IOM report *Injury in America: A Continuing Public Health Problem* (NRC and IOM, 1985) led to the Injury Control Act of 1990, which elevated CDC's Division of Injury Epidemiology and Control to NCIPC. NCIPC includes three divisions: Unintentional Injury Prevention, Violence Prevention, and Injury and Disability Outcomes. It operates much like an NIH center, with a focus on extramural research grants, plus cooperative agreements with states. NCIPC has nurtured biomechanics research and funded comprehensive Injury Control Research Centers. Some have argued that relative to NIH, CDC has funding limitations and lacks the infrastructure to pursue a strong basic and clinical research agenda (IOM, 1999). NCIPC supports no investigator training grants, but NIOSH does have a small number of pre- and postdoctoral training grants in occupational injury prevention. The IOM recommended that the center develop interdisciplinary training in epidemiology, biostatistics, biomechanics, and behavioral sciences through collaborations with NHTSA, HRSA, NIOSH, and others (IOM, 1999).

Other Agencies

With the exception of the NHTSA-supported CIREN program, described above, there is only limited support for trauma and injury research in other agencies. Most research in system design is sponsored by NCIPC and AHRQ, but health services research is not well funded in general, and trauma and injury represent a very small component of that research. HRSA's EMS and Trauma Systems Program supported the development and evaluation of trauma systems until it was defunded for fiscal year 2006.

Current and Future Research Directions

Current directions in trauma and injury research have been the subject of several recent reports. The NIH and DoD Working Group on Trauma Research Program was convened in 2003 and developed a report that identified and summarized current trauma research priorities (Hoyt et al., 2004). It identified priorities in three key areas: basic science, clinical trials, and clinical research. In basic sciences, it identified cellular injury (immune response following injury), bleeding and thrombosis, central nervous system injuries, and multiple organ failure. Areas in need of clinical trials to establish efficacy included airway management, fluid resuscitation, therapies for controlling bleeding, adjuvants to control postinjury immune response, and body temperature management. The three top areas for clinical research were physiological monitoring, automated clinical data collection, and development of large-scale longitudinal datasets for research. The report cited the continuing lack of an organized infrastructure as an impediment to progress in resolving a number of key issues and addressed ways to build this infrastructure for resuscitation research, including development of a consistent informed consent process (for multicenter trials), formation of an animal model consortium, increased use of multicenter trials, centralized tissue banks, and standardized data collection and analysis.

In 2002, NCIPC developed a research agenda that addressed the following broad injury categories: injuries at home, sports, transportation, domestic violence, suicide, youth violence, acute care, disability, and rehabilitation. The agenda also identified four cross-cutting research priorities: translating research into programs and policies, improving parenting and controlling alcohol abuse, identifying the costs and consequences of injury, and building the research infrastructure.

In 2005, CDC updated the acute care chapter of the 2002 agenda. This revision identified seven research priorities:

- Better translation of findings into patient care through guidelines
- Evidence-based protocols
- How trauma systems improve care
- How mass casualty impacts acute care
- Clinical prevention
- Psychosocial impact of injury
- Development of short- and long-term outcome measures

The report also called for enhancing research capacity through four actions: the development of acute care injury research networks; the conduct of research by mining current and future databases; the development of new investigators though training grants; and reductions in institutional barriers to research, such as Emergency Medical Treatment and Active Labor Act

(EMTALA) regulations. Finally, the report noted the need for more research on morbidity and disability outcomes (National Center for Injury Prevention and Control, 2005).

BARRIERS TO EMERGENCY CARE RESEARCH

There are unique logistical problems associated with conducting emergency care research, such as lack of a coordinating funding structure; the difficulty of establishing informed consent in emergency care situations; and the challenge of linking medical records to reconstruct an episode of care across prehospital, ED, and inpatient settings.

Organization and Funding of Emergency Care Research

Taken as a whole, the emergency care research enterprise has accomplished a great deal. Many of these accomplishments have been made with bootstrap funding and by poorly supported researchers in a disconnected fashion. But the field has reached a level of maturity that requires a new approach. There are well-defined areas of critical inquiry that require a coordinated and well-funded approach. In addition, there is a crucial need for an integrated research effort across disease lines that breaks down departments and requires multidisciplinary approaches to achieve effective translational research. This effort must include a wide range of disciplinary strengths—from epidemiology, pathophysiology, and toxicology to surgery, psychology, and biomechanics—to integrate the wide range of interrelated medical and sociological issues faced by the modern ED. It should be clear that the current uncoordinated approach to organizing and funding emergency and trauma care is ineffective. Therefore, the committee recommends that **the Secretary of the Department of Health and Human Services conduct a study to examine the gaps and opportunities in emergency and trauma care research, and recommend a strategy for the optimal organization and funding of the research effort (8.2).** This study should include consideration of training of new investigators, development of multicenter research networks, funding of General Clinical Research Centers that specifically include an emergency and trauma care component, involvement of emergency and trauma care researchers in the grant review and research advisory processes, and improved research coordination through a dedicated center or institute **(8.2a). Congress and federal agencies involved in emergency and trauma care research (including the Department of Transportation, the Department of Health and Human Services, the Department of Homeland Security, and the Department of Defense) should implement the study's recommendations (8.2b).** This study should encompass the broad range of emergency care research, including emergency medicine, trauma, and injury and basic, science, clinical research and health services research, and should consider ways to enhance the coordination of emergency care research across topics, disciplines, and agencies.

The inclusion of emergency care researchers on advisory and review committees has special merit in the committee's view. NIH, for example, uses a wide variety of advisory committees: (1) initial review groups (IRGs, also known as study sections) and special emphasis panels (SEPs), (2) national advisory councils, (3) boards of scientific counselors, and (4) program advisory committees. The IRGs and SEPs perform the first level of peer review, scoring grant applications on technical and scientific merit. The national advisory councils perform a second level of peer review, providing advice to the institute or center both on the funding of individual applications and on more general issues related to the mission and goals of the institute or center. The combined review by the IRGs/SEPs and the national advisory councils is commonly termed the "dual review system" (IOM, 2003). The boards of scientific counselors perform retrospective reviews of intramural research programs and are not discussed further here. The program advisory committees provide input on research programs, future research directions, and the development of extramural research initiatives (IOM, 2003). The vast majority of members of advisory committees are appointed by either the NIH director or the directors of the individual institutes or centers.

Emergency care providers often have a unique perspective on the evaluation and management of specific syndromes and diseases, as they routinely manage the most acute and extreme manifestations of those conditions and must often act decisively with only preliminary clinical information. Thus, emergency care providers can provide important complementary perspectives during the framing of clinical research questions to be addressed by interdisciplinary clinical research teams and during the evaluation of research applications and proposals. These perspectives can be particularly valuable for judging proposals that require the timely recruitment of research subjects in acute care situations and for addressing the logistical challenges of conducting well-controlled clinical research in EDs, trauma centers, and other acute care environments.

General Clinical Research Centers (GCRCs) play a critical role in supporting the clinical research enterprise and serving as a fertile ground for the development and training of young clinical investigators. There are currently 87 GCRCs supported by the National Center for Research Resources, which include both inpatient facilities and ambulatory research clinics associated with academic health centers. These facilities are potentially valuable in providing mentorship to new clinical investigators and junior faculty and in facilitating the enrollment of subjects into clinical research studies. However, GCRCs rarely if ever support clinical research conducted in the ED, much less in out-of-hospital settings. Thus, emergency care investigators have not had access to an important national resource. One reason is that most GCRCs are funded to conduct scheduled clinical research protocols. They are not well staffed, if staffed at all, to conduct emergency and trauma care research on a full-time basis. While it would be neither feasible nor perhaps prudent to staff all GCRCs in this way, a subset of GCRCs, particularly those based in hospitals with a major ED and level I trauma center, might be encouraged to compete for supplemental awards to support time-critical clinical trials on resuscitation and trauma care research.[3]

Protection of Human Research Subjects

Federal rules govern the protection of human research subjects, and these rules are enforced by institutional review boards (IRBs). Additional rules to protect the privacy of human subjects are defined in the Privacy Rule of the Health Insurance Portability and Accountability Act (HIPAA). The Office for Human Research Protections (OHRP) within the Department of Health and Human Services is the agency assigned to enforce protections for human subjects. The rules attempt to balance the value of important research against the potential harm to patients resulting from that research. Some have argued that the current rules overly restrict critically important research, particularly in emergency and trauma care (Newgard et al., 2005).

Informed consent requirements represent an important tool for evaluating new and promising therapies in an ethical and publicly transparent manner; however, complying with the requirements can be overly burdensome for emergency care researchers. Patients treated in the emergency care setting frequently have suffered acute, debilitating illnesses or injuries (e.g., cardiac arrest, traumatic brain injury) that affect their capacity to make informed decisions. Thus, potential research subjects often cannot participate in the informed consent process before participating in an interventional clinical trial, even when the investigational therapy offers the prospect of direct benefit to the individual subject. It is also difficult to secure informed consent because care must often be administered immediately. Currently, federal regulations (21 Code of Federal Regulations §50.24) allow a narrow exception to the general requirement for prospective, written informed consent for participation in research studies in the setting of an acute, debilitating illness or injury for which there is no accepted effective therapy (Biros et al., 1995, 1998, 1999; Baren et al., 1999; Sloan et al., 1999b; Lewis et al., 2001). Under this exception, however, it remains difficult to comply with the rules in many situations (NHTSA, 2001). As noted by Mann and colleagues

---

[3]Under the NIH's Roadmap Initiative, Clinical Translational Science Awards (CTSAs) are replacing GCRCs as the principal mechanism for supporting institutional clinical research. The Committee's concerns about support for emergency care also apply to CTSAs.

(2005, p. 1078), ". . . the logistical application of these ethical standards across institutions or among different research studies remains complex and variable." Furthermore, state regulations occasionally preempt the federal exception for emergency care research. Active guidance from OHRP to states and individual IRBs could eliminate some of the current obstacles that discourage innovation in treatment approaches of potential benefit to critically ill or injured patients. The committee therefore recommends that **states ease their restrictions on informed consent to match federal law (8.3).**

Patient Confidentiality Protection

Under new rules established in 2000, all entities participating in federally funded research must obtain a federalwide assurance (FWA) from OHRP. The FWA is a document that ensures the intent of the research organization to comply with applicable federal laws and standards for the protection of human research subjects. The FWA program was intended to streamline the previous, more cumbersome system of single- and multiple-project assurances. But many patients seen in the emergency care setting, either those initially treated by EMS or those treated in community EDs, produce important health care utilization and outcome data that are stored at nonacademic community-based medical facilities. These facilities are unlikely to participate in federally supported research in general and therefore generally do not have an FWA in place. Newgard and colleagues (2005) examined the difficulties associated with effecting FWA agreements with community hospitals to obtain patient-level outcome data from a low-risk EMS study. The study involved an attempt to validate a triage rule for children seriously injured during automobile crashes through a retrospective chart review of cases at 27 pediatric receiving hospitals in Los Angeles County. The researchers were unable to achieve participation from all 27 hospitals, which they attributed to the complexity and risk of the FWA requirement. All 27 hospitals had agreed to participate in an interventional randomized controlled trial of airway management in children several years earlier, before the FWA requirement was in place (Gausche, 2000). To have robust and generalizable results, it is important to include outcome information from the full range of receiving facilities to which the EMS system delivers patients. The NIH Roadmap itself cites the need to remove barriers to collaborative clinical research between community-based providers and academic researchers (Zerhouni, 2003).

In addition, there is limited guidance regarding FWAs in EMS research. In the Field Administration of Stroke Therapy–Magnesium (FAST–MAG) trial, a $16 million NIH grant, investigators had to seek help from OHRP. It was finally decided that hospitals had to either have an FWA, apply to have an FWA, or use an academic medical center as a "parent FWA" and sign a written agreement with the parent for their IRB to ensure protection of human subjects. Further, all of the 41 EMS agencies in Los Angeles County had to sign an agreement with the Los Angeles EMS Agency to allow the agency to serve as their FWA and oversee protection of human subjects. While for the most part successful, this effort has taken 2 years. To make it possible to conduct important emergency care research on representative populations in the community, the committee recommends that **Congress modify Federalwide Assurance Program regulations to allow the acquisition of limited, linked, patient outcomes data without the existence of a Federalwide Assurance Program (8.4).** One approach that has been suggested is to allow an experienced academic medical center IRB to serve as a regional IRB for community hospitals within a certain area, at least for minimum-risk research (Christian et al., 2002; Newgard et al., 2005).

SUMMARY OF RECOMMENDATIONS

8.1: Academic medical centers should support emergency and trauma care research by providing research time and adequate facilities for promising emergency care and trauma investigators, and by strongly considering the establishment of autonomous departments of emergency medicine.

8.2: The Secretary of the Department of Health and Human Services should conduct a study to examine the gaps and opportunities in emergency and trauma care research, and recommend a strategy for the optimal organization and funding of the research effort.

> **8.2a:** This study should include consideration of training of new investigators, development of multicenter research networks, funding of General Clinical Research Centers that specifically include an emergency and trauma care component, involvement of emergency and trauma care researchers in the grant review and research advisory processes, and improved research coordination through a dedicated center or institute.

> **8.2b:** Congress and federal agencies involved in emergency and trauma care research (including the Department of Transportation, the Department of Health and Human Services, the Department of Homeland Security, and the Department of Defense) should implement the study's recommendations.

8.3: States should ease their restrictions on informed consent to match federal law.

8.4: Congress should modify Federalwide Assurance Program regulations to allow the acquisition of limited, linked, patient outcomes data without the existence of a Federalwide Assurance Program.

REFERENCES

Abella BS, Zhao D, Alvarado J, Hamann K, Vanden Hoek TL, Becker LB. 2004. Intra-arrest cooling improves outcomes in a murine cardiac arrest model. *Circulation* 109(22): 2786–2791.

ACEP (American College of Emergency Physicians). 1986. *Guidelines for Trauma Care Systems.* Dallas, TX: ACEP.

ACEP. 2005. *Emergency Medicine Foundation.* [Online]. Available: http://www.acep.org/webportal/Education/EMF/ [accessed August 1, 2005].

ACEP Research Committee. 2005. *Report on Emergency Medicine Research.* Dallas, TX: ACEP.

ACS (American College of Surgeons). 1987. *Consultation for Trauma Systems.* Chicago, IL: ACS.

ACS. 2005. *National Trauma Data Bank Report 2005, Dataset Version 5.0.* Chicago, IL: ACS.

ACS COT (ACS, Committee on Trauma). 1976. Optimal hospital resources for care of the seriously injured. *Bulletin of the American College of Surgeons* 61:15–22.

Aghababian RV, Barsan WG, Bickell WH, Biros MH, Brown CG, Cairns CB, Callaham ML, Carden DL, Cordell WH, Dart RC, Dronen SH, Garrison HG, Goldfrank LR, Hedges JR, Kelen GD, Kellermann AL, Lewis LM, Lewis RG, Ling LJ, Marx JA, McCabe JB, Sanders AB, Schriger DL, Sklar DP. 1996. Research directions in emergency medicine. *American Journal of Emergency Medicine* 14(7):681–683.

AHRQ (Agency for Healthcare Research and Quality). 2004. *Funding Opportunities.* [Online]. Available: http://www.ahrq.gov/fund/funding.htm [accessed January 22, 2004].

AHRQ. 2006. *Costs of Treating Trauma Disorders Now Comparable to Medical Expenses for Heart Disease.* [Online]. Available: http://www.ahrq.gov/news/nn/nn012506.htm [accessed May 16, 2006].

Angle N, Hoyt DB, Coimbra R, Liu F, Herdon-Remelius C, Loomis W, Junger WG. 1998. Hypertonic saline resuscitation diminishes lung injury by suppressing neutrophil activation after hemorrhagic shock. *Shock* 9(3):164–170.

Auf der Heide TP, Sigurdsson G, Pirrallo RG, Yannopoulos D, McKnite S, von Briesen C, Sparks CW, Conrad CJ, Provo TA, Lurie KG. 2004. Hyperventilation-induced hypotension during cardiopulmonary resuscitation. *Circulation* 109(16):1960–1965.

Baren JM, Anicetti JP, Ledesma S, Biros MH, Mahabee-Gittens M, Lewis RJ. 1999. An approach to community consultation prior to initiating an emergency research study incorporating a waiver of informed consent. *Academic Emergency Medicine* 6(12):1210–1215.

Becker LB, Weisfeldt ML, Weil MH, Budinger T, Carrico J, Kern K, Nichol G, Shechter I, Traystman R, Webb C, Wiedemann H, Wise R, Sopko G. 2002. The pulse initiative: Scientific priorities and strategic planning for resuscitation research and life saving therapies. *Circulation* 105(21):2562–2570.

Bernard SA, Gray TW, Buist MD, Jones BM, Silvester W, Gutteridge G, Smith K. 2002. Treatment of comatose survivors of out-of-hospital cardiac arrest with induced hypothermia. *New England Journal of Medicine* 346(8):557–563.

Bickell WH, Bruttig SP, Millnamow GA, O'Benar J, Wade CE. 1992. Use of hypertonic saline/dextran versus lactated Ringer's solution as a resuscitation fluid after uncontrolled aortic hemorrhage in anesthetized swine. *Annals of Emergency Medicine* 21(9):1077–1085.

Biros MH, Lewis RJ, Olson CM, Runge JW, Cummins RO, Fost N. 1995. Informed consent in emergency research. Consensus statement from the coalition conference of acute resuscitation and critical care researchers. *Journal of the American Medical Association* 273(16):1283–1287.

Biros MH, Runge JW, Lewis RJ, Doherty C. 1998. Emergency medicine and the development of the Food and Drug Administration's final rule on informed consent and waiver of informed consent in emergency research circumstances. *Academic Emergency Medicine* 5(4):359–368.

Biros MH, Fish SS, Lewis RJ. 1999. Implementing the Food and Drug Administration's final rule for waiver of informed consent in certain emergency research circumstances. *Academic Emergency Medicine* 6(12):1272–1282.

Brown MD, Vance SJ, Kline JA. 2005. An emergency department guideline for the diagnosis of pulmonary embolism: An outcome study. *Academic Emergency Medicine* 12(1):20–25.

Calvano SE, Xiao W, Richards DR, Felciano RM, Baker HV, Cho RJ, Chen RO, Brownstein BH, Cobb JP, Tschoeke SK, Miller-Graziano C, Moldawer LL, Mindrinos MN, Davis RW, Tompkins RG, Lowry SF. 2005. A network-based analysis of systemic inflammation in humans. *Nature* 437(7061):1032–1037.

Christian MC, Goldberg JL, Killen J, Abrams JS, McCabe MS, Mauer JK, Wittes RE. 2002. A central institutional review board for multi-institutional trials. *New England Journal of Medicine* 346(18):1405–1408.

Coimbra R, Hoyt DB, Junger WG, Angle N, Wolf P, Loomis W, Evers MF. 1997. Hypertonic saline resuscitation decreases susceptibility to sepsis after hemorrhagic shock. *The Journal of Trauma* 42(4):602–660; discussion 606–607.

Cooper RJ. 2004. Emergency department triage: Why we need a research agenda. *Annals of Emergency Medicine* 44(5):524–526.

Courtney DM, Kline JA. 2005. Prospective use of a clinical decision rule to identify pulmonary embolism as likely cause of outpatient cardiac arrest. *Resuscitation* 65(1):57–64.

Cydulka RK, Rowe BH, Clark S, Emerman CL, Camargo CA Jr, MARC Investigators. 2003. Emergency department management of acute exacerbations of chronic obstructive pulmonary disease in the elderly: The multicenter airway research collaboration. *Journal of the American Geriatrics Society* 51(7):908–916.

Eisenberg M, Damon S, Mandel L, Tewodros A, Meischke H, Beaupied E, Bennett J, Guildner C, Ewell C, Gordon M. 1995. CPR instruction by videotape: Results of a community project. *Annals of Emergency Medicine* 25(2):198–202.

EMNet. 2005. *Emergency Medicine Network*. [Online]. Available: http://www.emnet–usa.org [accessed April 16, 2005].

Fine MJ, Auble TE, Yealy DM, Hanusa BH, Weissfeld LA, Singer DE, Coley CM, Marrie TJ, Kapoor WN. 1997. A prediction rule to identify low-risk patients with community-acquired pneumonia. *New England Journal of Medicine* 336(4):243–250.

GAO (U.S. Government Accountability Office). 1991. *Trauma Care: Lifesaving System Threatened by Unreimbursed Costs and Other Factors*. Washington, DC: GAO.

Gausche M. 2000. Effect of out-of-hospital pediatric endotracheal intubation on survival and neurologic outcome: A controlled clinical trial. *Journal of the American Medical Association* 283(6):783–790.

Goldman E, Marshall E. 2002. Research funding. NIH grantees: Where have all the young ones gone? *Science* 298(5591):40–41.

Haddon W Jr. 1968. The changing approach to the epidemiology, prevention, and amelioration of trauma: The transition to approaches etiologically rather than descriptively based. *American Journal of Public Health & the Nation's Health* 58(8):1431–1438.

Hoffman JR, Wolfson AB, Todd K, Mower WR. 1998. Selective cervical spine radiography in blunt trauma: Methodology of the national emergency x-radiography utilization study (NEXUS). *Annals of Emergency Medicine* 32(4):461–469.

Hoffman JR, Mower WR, Wolfson AB, Todd KH, Zucker MI. 2000. Validity of a set of clinical criteria to rule out injury to the cervical spine in patients with blunt trauma. National emergency x-radiography utilization study group. *New England Journal of Medicine* 343(2):94–99.

Hoyt DB, Holcomb J, Abraham E, Atkins J, Sopko G, Working Group on Trauma Research. 2004. Working Group on Trauma Research Program Summary Report: National Heart Lung Blood Institute (NHLBI), National Institute of General Medical Sciences (NIGMS), and National Institute of Neurological Disorders and Stroke (NINDS) of the National Institutes of Health (NIH), and the Department of Defense (DoD). *Journal of Trauma-Injury Infection & Critical Care* 57(2):410–415.

The Hypothermia After Cardiac Arrest Study Group. 1921. Mild therapeutic hypothermia to improve the neurologic outcome after cardiac arrest. *New England Journal of Medicine* 346(8):549–556.

IOM (Institute of Medicine). 1999. *Reducing the Burden of Injury.* Washington, DC: National Academy Press.

IOM. 2003. *Enhancing the Vitality of the National Institutes of Health: Organizational Change to Meet New Challenges.* Washington, DC: The National Academies Press.

IOM. 2004. *NIH Extramural Center Programs: Criteria for Initiation and Evaluation.* Washington, DC: The National Academies Press.

Josiah Macy, Jr. Foundation. 1995. *The Role of Emergency Medicine in the Future of American Medical Care.* New York: Josiah Macy, Jr. Foundation.

Kellermann AL, Hackman BB, Somes G. 1989. Dispatcher-assisted cardiopulmonary resuscitation. Validation of efficacy. *Circulation* 80(5):1231–1239.

Kim S, Emerman CL, Cydulka RK, Rowe BH, Clark S, Camargo CA, MARC Investigators. 2004. Prospective multicenter study of relapse following emergency department treatment of COPD exacerbation. *Chest* 125(2):473–481.

Kline JA, Wells PS. 2003. Methodology for a rapid protocol to rule out pulmonary embolism in the emergency department. *Annals of Emergency Medicine* 42(2):266–275.

Kline JA, Webb WB, Jones AE, Hernandez-Nino J. 2004. Impact of a rapid rule-out protocol for pulmonary embolism on the rate of screening, missed cases, and pulmonary vascular imaging in an urban U.S. emergency department. *Annals of Emergency Medicine* 44(5):490–502.

Kline JA, Novobilski AJ, Kabrhel C, Richman PB, Courtney DM. 2005. Derivation and validation of a bayesian network to predict pretest probability of venous thromboembolism. *Annals of Emergency Medicine* 45(3):282–290.

Lewis RJ. 2004. Academic emergency medicine and the "tragedy of the commons" defined. *Academic Emergency Medicine* 11(5):423–427.

Lewis RJ, Berry DA, Cryer H III, Fost N, Krome R, Washington GR, Houghton J, Blue JW, Bechhofer R, Cook T, Fisher M. 2001. Monitoring a clinical trial conducted under the Food and Drug Administration regulations allowing a waiver of prospective informed consent: The diaspirin cross-linked hemoglobin traumatic hemorrhagic shock efficacy trial. *Annals of Emergency Medicine* 38(4):397–404.

Maio RF, Garrison HG, Spaite DW, Desmond JS, Gregor MA, Cayten CG, Chew JL Jr, Hill EM, Joyce SM, MacKenzie EJ, Miller DR, O'Malley PJ, Stiell IG. 1999. Emergency Medical Services Outcomes Project I (EMSOP I): Prioritizing conditions for outcomes research. *Annals of Emergency Medicine* 33(4):423–432.

Mann NC, Schmidt TA, Richardson LD. 2005. Confronting the ethical conduct of resuscitation research: A consensus opinion. *Academic Emergency Medicine* 12(11):1078–1081.

Moran GJ, Talan DA, Mower W, Newdow M, Ong S, Nakase JY, Pinner RW, Childs JE. 2000. Appropriateness of rabies postexposure prophylaxis treatment for animal exposures. Emergency ID Net Study Group. *Journal of the American Medical Association* 284(8):1001–1007.

Morris D, Manning J. 2004. *Research in Academic Emergency Medicine.* [Online]. Available: www.saem.org/publicat/chap6.htm [accessed November 3, 2004].

NAS, NRC (National Academy of Sciences, National Research Council). 1966. *Accidental Death and Disability: The Neglected Disease of Modern Society.* Washington, DC: National Academy Press.

National Center for Injury Prevention and Control. 2005. *CDC Acute Injury Care Research Agenda: Guiding Research for the Future.* Atlanta, GA: Centers for Disease Control.

Neumar RW. 2000. Molecular mechanisms of ischemic neuronal injury. *Annals of Emergency Medicine* 36(5):483–506.

Newgard CD, Hui SH, Stamps-White P, Lewis RJ. 2005. Institutional variability in a minimal risk, population-based study: Recognizing policy barriers to health services research. *Health Services Research* 40(4):1247–1258.

NHTSA (National Highway Traffic Safety Administration). 2001. *National EMS Research Agenda.* Washington, DC: U.S. Department of Transportation.

NHTSA and CIREN Center Staffs. 2003. *NHTSA Crash Injury Research and Engineering Network (CIREN) Program Report, 2002.* Washington DC: NHTSA.

NIH (National Institutes of Health). 1994. *Report of the Task Force on Trauma Research.* Bethesda, MD: NIH.

NIH. 2003. *Ruth L. Kirschstein National Research Service Awards for Individual Postdoctoral Fellow (F32).* [Online]. Available: http://grants1.nih.gov/grants/guide/pa–files/PA–03–067.html [accessed April 17, 2005].

Nolan JP, Morley PT, Vanden Hoek TL, Hickey RW, Kloeck WG, Billi J, Bottiger BW, Morley PT, Nolan JP, Okada K, Reyes C, Shuster M, Steen PA, Weil MH, Wenzel V, Hickey RW, Carli P, Vanden Hoek TL, Atkins D, International Liaison Committee on Resuscitation. 2003. Therapeutic hypothermia after cardiac arrest: An advisory statement by the advanced life support task force of the International Liaison Committee on Resuscitation. *Circulation* 108(1):118–121.

NRC, IOM (National Research Council, Institute of Medicine). 1985. *Injury in America: A Continuing Public Health Problem.* Washington, DC: National Academy Press.

PECARN (Pediatric Emergency Care Applied Research Network). 2003. The Pediatric Emergency Care Applied Research Network (PECARN): Rationale, development, and first steps. *Academic Emergency Medicine* 10(6):661–668.

PECARN. 2005. *About PECARN.* [Online]. Available: http://www.pecarn.org/about_pecarn.htm [accessed April 16, 2005].

Pollack CV Jr, Cairns CB. 1999. The emergency medicine foundation: 25 years of advancing education and research. *Annals of Emergency Medicine* 33(4):448–450.

Pollack C, Hollander J, O'Neil B, Neumar R, Summers R, Camargo C, Younger J, Callaway C, Gallagher E, Kellermann A, Krause G, Schafermeyer R, Sloan E, Stern S. 2003. Status report: Development of emergency medicine research since the Macy report. *Annals of Emergency Medicine* 42(1):66–80.

Sayre MR, White LJ, Brown LH, McHenry SD, National EMS Research Strategic Plan Writing Team. 2005. The national EMS research strategic plan. *Prehospital Emergency Care* 9(3):255–266.

Seidel J, Henderson D, Tittle S, Jaffe D, Spaite D, Dean J, Gausche M, Lewis R, Cooper A, Zaritsky A, Espisito T, Maederis D. 1999. Priorities for research in emergency medical services for children: Results of a consensus conference. *Annals of Emergency Medicine* 33(2):206–210.

Sloan EP, Koenigsberg M, Gens D, Cipolle M, Runge J, Mallory MN, Rodman G Jr. 1999a. Diaspirin cross-linked hemoglobin (DCLHB) in the treatment of severe traumatic hemorrhagic shock: A randomized controlled efficacy trial. *Journal of the American Medical Association* 282(19):1857–1864.

Sloan EP, Koenigsberg M, Houghton J, Gens D, Cipolle M, Runge J, Mallory MN, Rodman G Jr, DCLHB Traumatic Hemorrhagic Shock Study Group. 1999b. The informed consent process and the use of the exception to informed consent in the clinical trial of diaspirin cross-linked hemoglobin (DCLHB) in severe traumatic hemorrhagic shock. *Academic Emergency Medicine* 6(12):1203–1209.

Stern SA. 2001. *Fellowship Training: A Necessity in Today's Academic World*. [Online]. Available: http://www.saem.org/newsltr/2001/july–august/stern.htm [accessed April 17, 2005].

Stern SA, Zink BJ, Mertz M, Wang X, Dronen SC. 2000. Effect of initially limited resuscitation in a combined model of fluid-percussion brain injury and severe uncontrolled hemorrhagic shock. *Journal of Neurosurgery* 93(2):305–314.

Sung NS, Crowley WF Jr, Genel M, Salber P, Sandy L, Sherwood LM, Johnson SB, Catanese V, Tilson H, Getz K, Larson EL, Scheinberg D, Reece EA, Slavkin H, Dobs A, Grebb J, Martinez RA, Korn A, Rimoin D. 2003. Central challenges facing the national clinical research enterprise. *Journal of the American Medical Association* 289(10):1278–1287.

Talan D, Moran G, Mower W, Newdow M, Ong S, Slutsker L, Jarvis W, Conn L, Pinner R. 1998. EMERGEncy ID NET: An emergency department-based emerging infections sentinel network. *Annals of Emergency Medicine* 32(6):703–711.

Talan DA, Citron DM, Abrahamian FM, Moran GJ, Goldstein EJ, Emergency Medicine Animal Bite Infection Study Group. 1999. Bacteriologic analysis of infected dog and cat bites. *New England Journal of Medicine* 340(2):85–92.

Talan DA, Abrahamian FM, Moran GJ, Citron DM, Tan JO, Goldstein EJ, Emergency Medicine Human Bite Infection Study Group. 2003. Clinical presentation and bacteriologic analysis of infected human bites in patients presenting to emergency departments. *Clinical Infectious Diseases* 37(11):1481–1489.

Todd KH, Braslow A, Brennan RT, Lowery DW, Cox RJ, Lipscomb LE, Kellermann AL. 1998. Randomized, controlled trial of video self-instruction versus traditional CPR training. *Annals of Emergency Medicine* 31(3):364–369.

Todd KH, Heron SL, Thompson M, Dennis R, O'Connor J, Kellermann AL. 1999. Simple CPR: A randomized, controlled trial of video self-instructional cardiopulmonary resuscitation training in an African American church congregation. *Annals of Emergency Medicine* 34(6):730–737.

Trunkey DD. 1981. Regionalization of trauma care. *Topics in Emergency Medicine* 3(2):91–96.

Wadman MC, Muelleman RL, Coto JA, Kellermann AL. 2003. The pyramid of injury: Using ecodes to accurately describe the burden of injury. *Annals of Emergency Medicine* 42(4):468–478.

Wright DW, Ritchie JC, Mullins RE, Kellermann AL, Denson DD. 2005. Steady-state serum concentrations of progesterone following continuous intravenous infusion in patients with acute moderate to severe traumatic brain injury. *Journal of Clinical Pharmacology* 45(6):640–648.

Wright S, Wrenn K. 1994. Funding in the emergency medicine literature: 1985 to 1992. *Annals of Emergency Medicine* 23(5):1077–1081.

Zerhouni E. 2003. Medicine. The NIH roadmap. *Science* 302(5642):63–72.

Zisson S. 2001. Anticipating a clinical investigator shortfall. *CenterWatch* 8(1).

APPENDIX
A

Committee and Subcommittee Membership

322

Gail Warden, MHA, *Chair*

SUBCOMMITTEES			MAIN COMMITTEE	SUBCOMMITTEE ONLY
Pediatric Emergency Care (PEDS)	Prehospital Emergency Medical Services (EMS)	Hospital-Based Emergency Care (ED)		
David Sundwall, MD (Chair)	Shirley Gamble, MBA (Chair)	Benjamin Chu, MD, MPH (Chair)	Thomas Babor, PhD, MPH	
George Foltin, MD	Robert Bass, MD	Stuart Altman, PhD	Robert Gates, MPA	
Darrell Gaskin, PhD	Brent Eastman, MD	Brent Asplin, MD, MPH	William Kelley, MD	
Marianne Gausche-Hill, MD	Arthur Kellermann, MD, MPH	John Halamka, MD	Mark Smith, MD, MBA	
Richard Orr, MD	Jerry Overton, MA	Mary Jagim, RN		
	Nels Sanddal, MS, REMT-B	Peter Layde, MD, MSc		
		Eugene Litvak, PhD		
		John Prescott, MD		
		William Schwab, MD		
Rosalyn Baker	Kaye Bender, PhD, RN	Kenneth Kizer, MD		
Mary Fallat, MD	Herbert Garrison, MD	John Lumpkin, MD		
Jane Knapp, MD	Mary Beth Michos, RN	Daniel Manz, EMT		
Thomas Loyacono, EMT-P	Fred Neis, RN	Joseph Wright, MD		
Milap Nahata, PharmD	Daniel Spaite, MD			
Donna Ojanen Thomas, RN				

APPENDIX
B

Biographical Information for Main Committee and Hospital-Based Emergency Care Subcommittee

Gail L. Warden, M.H.A., F.A.C.H.E., *Main Committee Chair,* is president emeritus of Henry Ford Health System in Detroit, Michigan, one of the nation's leading vertically integrated health care systems. He is an elected member of the Institute of Medicine (IOM) of the National Academy of Sciences and served on its Board of Health Care Services and Committee on Quality Health Care in America, as well as serving its two terms on its Governing Council. He chairs the Board of the National Quality Forum, the Healthcare Research and Development Institute, and the newly created National Center for Healthcare Leadership. Mr. Warden cochairs the National Advisory Committee on Pursuing Perfection: Raising the Bar for Health Care Performance. He is a member of The Robert Wood Johnson Foundation Board of Trustees, the Institute for Healthcare Improvement Board, and the RAND Health Board of Advisors. He is director emeritus and past chair of the Board of the National Committee on Quality Assurance. In 1997 President Clinton appointed him to the Federal Advisory Commission on Consumer Protection and Quality in the Health Care Industry. In 1995 Mr. Warden served as chair of the American Hospital Association Board of Trustees. He served as a member of the Pew Health Professions Commission and the National Commission on Civic Renewal, and is past chair of the Health Research and Education Trust Board of Directors. Mr. Warden served as president and chief executive officer of Henry Ford Health System from April 1988 until June 2003. Previously, he served as president and chief executive officer of Group Health Cooperative of Puget Sound in Seattle from 1981 to 1988. Prior to that he was executive vice president of the American Hospital Association from 1976 to 1981, and from 1965 to 1976 he served as executive vice president and chief operating officer of Rush-Presbyterian-St. Luke's Medical Center in Chicago. Mr. Warden is a graduate of Dartmouth College and holds an M.H.A. from the University of Michigan. He has an honorary doctorate in public administration from Central Michigan University and is a member of the faculty of the University of Michigan School of Public Health.

Benjamin K. Chu, M.D., M.P.H., *Hospital-Based Emergency Care Subcommittee Chair,* was appointed president, Kaiser Foundation Health Plan, Inc. and Kaiser Foundation Hospitals, Southern California Region, in February 2005. Before joining Kaiser Permanente, Dr. Chu was president of the New York City Health and Hospitals Corporation, with primary responsibility for management and policy implementation. Prior to that, he was senior associate dean at Columbia University College of Physicians and Surgeons. He has also served as associate dean and vice president for clinical affairs at the New York University Medical Center, managing and developing the clinical academic hospital network. Dr. Chu is a primary care internist by training, with extensive experience as a clinician, administrator, and policy advocate for the public hospital sector. He was senior vice president for medical and professional affairs at the New York City Health and Hospitals Corporation from 1990 to 1994. During that period, he also served as acting commissioner of health for the New York City Department of Health and acting executive director for Kings County Hospital Center. Dr. Chu has extensive experience in crafting public policy. He served as legislative assistant for health for Senator Bill Bradley as a 1989–1990 Robert Wood Johnson Health Policy Fellow. Earlier in his career, he served as acting director of the Kings County Hospital Adult Emergency Department. His areas of interests include health care access and insurance, graduate medical education policy, primary care, and public health issues. He has served on numerous advisory and not-for-profit boards focused on health care policy issues. Dr. Chu received a masters in public health from the Mailman School at Columbia University and his doctorate of medicine at New York University School of Medicine.

Stuart H. Altman, Ph.D., is Sol C. Chaikin Professor of National Health Policy at the Heller Graduate School for Social Policy and Management. He served as dean of the Heller School from 1977 to a 1993. In August 2005 he again assumed the deanship of the Heller School. Dr. Altman has had extensive experience with the federal government, serving as deputy assistant secretary for planning and evaluation/health in the U.S. Department of Health, Education, and Welfare, 1971–1976; chair of the congressionally mandated Prospective Payment Assessment Commission, 1983–1996; and a member of the Bipartisan Commission on the Future of Medicare, 1999–2001. In addition, from 1973 to 1974 he served as deputy director for health of the President's Cost-of-Living Council and was responsible for developing the council's program on health care cost containment. Dr. Altman has testified before various congressional committees on the problems of rising health care costs, Medicare reform, and the need to create a national health insurance program for the United States. He chaired the IOM's Committee on the Changing Market, Managed Care, and the Future Viability of Safety Net Providers. His research activities include several studies concerning the factors responsible for the recent increases in the use of emergency departments. He holds a Ph.D. in economics from the University of California, Los Angeles, and has taught at Brown University and the University of California, Berkeley.

Brent R. Asplin, M.D., M.P.H., F.A.C.E.P., is department head of emergency medicine at Regions Hospital and HealthPartners Research Foundation in St. Paul, Minnesota, and is an associate professor and vice chair of the Department of Emergency Medicine at the University of Minnesota. After receiving his degree from Mayo Medical School, he completed the University of Pittsburgh's Affiliated Residency in Emergency Medicine. To develop his interests in research and health care policy, Dr. Asplin completed The Robert Wood Johnson Clinical Scholars Program at the University of Michigan, where he obtained an M.P.H. in health management and policy. He is currently studying methods for enhancing the reliability and efficiency of health care operations, particularly strategies for improving patient flow in hospital settings.

Thomas F. Babor, Ph.D., M.P.H., spent several years in postdoctoral research training in social psychiatry at Harvard Medical School, and subsequently served as head of social science research at McLean Hospital's Alcohol and Drug Abuse Research Center in Belmont, Massachusetts. In 1982 he moved to the University of Connecticut School of Medicine, where he has served as scientific director at the Alcohol Research Center and interim chair of the Psychiatry Department. Dr. Babor's primary interests are psychiatric epidemiology and alcohol and drug abuse. In 1998 he became chair of the Department of Community Medicine and Health Care at the University of Connecticut School of Medicine, where he directs an active research program. Dr. Babor is regional editor of the international journal *Addiction*. He previously served on two IOM committees—Prevention and Treatment of Alcohol-Related Problems: An Update on Research Opportunities, and Treatment of Alcohol Problems.

Robert R. Bass, M.D., F.A.C.E.P., received his undergraduate and medical degrees from the University of North Carolina at Chapel Hill in 1972 and

1975, respectively. Prior to completing his undergraduate education, he was employed as a police officer in Chapel Hill, North Carolina, and served as a volunteer member of the South Orange Rescue Squad. Dr. Bass completed an internship and residency in the Navy and is currently board certified in both emergency medicine and family medicine. He has served as a medical director for emergency medical services (EMS) systems in Charleston, South Carolina; Houston, Texas; Norfolk, Virginia; and Washington, D.C. Since 1994, Dr. Bass has been executive director of the Maryland Institute for EMS Systems, the state agency responsible for the oversight of Maryland's EMS and trauma system. He is clinical associate professor of surgery (emergency medicine) at the University of Maryland at Baltimore and is associate professor in the Emergency Health Services Program at the University of Maryland, Baltimore County. Dr. Bass is the immediate past president of the National Association of State EMS Officials and a founding member and the immediate past president of the National Association of EMS Physicians. Additionally, he serves on the board of directors of the American Trauma Society and the University of Maryland Medical System, and is past chair of the EMS Committee of the American College of Emergency Physicians.

A. Brent Eastman, M.D., joined Scripps Memorial Hospital La Jolla in 1984 as director of trauma services and was appointed chief medical officer in 1998. He continues to serve in the role of director of trauma. Dr. Eastman received his medical degree from the University of California, San Francisco, where he also did his general surgical residency and served as chief surgical resident. He spent a year abroad in surgical training in England at Norfolk and Norwich Hospitals. Dr. Eastman served as chair of the Committee on Trauma for the American College of Surgeons from 1990 to 1994. This organization sets the standards for trauma care in the United States and abroad. The position led to his involvement nationally and internationally in the development of trauma systems in the United States, Canada, England, Ireland, Australia, Brazil, Argentina, Mexico, and South Africa. Dr. Eastman has authored or coauthored more than 25 publications and chapters relating principally to trauma. He has held numerous appointments and chairmanships over the last two decades, including chair, Trauma Systems Committee, for the U.S. Department of Health and Human Services; member of the board of directors, American Association for the Surgery of Trauma; and chair, Grant Review Committee, Center for Injury Prevention and Control at the U.S. Centers for Disease Control and Prevention.

George L. Foltin, M.D., F.A.A.P., F.A.C.E.P., began his involvement with the Emergency Medical Services for Children (EMS-C) Program of the Health Resources and Services Administration in 1985. He is board certified in pediatrics, emergency medicine, and pediatric emergency medicine. Dr. Foltin served on the Medical Oversight Committee for the EMT-Basic National Standard Curriculum project and was a subject expert for the Project to Revise EMT-Intermediate and Paramedic National Standard Curriculum. He is a former board member of the National Association of EMS Physicians and served on the Committee on Pediatric Emergency Medicine of the American Academy of Pediatrics (AAP). Currently Dr. Foltin cochairs the Statewide AAP Committee on Pediatric Emergency Medicine and sits on the Regional Medical Advisory Committee of New York City. He has published extensively in the field of EMS for children, has been principal investigator for several federal grants, and serves as a consultant to the New York City and State departments of health, as well as to federal programs such as those of the Maternal and Child Health Bureau, the Agency for Healthcare Research and Quality, and the National Highway Traffic Safety Administration.

Shirley Gamble, M.B.A., served as senior advisor to The Robert Wood Johnson Foundation's Urgent Matters initiative, which is working to help hospitals eliminate emergency department crowding and help communities understand the challenges facing the health care safety net. Ms. Gamble has over 20 years of experience in the health care industry, serving as an executive with Incarnate Word Health Services, Texas Health Plans HMO, and Tampa General Hospital. As a partner in Phase 2 Consulting, a health care management and economic consulting firm, Ms. Gamble led performance improvement and strategic planning efforts for major hospital systems, managed care entities, and university faculty practice plans. She currently is chief operating officer for the United Way Capital Area in Austin, Texas. She holds an M.B.A. and B.A. from the University of Texas at Austin.

Darrell J. Gaskin, Ph.D., M.S., is associate professor of health policy and management at The Johns Hopkins Bloomberg School of Public Health and deputy director of the Morgan-Hopkins Center for Health Disparities Solutions. Dr. Gaskin's research focuses on health care disparities and access to care for vulnerable populations. Dr. Gaskin was awarded the Academy Health 2002 Article-of-the-Year Award for his *Health Services Research* article entitled "Are Urban Safety-Net Hospitals Losing Low-Risk Medicaid Maternity Patients?" Dr. Gaskin is active in professional organizations. He is a member of Academy Health, the American Economic Association, the National Economics Association (NEA), the International Health Economics Association, the American Society of Health Economists, and the American Public Health Association (APHA). He has served as a member of the board of directors of the NEA. He has been a member of the Governing Council of the APHA and is currently solicited program chair and section councilor for the APHA's Medical Care Section. He has chaired the disparities program committee for Academy Health. He is a member of the board of directors for the Maryland Citizen's Health Initiative. Dr. Gaskin earned his Ph.D. in health economics at The Johns Hopkins University, a master's degree in economics from the Massachusetts Institute of Technology, and a bachelor's degree in economics from Brandeis University.

Robert C. Gates, M.P.A., began his career in the County of Los Angeles Chief Administrative Office, where he was principal budget analyst for the public health, hospital, and mental health departments. He left Los Angeles to become chief operating officer for the University of California, Irvine, Medical Center in Orange County. While in Orange County, he was instrumental in creating its paramedic system. Mr. Gates then returned to Los Angeles County and spent 6 years as chief deputy director of the Department of Health Services, guiding the creation of the Los Angeles County Trauma Center system. He was then appointed director of health services for Los Angeles County and served in that capacity for over 11 years. Mr. Gates is currently serving as medical services for indigents project director for the Orange County Health Care Agency.

Marianne Gausche-Hill, M.D., F.A.C.E.P., F.A.A.P., serves as professor of clinical medicine at the David Geffen School of Medicine at the University of California, Los Angeles (UCLA). She is director of EMS and EMS fellowship and director of pediatric emergency medicine fellowship at Harbor-UCLA Medical Center. Dr. Gausche-Hill also serves as director of pediatric emergency medicine at the Little Company of Mary Hospital in Torrance, California. Board certified in both emergency medicine and pediatric emergency medicine, she earned her medical degree and completed her residency at UCLA. Dr. Gausche-Hill is the first emergency physician in the United States to have completed a pediatric emergency fellowship and passed the sub-board examination. She has done extensive research on prehospital pediatric care, authoring *Pediatric Advanced Life Support: Pearls of Wisdom* in 2001 and *Pediatric Airway Management for the Prehospital Professional* in 2004. Her research tracking the results of the use of the windpipe tube method versus the traditional bag-and-pump method as oxygen treatment for pediatric emergencies was published in the *Journal of the American Medical Association* and in *Annals of Emergency Medicine*. In May 1999, her work earned the prestigious Best Clinical Science Presentation award from the Society for Academic Emergency Medicine.

John D. Halamka, M.D., M.S., is chief information officer of the CareGroup Health System, chief information officer and associate dean for educational technology at Harvard Medical School, chair of the New England Health Electronic Data Interchange Network (NEHEN), acting chief executive officer of MA-Share, chief information officer of the Harvard Clinical Research Institute, and a practicing emergency physician. As chief information officer at CareGroup, he is responsible for all clinical, financial, administrative, and academic information technology serving 3,000 doctors, 12,000 employees, and 1 million patients. As chief information officer and associate dean for educational technology at Harvard Medical School, he oversees all educational, research, and administrative computing for 18,000 faculty and 3,000 students. As chair of NEHEN, he oversees administrative data exchange in Massachusetts. As chief executive officer of MA-Share, he oversees the clinical data exchange efforts in Massachusetts. As chair of the Healthcare Information Technology Standards Panel, he coordinates the process of harmonization of electronic standards among all stakeholders nationwide.

Mary M. Jagim, R.N., B.S.N., C.E.N., F.A.E.N., is an experienced emergency/trauma nurse with extensive leadership background in program development and implementation, emergency department management and nursing workforce issues, emergency preparedness, government affairs, and community-based injury prevention. She is currently internal consultant for emergency preparedness and pandemic planning for MeritCare Health System in Fargo, North Dakota. Well versed in current issues affecting emergency/trauma nursing and emergency care, Ms. Jagim has served on the Emergency Nurses Association board of directors, for which she was national president in 2001. She currently serves as chair of the Emergency Nurses Association Foundation, is a member of the faculty for Key Concepts in Emergency Department Management, and is a fellow in the Academy of Emergency Nursing. She also served on the Centers for Disease Control and Prevention's (CDC) National Strategies for Advancing Child Pedestrian Safety Panel to Prevent Pedestrian Injuries and currently is cochair for Advocates for Highway and Auto Safety. Ms. Jagim received her B.S.N. from the University of North Dakota in 1984.

Arthur L. Kellermann, M.D., M.P.H., is professor and chair of the Department of Emergency Medicine at the Emory University School of Medicine and director of the Center for Injury Control at the Rollins School of Public Health at Emory University. His primary research focus is injury prevention and control. He has also conducted landmark research on prehospital cardiac care, use of diagnostic technology in emergency departments, and health care for the poor. His papers have been published in many of the nation's leading medical journals. He is a recipient of the Hal Jayne Academic Excellence Award from the Society for Academic Emergency Medicine, the Excellence in Science Award from the Injury Control and Emergency Health Services Section of the American Public Health Association, and the

Scholar/Teacher Award from Emory University. A member of the IOM, Dr. Kellermann served as cochair of the IOM's Committee on the Consequences of Uninsurance from 2001 to 2004.

William N. Kelley, M.D., currently serves as professor of medicine, biochemistry, and biophysics at the University of Pennsylvania School of Medicine. Previously, he served as chief executive officer of the University of Pennsylvania Medical Center and Health System and dean of the School of Medicine from 1989 to February 2000. At the University of Pennsylvania, Dr. Kelley led the development of one of the first academic fully integrated delivery systems in the nation. He also built and implemented the largest health and disease management program in the country, with over 500 physicians and staff and 60 separate clinical sites engaged in implementing the program. Dr. Kelley holds a patent in a frequently used gene transfer technique that has allowed for numerous advances in the application of gene therapy. He received his M.D. from Emory University School of Medicine and completed his residency in internal medicine at Parkland Memorial Hospital in Dallas. After a fellowship with the National Institutes of Health and a teaching fellowship at Harvard Medical School, he began his academic career as assistant professor of medicine at Duke University School of Medicine, moving on to head Duke's Division of Rheumatic and Genetic Diseases before becoming chair of internal medicine at the University of Michigan Medical School.

Kenneth W. Kizer, M.D., M.P.H., expanded his role as chairman of the board for Medsphere Systems Corporation to become its chief executive officer in December 2005. He joined Medsphere after serving as president and chief executive officer of the National Quality Forum (NQF), a private, nonprofit, voluntary consensus standards-setting organization established in Washington, D.C., in 1999, pursuant to a presidential commission. Prior to that, he served for 5 years as under secretary for health in the U.S. Department of Veterans Affairs. In this capacity, he was the highest-ranking physician in the federal government and chief executive officer of the veterans health care system, the largest integrated health care system in the United States. Dr. Kizer also served as director of the California Department of Health Services and was California's top health official for over 6 years. Prior to that, he was chief of public health for California and director of California's Emergency Medical Services Authority. He practiced emergency medicine and toxicology in both private and academic settings for over 15 years. Dr. Kizer is an honors graduate of Stanford University and UCLA. He is board certified in six medical specialties and/or subspecialties and has authored more than 350 original articles, book chapters, and other publications in the medical literature. He is a fellow of numerous professional societies and a member of the Alpha Omega Alpha National Honor Medical Society, the Delta Omega National Honorary Public Health Society, and the IOM.

Peter M. Layde, M.D., M.Sc., is professor and interim director of the Health Policy Institute at the Medical College of Wisconsin. He has been an epidemiologist for over 25 years and an active injury control researcher for over 20 years. He has published extensively on agricultural injuries and methods for injury epidemiology, including early work on the use of case-control studies for homicide and on the epidemiological representativeness of trauma center–based studies. He has been an ad hoc reviewer for the Injury Grant Review Committee for over 10 years and served as a member of that committee from 1997 to 2000. Dr. Layde serves as codirector of the Injury Research Center at the Medical College of Wisconsin and as director of its Research Development and Support Core. He is also principal investigator for the Risk Factors for Medical Injury research project.

Eugene Litvak, Ph.D., is cofounder and director of the Program for the Management of Variability in Health Care Delivery at the Boston University Health Policy Institute. He is also a professor at the Boston University School of Management. He received his doctorate in operations research from the Moscow Institute of Physics and Technology in 1977. In 1990, he joined the faculty of the Harvard Center for Risk Analysis in the Department of Health Policy and Management at the Harvard School of Public Health, where he still teaches as adjunct professor of operations management. Prior to that time he was chief of the Operations Management Group at the Computing Center in Kiev, Ukraine. His research interests include operations management in health care delivery organizations, cost-effective medical decision making, screening for HIV and other infectious diseases, and operations research. He was the leading author of cost-effective protocols for screening for HIV and is the principal investigator from the United States for an international trial of these protocols, which is supported by the U.S. Agency for International Development. Dr. Litvak was also principal investigator for the Emergency Room Diversion Study, supported by a grant from the Massachusetts Department of Public Health. He serves as a consultant on operations improvement to several major hospitals and is on the faculty of the Institute for Health Care Improvement.

John R. Lumpkin, M.D., M.P.H., is senior vice president and director, Health Care Group at The Robert Wood Johnson Foundation. Dr. Lumpkin joined the Illinois Department of Public Health (IDPH) in 1985 as associate director of IDPH's Office of Health Care Regulations, and later became the first African American to hold the position of director. Dr. Lumpkin served

6 years as chair of the National Committee for Vital and Health Statistics, advising the Secretary of the U.S. Department of Health and Human Services on health information policy. He received his medical degree in 1974 from Northwestern University Medical School. He trained in emergency medicine at the University of Chicago and earned his M.P.H. from the University of Illinois at Chicago, School of Public Health. Dr. Lumpkin is past president of the Association of State and Territorial Health Officials, a former member of the board of trustees of the Foundation for Accountability, former commissioner of the Pew Commission on Environmental Health, former board member of the National Forum for Health Care Quality Measurement and Reporting, past board member of the American College of Emergency Physicians, and past president of the Society of Teachers of Emergency Medicine. He has been the recipient of the Bill B. Smiley Award, Alan Donaldson Award, and African American History Maker Award, and was named Public Health Worker of the Year.

W. Daniel Manz, B.S., is director of EMS for the Vermont Department of Health. He has been involved in EMS for more than 25 years and worked as an emergency medical technician (EMT), volunteer squad leader, hospital communications technician, EMS regional coordinator, EMS trainer, and state EMS director. Much of his work has been in rural areas, including Maine and Saudi Arabia. Mr. Manz has been active in the National Association of State EMS Directors, serving as its president for 2 years and representing the association on several national projects, including the Emergency Medical Services Agenda for the Future, the Health Care Financing Administration's Negotiated Rule Making process, and the recently completed National EMS Scope of Practice Model. Mr. Manz remains active as a volunteer EMT-Intermediate with the local ambulance service in his community. In his spare time he enjoys running, fishing, and sheep farming.

Richard A. Orr, M.D., serves as professor at the University of Pittsburgh School of Medicine, associate director of the Cardiac Intensive Care Unit at the Children's Hospital of Pittsburgh, and medical director of the Children's Hospital Transport Team of Pittsburgh, Pennsylvania. Dr. Orr has devoted much of his career to interfacility transportation problems of infants and children in need of tertiary care. He is a member of many professional organizations and societies and has authored numerous articles regarding the safe and effective air and surface transport of the critically ill and injured pediatric patient. Dr. Orr is also a noted lecturer to the air and ground transport community, both nationally and internationally. He is editor of *Pediatric Transport Medicine*, a unique 700-page book published in 1995. He is the 2001 recipient of the Air Medical Physician Association (AMPA) Distinguished Physician Award and a founding member of AMPA.

Jerry L. Overton, M.A., serves as executive director, Richmond Ambulance Authority, Richmond, Virginia, and has overall responsibility for the Richmond EMS system. His duties extend to planning and administering the high-performance system's design, negotiating and implementing performance-based contracts, maximizing fee-for-service revenues, developing advanced patient care protocols, and employing innovative equipment and treatment modalities. Mr. Overton was previously executive director of the Kansas City, Missouri, EMS system. In addition, he has provided technical assistance to EMS systems throughout the United States and Europe, Russia, Asia, Australia, and Canada. He designed an implementation plan for an emergency medical transport program in Central Bosnia–Herzegovina. Mr. Overton is a faculty member of the Emergency Medical Department of the Medical College of Virginia, Virginia Commonwealth University, and the National EMS Medical Directors Course, National Association of EMS Physicians. He is past president of the American Ambulance Association and serves on the board of directors of the North American Association of Public Utility Models.

John E. Prescott, M.D., is dean of the West Virginia University (WVU) School of Medicine, and received both his B.S. and M.D. degrees at Georgetown University. He completed his residency training in emergency medicine at Brooke Army Medical Center, San Antonio, and was then assigned to Fort Bragg, North Carolina, where he was actively engaged in providing both operational and hospital emergency care in a variety of challenging situations. In 1990 he joined WVU and soon assumed leadership of the Section of Emergency Medicine. During that same year, he founded and became the first director of WVU's Center for Rural Emergency Medicine. In 1993 he became the first chair of WVU's newly established Department of Emergency Medicine. Dr. Prescott is a past recipient of major CDC and private foundation grants. His research and scholarly interests include rural emergency care, injury control and prevention, medical response to disasters and terrorism, and academic and administrative medicine. In 1999 Dr. Prescott became WVU's associate dean for the clinical enterprise and president/chief executive officer of University Health Associates, WVU's physician practice plan. In 2003 he was named senior associate dean; he was appointed dean of the WVU School of Medicine in 2004. He has been a fellow of the American College of Emergency Physicians since 1987 and is the recipient of WVU's Presidential Heroism Award.

Nels D. Sanddal, M.S., REMT-B, is president of the Critical Illness and Trauma Foundation (CIT) in Bozeman, Montana, and is currently on detachment as director of the Rural Emergency Medical Services and Trauma Technical Assistance Center. Mr. Sanddal has been involved in EMS since the 1970s and has held many state, regional, and national positions in organizations furthering EMS causes, including president of the Intermountain Regional EMS for Children Coordinating Council and core faculty for the Development of Trauma Systems Training Programs for the U.S. Department of Transportation. He is a nationally registered EMT-Basic, volunteers with a local fire department, and has been involved with CIT since its inception in 1986. He holds an M.S. in psychology and is currently pursuing a Ph.D. in health services.

C. William Schwab, M.D., F.A.C.S., is professor of surgery and chief of the Division of Traumatology and Surgical Critical Care at the University of Pennsylvania. His surgical practice reflects his expertise in trauma systems, including caring for the severely injured patient and incorporating the most advanced techniques into trauma surgery. He is director of the Firearm and Injury Center at Penn and holds several grants supporting work on reducing firearm and nonfirearm injuries and other repercussions. He has served as a trauma systems consultant to CDC, New York State, and several state health departments. He has established trauma centers and hospital-based aeromedical programs in Virginia, New Jersey, and Pennsylvania. He currently directs a network of three regional trauma centers throughout southeastern Pennsylvania. He has been president of the Eastern Association for the Surgery of Trauma and vice chair of the American College of Surgeons Committee on Trauma and currently serves as president of the American Association for the Surgery of Trauma.

Mark D. Smith, M.D., M.B.A., has led the California HealthCare Foundation in developing research and initiatives aimed at improving California's health care financing and delivery systems since the foundation's formation in 1996. Prior to joining the foundation, he was executive vice president at the Henry J. Kaiser Family Foundation and served as associate director of the AIDS Service and assistant professor of medicine and health policy and management at The Johns Hopkins University. Dr. Smith is a member of the IOM and is on the board of the National Business Group on Health. Previously, he served on the Performance Measurement Committee of the National Committee for Quality Assurance and the editorial board of the *Annals of Internal Medicine.* A board-certified internist, Dr. Smith is a member of the clinical faculty at the University of California, San Francisco, and an attending physician at the AIDS clinic at San Francisco General Hospital.

David N. Sundwall, M.D., was nominated by Governor Jon Huntsman Jr. to serve as executive director of the Utah State Department of Health in January 2005 and was subsequently confirmed for this position by the Utah

Senate. In this capacity, he supervises a workforce of almost 1,400 employees and a budget of almost $1.8 billion. Previously, Dr. Sundwall served as president of the American Clinical Laboratory Association (ACLA) from September 1994 until he was appointed senior medical and scientific officer in May 2003. Prior to his position at ACLA, he was vice president and medical director of American Healthcare System (AmHS), at that time the largest coalition of not-for-profit multihospital systems in the country. Dr. Sundwall has extensive experience in federal government and national health policy, including serving as administrator, Health Resources and Services Administration; in the Public Health Service, U.S. Department of Health and Human Services (DHHS); and as assistant surgeon general in the Commissioned Corps of the U.S. Public Health Service (1986–1988). During this period, he had adjunct responsibilities at DHHS, including serving as cochair of the secretary's Task Force on Medical Liability and Malpractice and as the secretary's designee to the National Commission to Prevent Infant Mortality. Dr. Sundwall also served as director, Health and Human Resources Staff (Majority), U.S. Senate Labor and Human Resources Committee (1981–1986). He was in private medical practice in Murray, Utah, from 1973 to 1975. He has held academic appointments at the Uniformed Services University of the Health Sciences, Bethesda, Maryland; Georgetown University School of Medicine, Washington, D.C.; and the University of Utah School of Medicine. He is board certified in internal medicine and family practice. He is licensed to practice medicine in the District of Columbia, is a member of the American Medical Association and the American Academy of Family Physicians, and previously served as volunteer medical staff of Health Care for the Homeless Project.

Joseph L. Wright, M.D., M.P.H., is executive director of the Child Health Advocacy Institute at Children's National Medical Center in Washington, D.C. In that capacity, he provides strategic leadership for the organization's advocacy mission and community partnership initiatives. He is professor and vice chair in the Department of Pediatrics, as well as professor of emergency medicine and prevention and community health at The George Washington University Schools of Medicine and Public Health. He has been attending faculty in the Division of Emergency Medicine at Children's Hospital since 1993 and was recently appointed interim executive director for hospital-based specialties at the institution. Dr. Wright is founding director of the Center for Prehospital Pediatrics at Children's and serves as the State EMS Medical Director for Pediatrics within the Maryland Institute for Emergency Medical Services Systems. His major areas of scholarly interest include EMS for children, injury prevention, and the needs of underserved communities. Dr. Wright received the Shining Star award from the Los Angeles-based Starlight Foundation for outstanding community service;

was inducted into Delta Omega, the nation's public health honor society; and was elected to membership in Leadership Greater Washington. He has been appointed over the years to several national advisory bodies, including the National Association of Children's Hospitals and Related Institutions and the American Academy of Pediatrics, where he serves as chair of the Subcommittee on Violence.

APPENDIX
C

List of Presentations to the Committee

February 2–4, 2004

Overview of Emergency Care in the U.S. Health System
- Overview of the Emergency Care System
  Arthur L. Kellermann (Emory University School of Medicine)
- Emergency Care Supply and Utilization
  Charlotte S. Yeh (Centers for Medicare and Medicaid Services)
- Rural Issues in Emergency Care
  John E. Prescott (West Virginia University)

Major Emergency Care Issue Areas
- Patient Flow and Emergency Department Crowding
  Brent R. Asplin (University of Minnesota)
- Evolution of the Emergency Department (circa 2004): A Systems Perspective
  Eric B. Larson (Group Health Cooperative)
- Mental Health and Substance Abuse Issues
  Michael H. Allen (University of Colorado Health Sciences Center)
- Workforce Education and Training
  Glenn C. Hamilton (Wright State University School of Medicine)
- Information Technology in Emergency Care
  Larry A. Nathanson (Beth Israel Deaconess Medical Center)

Prehospital Care, Public Health, and Emergency Preparedness
- Emergency Care and Public Health
  Daniel A. Pollock (Centers for Disease Control and Prevention)
- Overview of the Issues Facing Prehospital EMS
  Robert R. Bass (Maryland Institute for Emergency Medical Services Systems)
- Emergency Preparedness
  Joseph F. Waeckerle (University of Missouri Baptist Medical Center)

Research Agenda
- Overview of Research in Emergency Care
  E. John Gallagher (Montefiore Medical Center)
- Research Needs for the Future
  Robin M. Weinick (Agency for Healthcare Research and Quality)

June 9–11, 2004

Overview of Emergency Medical Services for Children
- The EMS-C Program: History and Current Challenges
  Jane Ball (The EMSC National Resource Center)
- The 1993 IOM Report: Promise and Progress
  Megan McHugh (IOM Staff)

Issues in Pediatric Emergency Care
- Pediatric Equipment and Care Management
  Marianne Gausche-Hill (Harbor-UCLA Medical Center)
- Special Problems in Pediatric Medication
  Milap Nahata (Ohio State University Schools of Pharmacy and Medicine)
- Training and Skills Maintenance
  Cynthia Wright-Johnson (Maryland Institute for EMS Systems)
- Emergency Research and Data Issues
  David Jaffe (Washington University in St. Louis)

Pediatric Disaster Preparedness
- *George Foltin (New York University Bellevue Hospital Center)*

Organization and Delivery of Emergency Medical Services
- System-Wide EMS and Trauma Planning and Coordination
  Stephen Hise (National Association of State EMS Directors)
- Fire Perspective on EMS
  John Sinclair (International Association of Fire Chiefs)
- Trauma Systems
  Alasdair Conn (Massachusetts General Hospital)
- Critical Care Transport
  Richard Orr (Children's Hospital of Pittsburgh)

History and Organization of EMS in the United States
- EMS System Overview and History
  Robert Bass (Maryland Institute for Emergency Medical Services Systems)
- Overview of Local EMS Systems
  Mike Williams (Abaris Group)

- Issues Facing Rural Emergency Medical Services
  Fergus Laughridge (Emergency Medical Services, Nevada State Health Division)

Prehospital EMS Issue Areas
- EMS Financing and Reimbursement
  Jerry Overton (Richmond Ambulance Authority)
- EMS Quality Improvement and Patient Safety
  Robert A. Swor (William Beaumont Hospital)
- Overview of the EMS Agenda for the Future
  Ted Delbridge (University of Pittsburgh)
- EMS Data Needs
  Greg Mears (University of North Carolina-Chapel Hill)
- Overview of Current EMS Research
  Ron Maio (University of Michigan)

Agency Reaction Panel
- Health Resources and Services Administration, Maternal and Child Health Bureau
  Dave Heppel (Division of Child, Adolescent, and Family Health) and/or Dan Kavanaugh (EMSC-Program)
- National Highway Traffic Safety Administration
  Drew Dawson (EMS Division)
- Agency for Healthcare Research and Quality
  Robin Weinick (Safety Nets and Low Income Populations and Intramural Research)
- Centers for Disease Control and Prevention, National Center for Injury Prevention and Control
  Rick Hunt (Division of Injury and Disability Outcomes and Programs)
- Health Resources and Services Administration, Office of Rural Health Policy
  Evan Mayfield (U.S. Public Health Service and Public Health Analyst)

June 24–25, 2004

Workforce Issues in the Emergency Department
- Issues Facing the Emergency Care Nursing Workforce
  Mary Jagim (MeritCare Hospital)
  Carl Ray (Bon Secours DePaul Medical Center)
  Kathy Robinson (Pennsylvania Department of Health)

Current Initiatives in Patient Flow
- Patient Flow Initiative Implemented at University of Utah
  Jadie Barrie (University of Utah)
  Pamela Proctor (University of Utah)
- Program for Management of Variability in Health Care Delivery
  Eugene Litvak (Boston University Health Policy Institute)

Luncheon Speaker—Medical Technology in Emergency Medicine
- *Michael Sachs (Sg2)*

September 20–21, 2004

Prehospital EMS Issue Areas
- International EMS Systems
  Jerry Overton (Richmond Ambulance Authority)
- Current Status of Federal Emergency Care Legislation and Funding
  Mark Mioduski (Cornerstone Government Affairs)
- Overview of EMS Workforce Issues
  John Becknell (Consultant)
- EMS System Design and Coordination
  Bob Davis (USA Today)

Reimbursement and Funding of Pediatric Emergency Care Services
- Reimbursement Issues in Pediatric Emergency Care
  Steven E. Krug (Northwestern University/Children's Memorial Hospital)
- Current Status of Federal Emergency Care Legislation and Funding
  Mark Mioduski (Cornerstone Government Affairs)

Issues Facing Pediatric Emergency Care
- Funding of Children's Hospitals
  Peter Holbrook (Children's National Medical Center)
- Survey on Pediatric Preparedness
  Marianne Gausche-Hill (Harbor-UCLA Medical Center)

October 4–5, 2004

No open sessions held.

March 2–4, 2005

Public Health Perspectives
- Overview of EMS and Trauma System Issues
  William Koenig (Emergency Medical Services Agency, LA County)

- The Hospital Perspective
  Doug Bagley (Riverside County Regional Medical Center)
- The Safety Net and Community Providers Perspective
  John Gressman (San Francisco Community Clinics Consortium)
- Mental Health and Substance Abuse
  Barry Chaitin (University of California—Irvine)
- The Patient Perspective
  Sandy Schuhmann-Atkins (University of California—Irvine)

On-Call Coverage Issues
- Survey of On-Call Coverage in California
  Mark Langdorf (University of California—Irvine)
- Specialty Physician Perspective—Orthopedics
  Nick Halikis (Little Company of Mary Hospital)
- Specialty Physician Perspective—Neurosurgery
  John Kusske (University of California—Irvine)

Issues in Rural Emergency Care
- The Family Practice Perspective
  *Arlene Brown (Southern New Mexico Family Medicine Residency
  and Family Practice Associates of Ruidoso, PC)*
- Telemedicine in Rural Emergency Care
  Jim Marcin (University of California—Davis)

APPENDIX
D

List of Commissioned Papers

1. The Role of the Emergency Department in the Health Care Delivery System
   Consultant: Eva Stahl, Brandeis University

2. Patient Safety and Quality of Care in Emergency Services
   Consultant: Jim Adams, Northwestern University

3. Patient Flow in Hospital-Based Emergency Services
   Consultant: Brad Prenny, Boston University, Health Policy Institute

4. Models of Organization, Delivery, and Planning for EMS and Trauma Systems
   Consultant: Tasmeen Singh, Children's National Medical Center

5. Information Technology in Emergency Care
   Consultant: Larry Nathanson, Harvard Medical School

6. Emergency Care in Rural America
   Consultant: Janet Williams, University of Rochester

7. The Emergency Care Workforce
   Consultant: Jean Moore, State University of New York School of Public Health

8. The Financing of EMS and Hospital-Based Emergency Services
   Consultants: John McConnell, Oregon Health and Sciences University
   David Gray, Medical University of South Carolina
   Richard Lindrooth, Medical University of South Carolina

9. **The Impact of New Medical Technologies on Emergency Care**
   Consultant: Sg2

10. **Mental Health and Substance Abuse in the Emergent Care Setting**
    Consultant: Linda Degutis, DrPH, Yale University

11. **Emergency Care Research Funding**
    Consultant: Roger Lewis, Harbor-UCLA Medical Center

APPENDIX
E

Statistics on Emergency and Trauma Care Utilization

Emergency departments (EDs) and trauma centers see an enormous variety of patients and conditions on a daily basis. Regardless of income, insurance status, age, or race, people rely on EDs for care in the event of a serious illness or injury, and increasingly for primary care. This appendix describes some of the key utilization trends in hospital-based emergency care. It is based largely on data from the Centers for Disease Control and Prevention's (CDC) National Hospital Ambulatory Health Care Survey for 2003, as reported by McCaig and Burt (2005), supplemented by other sources.

INJURIES AND CONDITIONS TREATED

In 2003, the most common medical diagnoses among ED patients, excluding injuries, were acute upper respiratory infections (5.7 percent), abdominal pain (3.9 percent), chest pain (3.7 percent), and spinal disorders (2.5 percent). About 40.2 million visits, or 35.3 percent of visits, were injury related. Of the visits related to injuries, 70 percent were for unintentional injuries, such as falls, being unintentionally struck by an object, motor vehicle crashes, and injuries from a piercing instrument or object. About 5 percent of injuries were intentional, including assaults and self-inflicted injuries (McCaig and Burt, 2005). Reasons for hospital ED visits are summarized in Table E-1.

There has also been a marked increase in the number of trauma visits, resulting in a significant increase in emergency workloads and contributing to the crowding problem (Reilly et al., 2005). During the 5 years between

TABLE E-1 ED Visits by 20 Leading Diagnoses

Principal Reason for Visit	Percent
Contusion with intact skin surface	4.2
Acute upper respiratory infections, excluding pharyngitis	4.0
Abdominal pain	3.9
Chest pain	3.7
Open wound, excluding head	3.6
Spinal disorders	2.5
Otitis media and eustachian tube disorders	2.3
Sprains and strains, excluding neck and back	2.2
Fractures, excluding lower limb	2.1
Open wound of head	2.0
Sprains and strains of neck and ankle and back	2.0
Acute pharyngitis	1.7
Urinary tract infection	1.6
Chronic and unspecified bronchitis	1.6
Superficial injuries	1.6
Cellulitis and abscess	1.6
Pyrexia of unknown origin	1.5
Asthma	1.5
Heart disease, excluding ischemic	1.5
Rheumatism, excluding back	1.5
All other	53.1
Total	99.7

SOURCE: McCaig and Burt, 2005.

1999 and 2003, trauma visits rose by 18.1 percent. Most of this increase reflects patients who were seen by the trauma team and released rather than admitted as patients. The authors suggest that overtriage, perhaps related to malpractice and Emergency Medical Treatment and Active Labor Act (EMTALA) concerns associated with treating injured patients at nontrauma centers, may be a major factor.

Over the past several years, increasingly complex cases have been seen in the ED. Patients are presenting with higher severity of illness, and many have comorbidities and chronic diseases (Derlet and Richards, 2000; Bazzoli et al., 2003). These patients require more complex and time-consuming workups and treatments.

In 2000, 45.4 percent of Americans had a chronic condition (see Figure E-1). That number is expected to grow to 47.7 percent by 2015 (Partnership for Solutions, 2002). Specifically, the prevalence of cardiovascular disease (CVD) will increase by 18 percent as a result of the aging of the population. In 2003, 71 million Americans had CVD (AHA, 2006); by 2010, it is projected that 69 million Americans will have the disease. Simi-

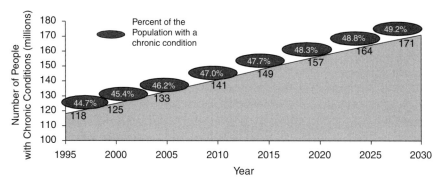

FIGURE E-1 Portion of the U.S. population with a chronic disease.
SOURCE: Partnership for Solutions, 2002.

larly, the prevalence of neurological diseases, particularly those associated with aging, such as Parkinson's disease, stroke, and Alzheimer's disease, will increase.

Increases in disease prevalence over the coming decade, especially of CVD and neurological disease, will also drive growth in ED use. The use of medical therapies will reduce ED visits in the near term, but those same patients will live longer, resulting in increased ED visits in the longer term. Implantable technologies for cardiac diseases will increase patient survival and the likelihood of increased ED visits later in patients' lives. A higher prevalence of chronic diseases, such as diabetes, asthma, and obesity, will also lead to higher ED utilization. Poor patient management of chronic diseases and polypharmacy issues—the unwanted duplication of drugs—will contribute to increased ED utilization as well.

ED VISITS BY AGE

Elderly

Older Americans (75+) have a much higher rate of ED visits than other age groups (see Table E-2). Care of the elderly presents unique challenges. This pool of patients tends to come to the ED with more severe medical-related conditions, to have a higher probability of being admitted to the hospital, and to consume more resources than other patients.

Elderly patients may not receive appropriate care, particularly when there is cognitive impairment (Sanders, 2002). Their problems tend to be

TABLE E-2 Visits and Visits per 100 by
Age, 2003

Age	Number of Visits in Thousands	Visits per 100 Persons
Under 15	24,733	40.8
15–24	17,731	44.2
25–44	32,906	40.0
45–64	20,992	30.8
65–74	7,153	39.5
75 and older	10,389	64.2

SOURCE: McCaig and Burt, 2005.

complex and time-consuming, and therefore have a disproportionate impact on emergency care services (Sanders, 2001). For older patients, workups are more difficult, and lengths of stay in the ED are greater; nearly half of older patients (65 and older) are admitted to the hospital, compared with 11 percent of younger adults (McNamara et al., 1992; Singal et al., 1992). More patients aged 75 and older arrive by emergency medical transport (40.9 percent, versus 4.2 percent of all patients), and patients 65 and older are most likely to be classified as emergent (25.5 percent, versus 15.2 percent of all patients) (McCaig and Burt, 2005). Utilization of the ED by elderly patients is likely to increase as the population ages over the next two decades; by 2050, individuals aged 65+ are expected to make up over 20 percent of the total U.S. population (U.S. Census Bureau, 2004).

Children

In 2003, children under age 15 made over 24 million visits to EDs, representing 22 percent of all ED visits. This equates to almost 4 visits for every 10 children under age 15 (McCaig and Burt, 2005). Despite the frequent use of emergency services by children, the training, equipment, medications, and technology of emergency care often fail to address their needs (Glaser et al., 1997; Moreland et al., 1998; Tamariz et al., 2000; Middleton and Burt, 2006). Children are different from adults in a wide range of clinically significant ways. For example, they have different metabolic and respiratory rates, different blood pressure levels, smaller airways, greater surface-to-body weight ratios, higher emotional sensitivity, and limited communication skills. The services, drugs, and equipment developed for use by adult patients in an emergency situation are often inappropriate for pediatric patients. The limited availability of pediatric equipment and supplies in ambulances and EDs has been well documented in several reports (IOM, 1993; Hamilton et al., 2003). One survey of EDs found that the average hospital in the

United States had about 80 percent of the American Academy of Pediatrics' (AAP) recommended pediatric supplies, and only 6 percent of hospitals had all of the recommended equipment (Middleton and Burt, 2006). And while children's hospitals are a unique resource for pediatric patients, most such patients are treated in general rather than children's hospitals (Gausche-Hill et al., 2004). Pediatric emergency care is dealt with comprehensively in the companion IOM report in this series titled *Emergency Care for Children: Growing Pains*.

ED VISITS BY RACIAL AND ETHNIC COMPOSITION

The 2002 utilization rate for African Americans was 71 percent higher than that for whites. In addition, African Americans had some of the largest increases in ED utilization rates during the 1990s. Particularly among those over 65, African Americans increased their ED utilization by 59 percent during that decade, while utilization among whites in the same age bracket remained relatively unchanged (McCaig and Ly, 2002).

Other minority populations, including Hispanic and non-English-speaking populations, also utilize the ED at higher rates than whites. The proportion of the population that said they spoke English less than "very well" grew from 4.8 percent in 1980 to 6.1 percent in 1990 and 8.1 percent in 2000 (U.S. Census Bureau, 2004). Language barriers can result in higher rates of resource utilization for diagnostic studies, increased ED visit times (Hampers et al., 1999), and lower satisfaction with care (Carrasquillo et al., 1999). In addition, non-English-speaking people may be less likely to trust the emergency system and more likely to be unfamiliar with 9-1-1 and to fail to understand which services are available to them and at what cost.

While racial disparities in health care have been well documented (IOM, 2002; AHRQ, 2003), the evidence for disparities in emergency services is limited. Studies have shown differences in wait times for Hispanic patients, insurer authorization for ED visits by African Americans (Lowe and Bindman, 1994), and administration of pain medication for African Americans (Todd et al., 2000).

FREQUENT USERS

One particularly challenging group of ED patients is those who make repeated visits. Estimates from different data sources indicate that 5 to 7 percent of the U.S. population will make two or more ED visits in a given year (Zuckerman and Shen, 2004). A smaller group of individuals, often referred to as "frequent flyers," visit the ED for care even more frequently. Frequent users tend to be in poor health, suffering from high rates of chronic illness, drug disorders, and mental illness (Sun et al., 2003; Washington

State Department of Social and Health Services, 2004). Many also suffer from socioeconomic distress (Sun et al., 2003). Frequent users are a challenge to ED staff because they require intensive resources, such as mental health, substance-abuse, and case management services, that often are not available at EDs.

REFERENCES

AHA (American Heart Association). 2006. *Heart Disease and Stroke Statistics—2006 Update.* Dallas, TX: AHA.

AHRQ (Agency for Healthcare Research and Quality). 2003. *National Healthcare Disparities Report.* Rockville, MD: U.S. Department of Health and Human Services.

Bazzoli GJ, Brewster LR, Liu G, Kuo S. 2003. Does U.S. hospital capacity need to be expanded? *Health Affairs* 22(6):40–54.

Carrasquillo O, Orav E, Brennan T, Burstin H. 1999. Impact of language barriers on patient satisfaction in an emergency department [Abstract]. *Journal of General Internal Medicine* 14(2):82–87.

Derlet RW, Richards JR. 2000. Overcrowding in the nation's emergency departments: Complex causes and disturbing effects. *Annals of Emergency Medicine* 35(1):63–68.

Gausche-Hill M, Lewis R, Schmitz C. 2004. *Survey of US Emergency Departments for Pediatric Preparedness—Implementation and Evaluation of Care of Children in the Emergency Department: Guidelines for Preparedness.* [unpublished].

Glaser NS, Kuppermann N, Yee CK, Schwartz DL, Styne DM. 1997. Variation in the management of pediatric diabetic ketoacidosis by specialty training. *Archives of Pediatrics & Adolescent Medicine* 151(11):1125–1132.

Hamilton S, Adler M, Walker A. 2003. Pediatric calls: Lessons learned from pediatric research. *JEMS: Journal of Emergency Medical Services* 28(7):56–63.

Hampers LC, Cha S, Gutglass DJ, Binns HJ, Krug SE. 1999. Language barriers and resource utilization in a pediatric emergency department. *Pediatrics* 103(6 Pt. 1):1253–1256.

IOM (Institute of Medicine). 1993. *Emergency Medical Services for Children.* Washington, DC: National Academy Press.

IOM. 2002. *Unequal Treatment: Confronting Racial and Ethnic Disparities in Health Care.* Washington, DC: The National Academies Press.

Lowe RA, Bindman AB. 1994. The ED and triage of nonurgent patients. *Annals of Emergency Medicine* 24(5):990–992.

McCaig LF, Burt CW. 2005. *National Hospital Ambulatory Medical Care Survey: 2003 Emergency Department Summary.* Hyattsville, MD: National Center for Health Statistics.

McCaig LF, Ly N. 2002. *National Hospital Ambulatory Medical Care Survey: 2000 Emergency Department Summary* (Advance Data from Vital and Health Statistics No. 326). Hyattsville, MD: National Center for Health Statistics.

McNamara RM, Rousseau E, Sanders AB. 1992. Geriatric emergency medicine: A survey of practicing emergency physicians. *Annals of Emergency Medicine* 21(7):796–801.

Middleton KR, Burt CW. 2006. *Availability of Pediatric Services and Equipment in Emergency Departments: United States, 2002–03.* Hyattsville, MD: National Center for Health Statistics.

Moreland JE, Sanddal ND, Sanddal TL, Pickert CB. 1998. Pediatric equipment in ambulances. *Pediatric Emergency Care* 14(1):84.

Partnership for Solutions. 2002. *Chronic Conditions: Making the Case for Ongoing Care.* Baltimore, MD: Johns Hopkins University.

Reilly PM, Schwab CW, Kauder DR, Dabrowski GP, Gracias V, Gupta R, Pryor JP, Braslow

BM, Kim P, Wiebe DJ. 2005. The invisible trauma patient: Emergency department discharges. *Journal of Trauma-Injury Infection & Critical Care* 58(4):675–683; discussion 683–685.

Sanders AB. 2001. Older persons in the emergency medical care system. *Journal of the American Geriatrics Society* 49(10):1390–1392.

Sanders AB. 2002. Quality in emergency medicine: An introduction. *Academic Emergency Medicine* 9:1064–1066.

Singal BM, Hedges JR, Rousseau EW, Sanders AB, Berstein E, McNamara RM, Hogan TM. 1992. Geriatric patient emergency visits. Part I: Comparison of visits by geriatric and younger patients. *Annals of Emergency Medicine* 21(7):802–807.

Sun BC, Burstin HR, Brennan TA. 2003. Predictors and outcomes of frequent emergency department users. *Academic Emergency Medicine* 10(4):320–328.

Tamariz VP, Fuchs S, Baren JM, Pollack ES, Kim J, Seidel JS. 2000. Pediatric emergency medicine education in emergency medicine training programs. SAEM pediatric education training task force. *Academic Emergency Medicine* 7(7):774–778.

Todd K, Deaton C, D'Adamo A, Goe L. 2000. Ethnicity and analgesic practice. *Annals of Emergency Medicine* 35(1):11–16.

U.S. Census Bureau. 2004. *The Face of Our Population*. [Online]. Available: http://factfinder.census.gov/jsp/saff/SAFFInfo.jsp?_pageId=tp9_race_ethnicity [accessed March 22, 2005].

Washington State Department of Social and Health Services. 2004. *Frequent Emergency Room Visits Signal Substance Abuse and Mental Illness DSHS Research and Data Analysis Division*. Olympia, WA: Washington State Department of Social and Health Services.

Zuckerman S, Shen Y-C. 2004. Characteristics of occasional and frequent emergency department users. *Medical Care* 42(2):176–182.

Historical Development of Hospital-Based Emergency and Trauma Care

HOSPITAL-BASED EMERGENCY CARE

The modern emergency department (ED) developed at a time when the specialization of medical practice swept the nation after World War II, and it reflects the general trend toward hospitals as a site of medical care rather than homes and physicians' offices. As the practice of generalist physicians making house calls declined, patients increasingly turned to the local hospital for treatment. This trend was reinforced by the development of private insurance plans, which geared payments toward hospitals and away from home visits (Rosen, 1995). The development of the ED also reflects the passage of the Hill-Burton Act of 1946, which gave states federal grants to build hospitals provided that the states met a variety of conditions, including a community service obligation. Among other things, the community service obligation requires hospitals receiving Hill-Burton funding to maintain an emergency room. This requirement applies to the vast majority of nonprofit U.S. hospitals in operation today (Rosenblatt et al., 2001).

But hospital-based emergency care was really spurred forward by developments in trauma care that resulted from America's wartime experiences. World War II saw the development of blood transfusions, resuscitation, rapid transport of injured patients to field hospitals, and advances in surgical care of injuries. Military medicine advanced further during the Korean and Vietnam wars with the introduction of medical evacuation by helicopter to mobile field hospitals. Modern emergency medical services (EMS) and trauma systems grew out of a growing recognition that these methods could also be applied to civilian populations back home (Boyd, 1983).

Coincident with developments in the treatment of injuries were advances in the treatment of acute coronary syndrome (ACS). In Belfast, Ireland, Dr. Frank Pantridge was demonstrating that a mobile coronary care unit could substantially reduce mortality among heart attack victims (Pantridge and Geddes, 1967). Following his lead, several medical centers in the United States began programs to deliver rapid emergency care to cardiac patients. William Grace, for example, established a mobile coronary care unit at St. Vincent's Hospital in New York City—the first of its kind in America—that transported physicians to the scene of patients experiencing ACS (Key et al., 2005). Other programs were started independently in Los Angeles, Seattle, Columbus, and Miami.

The recognition that injured or acutely ill people could be saved if they received treatment within a short span of time led to the development of prehospital EMS systems designed to get patients to the hospital quickly. This in turn stimulated the development of hospital-based emergency care and the specialty of emergency medicine. The introduction of new technologies that facilitated the rapid diagnosis and treatment of injuries and acute illnesses, such as the computed tomography (CT) scan and cardiac monitoring, contributed to this growth.

Public interest in the importance of emergency services was sparked by the 1966 landmark National Academy of Sciences/National Research Council (NAS/NRC) report *Accidental Death and Disability: The Neglected Disease of Modern Society* (NAS and NRC, 1966). The report described the epidemic of automobile and other injuries—due in part to the expansion of the interstate highway system—and the deplorable system for treating these injuries nationwide. At the time, most emergency rooms appeared to offer only advanced first aid; only a few facilities had the staff and equipment to provide complete care for seriously ill or injured patients. Patients who appeared at the hospital were often turned away if they did not have funds to pay for their care, and transfers to the city or county indigent care facility were conducted without concern for patients' well-being (Rosen, 1995). To many in the field, the 1966 NAS/NRC report marked the beginning of the modern emergency care system. Coupled with advances in military medicine and civilian cardiac care, this report led to the Highway Safety Act of 1966 (P.L. 89-564), which created the National Highway Traffic Safety Administration (NHTSA) within the Department of Transportation and required states to develop regional emergency care systems.

The growing demand for emergency care and the difficulty of finding physicians to provide it led hospitals to require that active medical staff take turns covering the ED at night and to hire additional ED staff, regardless of their skills or experience. Eventually, some physicians gave up their regular practices to work in the ED full time. One of the first to do so was James Mills, M.D., who started the Alexandria Plan in 1961, a group made up of physicians who worked only in the ED. Similar plans in Pontiac and Flint,

Michigan, soon followed. Because of the advantages to hospitals of having a steady, full-time team covering the ED, hospitals began contracting for emergency services, and an increasing number of physicians decided to work in EDs full time. Most private physicians entering this new field had no specialized medical training; they entered ED practice after completing only an internship (Rosen, 1995).

The Emergency Medical Services Systems Act of 1973 (P.L. 93-154) created a new grant program in the Division of EMS in the Department of Health, Education, and Welfare (DHEW) to foster the development of regional EMS systems. NHTSA simultaneously funded the prehospital components of EMS systems and oversaw the development of curricula and training for EMS professionals. A number of advances resulted from this confluence of efforts, including the establishment of state coordinating offices and local EMS planning councils, the proliferation of trained emergency medical technicians (EMTs), and the development of air transport services.

But while EMS systems benefited from an influx of federal funding in the 1970s, EDs received less support, and deficiencies remained. Throughout the 1970s, a pattern was established of soaring ED patient volumes along with relative neglect of the needs of EDs.

In the early 1980s, the period of strong federal leadership and funding for the development of emergency care came to an end with the passage of the Omnibus Reconciliation Act of 1981 (P.L. 97-35). This legislation replaced the categorical funding for EMS activities in the states with Preventive Health and Health Services Block Grants that allowed states to allocate federal EMS dollars to other programs. The act eliminated most emergent care activities under DHEW, and spending on EMS dropped dramatically. NHTSA therefore became the de facto federal lead agency for emergency care activities, although its emphasis was even more focused on prehospital activities than DHEW's, and even NHTSA's funding for EMS, provided through Section 402 of the State and Community Highway Safety Program, was reduced (IOM, 1993). A General Accounting Office (GAO) report found that funding fell by 34 percent between 1981 and 1983. Funding also shifted to the states: in 1981 about 27 percent of funding was from state and local funds; by 1988, the state and local share had increased to 82 percent (GAO, 1986).

Also in the 1980s, the importance of prevention of injury was becoming more widely recognized and was highlighted in the 1985 NAS/NRC report *Injury in America: A Continuing Health Problem* (NRC and IOM, 1985). This report led to the establishment of the Centers for Disease Control and Prevention's (CDC) National Center for Injury Prevention and Control in 1992. Also, a growing recognition of the unmet emergency care needs of children, particularly among professional organizations such as the American Academy of Pediatrics, the American College of Emergency Physicians (ACEP), the Society of Critical Care Medicine, and the National Association of EMS Physicians, led to the establishment of the Emergency Medical Services for Children (EMS-C) program within the Department of Health and Human Services (DHHS) as part of the Health Services, Preventive Health Services, and Home and Community Based Services Act of 1984 (P.L. 98-555). The EMS-C program, established as a demonstration grant program despite its longevity, has funded two resource centers and established grants to states for the development and implementation of EMS-C programs. While focused on pediatrics, the program has worked closely and jointly funded general projects with NHTSA and other federal partners to promote both general enhancements that will benefit children and the integration of children's issues into general emergency care planning and activities.

THE DEVELOPMENT OF TRAUMA CARE

Trauma represents a particular kind of medical emergency. It is typically defined as involving a physical wound caused by force or impact, such as a fall, automobile crash, or gunshot; burns and other severe wounds are also considered a form of trauma. Life-threatening emergencies caused by preexisting conditions, such as a heart attack, are generally not considered trauma. Trauma care is distinguished from care received in a general ED by the severity of the injury and the specialized diagnostic and treatment procedures necessary to care for the patient. Ideally, traumatically injured patients are cared for in a trauma center, a hospital that is able to receive such patients 24 hours a day, 7 days a week. Trauma centers are designed to meet the complex surgical needs of critically injured patients immediately. To qualify as a trauma center, a hospital must have a number of capabilities, including a resource-intensive ED, a high-quality intensive care ward, and an operating room that is functional at all times.

The development of trauma care mirrors the development of surgery in general and has been stimulated by wartime experiences. The seeds of the modern trauma system can be traced to the beginnings of the American College of Surgeons (ACS), which was founded in 1922 (Trunkey, 2000). The ACS established a Committee on Fractures, as well as the Hospital Standardization Program, which collected data on fracture injuries, thus becoming the first trauma registry. (This program later became the Joint Commission on Accreditation of Healthcare Organizations [JCAHO].) The ACS later formed the Board of Industrial Medicine and Traumatic Injury in 1926.

Rapid advances in medical treatment and in the rapid delivery of patients to hospitals occurred during World Wars I and II and the Korean and Vietnam wars, and the current conflict in Iraq continues this pattern, with a number of important advances being made. The modern era of trauma care is equally concerned with the development of trauma care systems. San Francisco General Hospital and Cook County Hospital in Chicago began the development of systematic approaches to trauma care. These efforts were closely followed by the development of Maryland's statewide trauma care system by R. Adams Crowley (Trunkey, 2000). In 1976, the American College of Surgeons Committee on Trauma (ACS COT) published formal criteria for trauma systems—*Optimal Criteria for the Care of the Injured Patient*—which included the categorization of trauma centers based on their capabilities in treating traumatic injuries (ACS COT, 1999).

Optimal Criteria for Care of the Injured Patient

The development of trauma systems, which was limited to a few states before 1990, accelerated greatly with the enactment of the Trauma Care Systems Planning and Development Act (P.L. 101-590) in 1990, and the number of trauma centers nationwide began to increase rapidly. This program was eliminated in 1995, leaving a gap in federal leadership on trauma system development until the creation of the Trauma/EMS Systems Program within the Healthcare Resources and Services Administration's (HRSA) Division of Healthcare Preparedness in 2001. This new program again provided national leadership for trauma care planning, infrastructure development, standards development, and coordination with other federal agencies until it, too, was zeroed out of the federal budget for fiscal year 2006.

A trauma system is a coordinated approach to trauma care and injury prevention. It is based on the premise that optimal care is delivered to injured patients when preconceived processes and resources are coordinated in an organizational plan. A well-organized trauma system allows patients to move seamlessly and expediently through the system. The formality of trauma systems varies by states. Almost all systems have standardized triage processes and constant oversight over trauma centers, but systems vary on many other factors, including designation processes and criteria for interfacility transfers.

The most recent nationwide inventory of trauma centers was published in 2003, based on data collected in 2001–2002. A total of 1,154 trauma centers were identified in the 50 states and the District of Columbia; an additional 31 trauma centers treat only children. Every state has at least one trauma center of some level, and all but Arkansas have at least one level I or level II (the most sophisticated).

An important aspect of trauma systems is the categorization of hospitals according to the level of trauma services they provide. This information is then used by regional EMS agencies and community hospitals to direct trauma patients to the most appropriate level of care given their condition and location. The process of categorizing hospitals was pioneered in 1976 by ACS COT, which today is the principal body for verifying that trauma centers meet accepted standards of trauma care. The Verification Review Committee, a subcommittee of ACS COT, was established in the late 1980s to conduct on-site consultations and verifications. Consultations are conducted at the request of a hospital, community, or state authority to prepare a facility for a verification review. Verification review is ACS COT's process of assessing the trauma care capabilities of a facility based on the criteria contained in *Resources for Optimal Care of the Injured Patient*. Through the verification review process, a facility is established as a level I, II, III, or IV trauma center based on a variety of factors, including the volume of severely injured patients, 24-hour availability of trauma surgeons and other specialists, whether these specialists are in house or on call, the surgical capabilities of the center, and the availability of specialized equipment. (See Box F-1.)

Designation is the process by which local governments designate specific facilities as trauma centers within their system, usually based on ACS COT verification. A minority of trauma centers are verified not by the ACS COT process, but by a state verification process. The criteria and categorization systems used by states that conduct verification can vary, and some states include a fifth level of triage designation. Level V trauma centers are not formally recognized by the ACS, but they are used by some states to further categorize hospitals providing life support prior to transfer.

Current Issues in Trauma Systems

Although trauma centers and trauma systems have developed extensively over the last two decades, a number of critical issues remain.

Lack of Regional Coordination

Ensuring that each patient is directed to the most appropriate setting for care requires that many elements within the regional system—community hospital, trauma centers, and particularly prehospital EMS—effectively coordinate the regional flow of patients. In addition to improving patient care, coordinating the regional flow of patients is a critical tool in reducing overcrowding in EDs. Few systems nationwide have effective coordination between EMS and hospital EDs and trauma centers and actively direct patients to the best location based on current availability of beds, operating rooms, specialists, and critical equipment.

BOX F-1
Classification System for Trauma Center Levels of the American College of Surgeons Committee on Trauma

Level I

Provides comprehensive trauma care; serves as a regional resource; and provides leadership in education, research, and system planning. A level I center is required to have trauma surgeons, anesthesiologists, physician specialists, nurses, and resuscitation equipment immediately available. Volume performance criteria further stipulate that level I centers must treat 1,200 admissions per year or 240 major trauma patients per year or an average of 35 major trauma patients per surgeon.

Level II

Provides comprehensive trauma care either as a supplement to a level I trauma center in a large urban area or as the lead hospital in a less population-dense area. Level II centers must meet essentially the same criteria as level I, but volume performance standards are not required and may depend on the geographic area served. Centers are not expected to provide leadership in teaching and research.

Level III

Provides prompt assessment, resuscitation, emergency surgery, and stabilization, with transfer to a level I or II center as indicated. Level III facilities typically serve communities that lack immediate access to a level I or II center.

Level IV

Provides advanced trauma life support prior to patient transfer in remote areas in which no higher level of care is available. The key role of a level IV center is to resuscitate and stabilize patients and arrange for their transfer to the closest and most appropriate level of facility.

Decreased Pool of Trauma Surgeons and Other Specialists

There is a declining pool of trauma surgeons and on-call specialists because of the large amount of uncompensated care they are required to provide, the extraordinary medical malpractice risk involved, and the lifestyle burdens associated with providing emergency call day and night.

Loss of Trauma Centers

Trauma care is expensive to provide and often is poorly compensated. As a result, level I trauma centers have been closing in major cities because of the financial pressure of caring for uninsured and underinsured patients. When a trauma center closes, nearby centers are under substantial pressure to take additional patients. The loss of regional trauma capacity can be perilous for patients, as it can increase the time required to reach definitive care.

MILITARY EMERGENCY AND TRAUMA CARE

Just as the U.S. civilian emergency care system benefited from advances made in military medicine during the Vietnam and Korean wars, the civilian system may benefit from further medical advances being made during the current U.S. military operations in Afghanistan and Iraq. Indeed, military medics and physicians today have better information and tools at their disposal relative to those involved in previous military engagements, and these advances are expected to reduce battlefield deaths considerably. The Iraq war has produced the lowest casualty fatality rate ever seen in combat among injured U.S. soldiers (Connolly, 2004). In many respects, military medicine is well ahead of the civilian trauma system in place today.

One important advance has been the development and implementation of a medical information management system for military forces. In past military engagements, soldiers carried paper medical cards to be inserted into their medical records at a later time. However, the cards would often get damaged or lost, leaving field medics with little information on wounded soldiers (Campbell, 2005). In 1999, the Department of Defense adopted Medical Communications for Combat Casualty Care (MC4), a system that contains digitally secure, accurate medical histories of soldiers and makes that information available to military clinicians around the world. The system incorporates information from pre- and postdeployment health surveys, and military medics enter additional information from the field using MC4 laptops and handheld devices if a soldier is wounded (Onley, 2003; Steen, 2005). Medics can also use the system to order supplies, find information on drug doses and physician references, and track the movement of patients as they receive higher levels of care (Onley, 2003). The central database allows medical specialists to track trends and conduct surveillance, with the hope of eliminating the phenomenon that occurred after the Gulf War, when soldiers came back with unusual symptoms, and there was no paper trail documenting what chemicals they were exposed to or what care they may have received. Although a number of brigades in Iraq are still using paper records, more than 10,000 deployable medical and ancillary professionals have been trained on the MC4, and the system is being used by more than 250 units in Iraq (Onley, 2003; Steen, 2006).

The military has also improved access to medical care so that wounded soldiers receive higher levels of care more quickly. To this end, the military has moved its medical assets closer to the front lines and improved air medical capabilities (Miles, 2005). The Marine Corps and the Navy introduced forward resuscitative surgery systems—small, mobile trauma surgical teams of eight individuals (two surgeons and support staff) designed to provide tactical surgical intervention for combat casualties in the forward area (Chambers et al., 2005). The units can erect a battlefield hospital with two operating tables and four ventilator-equipped beds in less than 1 hour (Gawande, 2004). New medical technologies, such as compact ultrasound and x-ray machines, generators that extract pure oxygen from the air, and computerized diagnostic equipment, have allowed the teams to provide fairly sophisticated care (Barnes et al., 2005). With these new surgical teams, however, the U.S. military's strategy is to conduct damage control in the field—stop bleeding, keep a patient warm—and leave definitive care to physicians at a hospital. Surgeons limit surgery to 2 hours or less and send the patient off to the next level of care.

Air medical evacuation procedures and equipment have improved to allow rapid transport of a critically injured solider. Thanks to those advances, the Air Force is transporting patients that it would have never considered moving in previous wars (Miles, 2005). From the field surgery teams, patients are brought by helicopter to a larger combat support hospital in Iraq. Air medical evacuations are now lighter and more adaptable; patient support pallets can be moved from one aircraft to the next, and medical teams carry much of their equipment in backpacks. If a soldier is critically wounded, a critical care air transport team joins in the air medical evacuation to help transport the patient to a combat hospital in Iraq, which has additional equipment.

Patient stays at military hospitals in Iraq are brief. Patients are transported as quickly as possible on an aircraft to a U.S. hospital in Germany. Today, the military is able to transport patients on a larger variety of aircraft than in the past, so there is no need to wait for a specific plane to arrive. One aircraft, the C-17 Globemaster III, has the ability to move 70 patients at a time, including 9 with critical injuries. The plane is quieter, vibrates less, and has more temperature control than its predecessors. With medical information systems in place, air medical evacuation teams have detailed information about patients' medical history, medications, medical conditions, and procedures already performed (Miles, 2005). Whereas it took an injured soldier in Vietnam 45 days to reach a U.S. facility, today soldiers go from the battlefield to a U.S. hospital in less than 4 days, and continuous medical care is provided throughout the journey (Gawande, 2004).

The training of medics has also advanced. In the past, medics learned from books and rarely practiced on live patients. Today, training is conducted using specially developed computer software that asks trainees to make critical-care decisions and then provides feedback on the impact of those decisions on the patient. The practice mannequins have mechanized lungs and vital signs controlled by computer (Online NewsHour, 2003).

Soldiers and medics also have new medical tools in Iraq. They carry a new tourniquet designed for one-handed application, so that a solider can apply the tourniquet to himself or herself if necessary (Crisp, 2005). Additionally, many soldiers and medics now carry bandages coated with blood clot–forming compounds that can stop life-threatening bleeding quickly. Anticlotting products are critical since profuse bleeding is a primary reason for casualties on the battlefield (Kolata, 2003). In the past, medics relied simply on gauze and tape (Mishra, 2003). Many special operations medics are carrying hetastarch instead of bulky bags of intravenous saline solution. Hetastarch is a more compact material, making it easier to carry, and it stays in the vascular system longer than saline, helping to maintain blood pressure (Barnes et al., 2005).

The armed forces continue to investigate new ways to improve survival rates in combat zones. As an example, the U.S. Army and Navy commissioned an outside firm to form an expert panel to review and rank research proposals for resuscitation fluids and therapies to determine which held the most promise for improving survival. A second expert panel was convened to examine and improve the ways in which the military obtains results from scientific research for military medicine (Krupa, 2005). Air Force officials report working daily to improve air medical communications, equipment, and procedures (Miles, 2005).

REFERENCES

ACS COT (American College of Surgeons Committee on Trauma). 1999. *Resources for Optimal Care of the Injured Patient*. Chicago: ACS.

Barnes J, Roane K, Szegedy-Maszak M. 2005, April 5. Stemming the fatalities with a modern touch. *Sydney Morning Herald*.

Boyd DR. 1983. The history of emergency medical services (EMS) systems in the United States of America. In: Boyd DR, Edlich RF, Micik SH, eds. *Systems Approach to Emergency Medical Care*. Norwalk, CT: Appleton-Century-Crofts.

Campbell P. 2005, December 12. APL helps Army choose systems for digitizing medical records. *The Johns Hopkins University Gazette*.

Chambers LW, Rhee P, Baker BC, Perciballi J, Cubano M, Compeggie M, Nace M, Bohman HR. 2005. Initial experience of U.S. Marine Corps forward resuscitative surgical system during Operation Iraqi Freedom. *Archives of Surgery* 140(1):26–32.

Connolly C. 2004, December 9. U.S. combat fatality rate lowest ever. *The Washington Post*.

Crisp JD. 2005, July 18. New tourniquet issued to deployed soldiers. *Defend America*.

Gawande A. 2004. Casualties of war: Military care for the wounded from Iraq and Afghanistan. *New England Journal of Medicine* 351(24):2471–2475.

GAO (U.S. General Accounting Office). 1986. *States Assume Leadership Role in Providing Emergency Medical Services* (GAO/HRD-86-41). Washington, DC: GAO.

IOM (Institute of Medicine). 1993. *Emergency Medical Services for Children.* Washington, DC: National Academy Press.

Key CB, Lewis R, Schaal S. 2005. How today's street medicine evolved form the Columbus Heartmobile & other pioneering projects. *Journal of Emergency Medical Services* 30(12):48–55.

Kolata G. 2003, March 30. Armed with new tools, doctors head to battle. *The New York Times.*

Krupa D. 2005. *Armed Forces Search for Ways to Improve Survival in the Combat Zone (Press Release).* Bethesda, MD: Life Sciences Research Office. [Online]. Available: http://www.lsro.org/newsroom/resuscitation_press_release_2005_07_25.pdf [accessed May 20, 3006].

Miles D. 2005, August 10. Aeromedical evacuation improvements saving lives. *DefenseLink News.*

Mishra R. 2003, March 25. Advances in battlefield medicine pay off immediately. *Boston Globe.*

NAS, NRC (National Academy of Sciences, National Research Council). 1966. *Accidental Death and Disability: The Neglected Disease of Modern Society.* Washington, DC: National Academy of Sciences.

NRC, IOM (National Research Council, Institute of Medicine). 1985. *Injury in America: A Continuing Public Health Problem.* Washington, DC: National Academy Press.

Onley D. 2003. Medics tap patient data. *Government Computer News* 22(7).

Online NewsHour. 2003. *Combat Medicine. A NewsHour with Jim Lehrer.* [Online]. Available: http://www.pbs.org/newshour/bb/military/jan-june03/medicine_3-29.html [accessed May 20, 2006].

Pantridge JF, Geddes JS. 1967. A mobile intensive-care unit in the management of myocardial infarction. *Lancet* 2(7510):271–273.

Rosen P. 1995. *History of Emergency Medicine.* New York: Josiah Macy, Jr. Foundation. Pp. 59–79.

Rosenblatt R, Law S, Rosenbaum S. 2001. *Law and the American Health Care System.* New York: Foundation Press.

Steen R. 2005. A gateway to medical information for deployed. *Military Medicine Technology* 9(4).

Steen R. 2006. *U.S. Embassy Clinic in Iraq Uses Digital Medical Recording System: Medical Communications for Combat Casualty Care Connects Clinic to Combat Support Hospital.* [Online]. Available: http://www.dcmilitary.com/army/standard/12_26/national_news/38937-1.html [accessed May 20, 2006].

Trunkey DD. 2000. History and development of trauma care in the United States. *Clinical Orthopaedics & Related Research* (374):36–46.

APPENDIX
G

Recommendations and Responsible Entities from the *Future of Emergency Care* Series

HOSPITAL-BASED EMERGENCY CARE: AT THE BREAKING POINT

	Congress	DHHS	DOT	DHS	DOD	States	Hospitals	EMS Agencies	Private Industry	Professional Organizations	Other
Chapter 2: The Evolving Role of Hospital-Based Emergency Care											
2.1 Congress should establish dedicated funding, separate from Disproportionate Share Hospital payments, to reimburse hospitals that provide significant amounts of uncompensated emergency and trauma care for the financial losses incurred by providing those services.	X	X									
2.1a Congress should initially appropriate $50 million for the purpose, to be administered by the Centers for Medicare and Medicaid Services.											
2.1b The Centers for Medicare and Medicaid Services should establish a working group to determine the allocation of these funds, which should be targeted to providers and localities at greatest risk; the working group should then determine funding needs for subsequent years.											
Chapter 3: Building a 21st-Century Emergency Care System											
3.1 The Department of Health and Human Services and the National Highway Traffic Safety Administration, in partnership with professional organizations, should convene a panel of individuals with multidisciplinary expertise to develop evidence-based categorization systems for emergency medical services, emergency departments, and trauma centers based on adult and pediatric service capabilities.		X	X							X	

3.2 The National Highway Traffic Safety Administration, in partnership with professional organizations, should convene a panel of individuals with multidisciplinary expertise to develop evidence-based model prehospital care protocols for the treatment, triage, and transport of patients.

3.3 The Department of Health and Human Services should convene a panel of individuals with emergency and trauma care expertise to develop evidence-based indicators of emergency and trauma care system performance.

3.4 The Department of Health and Human Services should adopt regulatory changes to the Emergency Medical Treatment and Active Labor Act and the Health Insurance Portability and Accountability Act so that the original goals of the laws will be preserved, but integrated systems can be further developed.

3.5 Congress should establish a demonstration program, administered by the Health Resources and Services Administration, to promote coordinated, regionalized, and accountable emergency care systems throughout the country, and appropriate $88 million over 5 years to this program.

	Congress	DHHS	DOT	DHS	DOD	States	Hospitals	EMS Agencies	Private Industry	Professional Organizations	Other
3.6 Congress should establish a lead agency for emergency and trauma care within 2 years of the release of this report. The lead agency should be housed in the Department of Health and Human Services, and should have primary programmatic responsibility for the full continuum of emergency medical services and emergency and trauma care for adults and children, including medical 9-1-1 and emergency medical dispatch, prehospital emergency medical services (both ground and air), hospital-based emergency and trauma care, and medical-related disaster preparedness. Congress should establish a working group to make recommendations regarding the structure, funding, and responsibilities of the new agency, and develop and monitor the transition. The working group should have representation from federal and state agencies and professional disciplines involved in emergency and trauma care.	X	X									

Chapter 4: Improving the Efficiency of Hospital-Based Emergency Care

	Congress	DHHS	DOT	DHS	DOD	States	Hospitals	EMS Agencies	Private Industry	Professional Organizations	Other
4.1 The Centers for Medicare and Medicaid Services should remove the current restrictions on the medical conditions that are eligible for separate clinical decision unit (CDU) payment.		X									
4.2 Hospital chief executive officers should adopt enterprisewide operations management and related strategies to improve the quality and efficiency of emergency care.							X				

4.3 Training in operations management and related approaches should be promoted by professional associations; accrediting organizations, such as the Joint Commission on Accreditation of Healthcare Organizations and the National Committee for Quality Assurance; and educational institutions that provide training in clinical, health care management, and public health disciplines.

4.4 The Joint Commission on Accreditation of Healthcare Organizations should reinstate strong standards designed to sharply reduce and ultimately eliminate ED crowding, boarding, and diversion.

4.5 Hospitals should end the practices of boarding patients in the emergency department and ambulance diversion, except in the most extreme cases, such as a community mass casualty event. The Centers for Medicare and Medicaid Services should convene a working group that includes experts in emergency care, inpatient critical care, hospital operations management, nursing, and other relevant disciplines to develop boarding and diversion standards, as well as guidelines, measures, and incentives for implementation, monitoring, and enforcement of these standards.

Chapter 5: Technology and Communications

5.1 Hospitals should adopt robust information and communications systems to improve the safety and quality of emergency care and enhance hospital efficiency.

Chapter 6: The Emergency Care Workforce

6.1 Hospitals, physician organizations, and public health agencies should collaborate to regionalize critical specialty care on-call services.

	Congress	DHHS	DOT	DHS	DOD	States	Hospitals	EMS Agencies	Private Industry	Professional Organizations	Other
6.2 Congress should appoint a commission to examine the impact of medical malpractice lawsuits on the declining availability of providers in high-risk emergency and trauma care specialties, and to recommend appropriate state and federal actions to mitigate the adverse impact of these lawsuits and ensure quality of care.	X										X
6.3 The American Board of Medical Specialties and its constituent boards should extend eligibility for certification in critical care medicine to all acute care and primary care physicians who complete an accredited critical care fellowship program.										X	
6.4 The Department of Health and Human Services, the Department of Transportation, and the Department of Homeland Security should jointly undertake a detailed assessment of emergency and trauma workforce capacity, trends, and future needs, and develop strategies to meet these needs in the future.		X	X	X							
6.5 The Department of Health and Human Services, in partnership with professional organizations, should develop national standards for core competencies applicable to physicians, nurses, and other key emergency and trauma professionals, using a national, evidence-based, multidisciplinary process.		X								X	
6.6 States should link rural hospitals with academic health centers to enhance opportunities for professional consultation, telemedicine, patient referral and transport, and continuing professional education.						X	X				

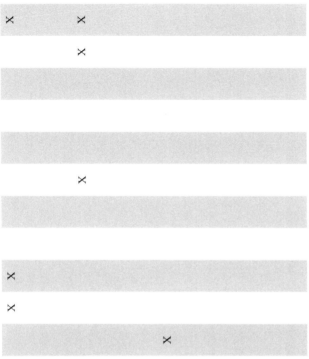

Chapter 7: Disaster Preparedness

7.1 The Department of Homeland Security, the Department of Health and Human Services, the Department of Transportation, and the states should collaborate with the Veterans Health Administration (VHA) to integrate the VHA into civilian disaster planning and management.

7.2 All institutions responsible for the training, continuing education, and credentialing and certification of professionals involved in emergency care (including medicine, nursing, emergency medical services, allied health, public health, and hospital administration) should incorporate disaster preparedness training into their curricula and competency criteria.

7.3 Congress should significantly increase total preparedness funding in fiscal year 2007 for hospital emergency preparedness in the following areas: strengthening and sustaining trauma care systems; enhancing emergency department, trauma center, and inpatient surge capacity; improving emergency medical services' response to explosives; designing evidence-based training programs; enhancing the availability of decontamination showers, standby intensive care unit capacity, negative pressure rooms, and appropriate personal protective equipment; and conducting international collaborative research on the civilian consequences of conventional weapons terrorism.

Chapter 8: Enhancing the Emergency Care Research Base

8.1 Academic medical centers should support emergency and trauma care research by providing research time and adequate facilities for promising emergency care and trauma investigators, and by strongly considering the establishment of autonomous departments of emergency medicine.

	Congress	DHHS	DOT	DHS	DOD	States	Hospitals	EMS Agencies	Private Industry	Professional Organizations	Other
8.2 The Secretary of the Department of Health and Human Services should conduct a study to examine the gaps and opportunities in emergency and trauma care research, and recommend a strategy for the optimal organization and funding of the research effort.	X	X	X	X	X						
8.2a This study should include consideration of training of new investigators, development of multicenter research networks, funding of General Clinical Research Centers that specifically include an emergency and trauma care component, involvement of emergency and trauma care researchers in the grant review and research advisory processes, and improved research coordination through a dedicated center or institute.											
8.2b Congress and federal agencies involved in emergency and trauma care research (including the Department of Transportation, the Department of Health and Human Services, the Department of Homeland Security, and the Department of Defense) should implement the study's recommendations.											
8.3 States should ease their restrictions on informed consent to match federal law.	X										
8.4 Congress should modify Federalwide Assurance Program regulations to allow the acquisition of limited, linked, patient outcome data without the existence of a Federalwide Assurance Program.											

EMERGENCY MEDICAL SERVICES AT THE CROSSROADS

	Congress	DHHS	DOT	DHS	DOD	States	Hospitals	EMS Agencies	Private Industry	Professional Organizations	Other
Chapter 3: Building a 21st-Century Emergency Care System											
3.1 The Department of Health and Human Services and National Highway Traffic Safety Administration, in partnership with professional organizations, should convene a panel of individuals with multidisciplinary expertise to develop evidence-based categorization systems for emergency medical services, emergency departments, and trauma centers based on adult and pediatric service capabilities.		X	X							X	
3.2 The National Highway Traffic Safety Administration, in partnership with professional organizations, should convene a panel of individuals with multidisciplinary expertise to develop evidence-based model prehospital care protocols for the treatment, triage, and transport of patients.			X							X	
3.3 The Department of Health and Human Services should convene a panel of individuals with emergency and trauma care expertise to develop evidence-based indicators of emergency and trauma care system performance.		X									
3.4 Congress should establish a demonstration program, administered by the Health Resources and Services Administration, to promote coordinated, regionalized, and accountable emergency and trauma care systems throughout the country, and appropriate $88 million over 5 years to this program.	X	X									

	Congress	DHHS	DOT	DHS	DOD	States	Hospitals	EMS Agencies	Private Industry	Professional Organizations	Other
3.5 Congress should establish a lead agency for emergency and trauma care within 2 years of the release of this report. This lead agency should be housed in the Department of Health and Human Services, and should have primary programmatic responsibility for the full continuum of emergency medical services and emergency and trauma care for adults and children, including medical 9-1-1 and emergency medical dispatch, prehospital emergency medical services (both ground and air), hospital-based emergency and trauma care, and medical-related disaster preparedness. Congress should establish a working group to make recommendations regarding the structure, funding, and responsibilities of the new agency, and design and monitor the transition to its assumption of the responsibilities outlined above. The working group should include representatives from federal and state agencies and professional disciplines involved in emergency and trauma care.	X	X									
3.6 The Department of Health and Human Services should adopt rule changes to the Emergency Medical Treatment and Active Labor Act and the Health Insurance Portability and Accountability Act so that the original goals of the laws will be preserved, but integrated systems can be further developed.		X									
3.7 The Centers for Medicare and Medicaid Services should convene an ad hoc working group with expertise in emergency care, trauma, and emergency medical services systems to evaluate the reimbursement of emergency medical services, and make recommendations with regard to including readiness costs and permitting payment without transport.		X									

Chapter 4: Supporting a High-Quality EMS Workforce

4.1 State governments should adopt a common scope of practice for emergency medical services personnel, with state licensing reciprocity.

4.2 States should require national accreditation of paramedic education programs.

4.3 States should accept national certification as a prerequisite for state licensure and local credentialing of emergency medical services providers.

4.4 The American Board of Emergency Medicine should create a subspecialty certification in emergency medical services.

Chapter 5: Advancing System Infrastructure

5.1 States should assume regulatory oversight of the medical aspects of air medical services, including communications, dispatch, and transport protocols.

5.2 Hospitals, emergency medical services agencies, public safety departments, emergency management offices, and public health agencies should develop integrated and interoperable communications and data systems.

5.3 The National Coordinator for Health Information Technology should fully involve prehospital emergency medical services leadership in discussions about design, deployment, and financing of the National Health Information Infrastructure.

	Congress	DHHS	DOT	DHS	DOD	States	Hospitals	EMS Agencies	Private Industry	Professional Organizations	Other
Chapter 6: Preparing for Disasters											
6.1 The Department of Health and Human Services, the Department of Transportation, the Department of Homeland Security, and the states should elevate emergency and trauma care to a position of parity with other public safety entities in disaster planning and operations.		X	X	X		X					
6.2 Congress should substantially increase funding for emergency medical services–related disaster preparedness through dedicated funding streams.	X										
6.3 Professional training, continuing education, and credentialing and certification programs for all the relevant professional categories of emergency medical services personnel should incorporate disaster preparedness into their curricula and require the maintenance of competency in these skills.			X			X				X	X
Chapter 7: Optimizing Prehospital Care Through Research											
7.1 Federal agencies that fund emergency and trauma care research should target an increased share of research funding at prehospital emergency medical services research, with an emphasis on systems and outcomes research.		X	X	X	X						X
7.2 Congress should modify Federalwide Assurance Program regulations to allow the acquisition of limited, linked patient outcome data without the existence of a Federalwide Assurance Program.	X										

7.3 The Secretary of the Department of Health and Human Services should conduct a study to examine the research gaps and opportunities in emergency and trauma care research, and recommend a strategy for the optimal organization and funding of the research effort. This study should include consideration of the training of new investigators, the development of multicenter research networks, the involvement of emergency medical services researchers in the grant review and research advisory processes, and improved research coordination through a dedicated center or institute. Congress and federal agencies involved in emergency and trauma care research (including the Department of Transportation, the Department of Health and Human Services, the Department of Homeland Security, and the Department of Defense) should implement the study's recommendations.

EMERGENCY CARE FOR CHILDREN: GROWING PAINS

Chapter 3: Building a 21st-Century Emergency Care System

3.1 The Department of Health and Human Services and the National Highway Traffic Safety Administration, in partnership with professional organizations, should convene a panel of individuals with multidisciplinary expertise to develop evidence-based categorization systems for emergency medical services, emergency departments, and trauma centers based on adult and pediatric service capabilities.

	Congress	DHHS	DOT	DHS	DOD	States	Hospitals	EMS Agencies	Private Industry	Professional Societies	Other
7.3	X	X	X		X						
3.1		X	X							X	

	Congress	DHHS	DOT	DHS	DOD	States	Hospitals	EMS Agencies	Private Industry	Professional Societies	Other
3.2 The National Highway Traffic Safety Administration, in partnership with professional organizations, should convene a panel of individuals with multidisciplinary expertise to develop evidence-based model prehospital care protocols for the treatment, triage, and transport of patients, including children.			X							X	
3.3 The Department of Health and Human Services should convene a panel of individuals with emergency and trauma care expertise to develop evidence-based indicators of emergency and trauma care system performance, including the performance of pediatric emergency care.		X									
3.4 Congress should establish a demonstration program, administered by the Health Resources and Services Administration, to promote coordinated, regionalized, and accountable emergency care systems throughout the country, and appropriate $88 million over 5 years to this program.	X	X									
3.5 The Department of Health and Human Services should adopt rule changes to the Emergency Medical Treatment and Active Labor Act and the Health Insurance Portability and Accountability Act so that the original goals of the laws are preserved, but integrated systems may further develop.		X									

3.6 Congress should establish a lead agency for emergency and trauma care within 2 years of the release of this report. The lead agency should be housed in the Department of Health and Human Services, and should have primary programmatic responsibility for the full continuum of emergency medical services and emergency and trauma care for adults and children, including medical 9-1-1 and emergency medical dispatch, prehospital emergency medical services (both ground and air), hospital-based emergency and trauma care, and medical-related disaster preparedness. Congress should establish a working group to make recommendations regarding the structure, funding, and responsibilities of the new agency, and design and monitor the transition to its assumption of the responsibilities outlined above. The working group should have representation from federal and state agencies and professional disciplines involved in emergency and trauma care.

3.7 Congress should appropriate $37.5 million per year for the next 5 years to the Emergency Medical Services for Children program.

Chapter 4: Arming the Emergency Care Workforce with Knowledge and Skills

4.1 Every pediatric- and emergency care–related health professional credentialing and certification body should define pediatric emergency care competencies and require practitioners to receive the level of initial and continuing education necessary to achieve and maintain those competencies.

4.2 The Department of Health and Human Services should collaborate with professional organizations to convene a panel of individuals with multidisciplinary expertise to develop, evaluate, and update clinical practice guidelines and standards of care for pediatric emergency care.

	Congress	DHHS	DOT	DHS	DOD	States	Hospitals	EMS Agencies	Private Industry	Professional Societies	Other
4.3 Emergency medical services agencies should appoint a pediatric emergency coordinator, and hospitals should appoint two pediatric emergency coordinators—one a physician—to provide pediatric leadership for the organization.							X	X			
Chapter 5: Improving the Quality of Pediatric Emergency Care											
5.1 The Department of Health and Human Services should fund studies of the efficacy, safety, and health outcomes of medications used for infants, children, and adolescents in emergency care settings in order to improve patient safety.		X									
5.2 The Department of Health and Human Services and the National Highway Traffic Safety Administration should fund the development of medication dosage guidelines, formulations, labeling, and administration techniques for the emergency care setting to maximize effectiveness and safety for infants, children, and adolescents. Emergency medical services agencies and hospitals should incorporate these guidelines, formulations, and techniques into practice.		X	X				X	X			
5.3 Hospitals and emergency medical services agencies should implement evidence-based approaches to reducing errors in emergency and trauma care for children.							X	X			
5.4 Federal agencies and private industry should fund research on pediatric-specific technologies and equipment used by emergency and trauma care personnel.		X	X	X					X		

5.5 Emergency medical services agencies and hospitals should integrate family-centered care into emergency care practice.

Chapter 6: Improving Emergency Preparedness and Response for Children Involved in Disasters

6.1 Federal agencies (the Department of Health and Human Services, the National Highway Traffic Safety Administration, and the Department of Homeland Security), in partnership with state and regional planning bodies and emergency care providers, should convene a panel with multidisciplinary expertise to develop strategies for addressing pediatric needs in the event of a disaster. This effort should encompass the following:

- Development of strategies to minimize parent–child separation and improved methods for reuniting separated children with their families.
- Development of strategies to improve the level of pediatric expertise on disaster medical assistance teams and other organized disaster response teams.
- Development of disaster plans that address pediatric surge capacity for both injured and noninjured children.
- Development of and improved access to specific medical and mental health therapies, as well as social services, for children in the event of a disaster.
- Development of policies to ensure that disaster drills include a pediatric mass casualty incident at least once every 2 years.

Chapter 7: Building the Evidence Base for Pediatric Emergency Care

	Congress	DHHS	DOT	DHS	DOD	States	Hospitals	EMS Agencies	Private Industry	Professional Societies	Other
7.1 The Secretary of Health and Human Services should conduct a study to examine the gaps and opportunities in emergency care research, including pediatric emergency care, and recommend a strategy for the optimal organization and funding of the research effort. This study should include consideration of the training of new investigators, development of multicenter research networks, involvement of emergency and trauma care researchers in the grant review and research advisory processes, and improved research coordination through a dedicated center or institute. Congress and federal agencies involved in emergency and trauma care research (including the Department of Transportation, Department of Health and Human Services, Department of Homeland Security, and Department of Defense) should implement the study's recommendations.		X	X	X	X						
7.2 Administrators of state and national trauma registries should include standard pediatric-specific data elements and provide the data to the National Trauma Data Bank. Additionally, the American College of Surgeons should establish a multidisciplinary pediatric specialty committee to continuously evaluate pediatric-specific data elements for the National Trauma Data Bank and identify areas for pediatric research.											X

Index

A

Academic health centers
  ED crowding in, 40
  linkage with rural EDs, 11, 250, 251
  recommendations for, 11, 250, 251,
    297, 315
  research support, 297, 315
Accidental Death and Disability: The
  Neglected Disease of Modern
  Society, 27, 82, 92, 305, 354
Accountability
  challenges in implementing, 94
  current efforts to improve local
    emergency care systems, 104, 105,
    106, 107
  importance of, 14, 94
  for patient flow management, 155–156
  shortcomings of current system, 14–15,
    22–23
  See also Performance measurement
Accrediting organizations, 95
Admissions, hospital ED
  admission/discharge unit, 151
  alcohol- and drug-related, 63–64
  automated triage systems, 182–184
  bedside registration, 150, 175
  bottlenecks, 136
  causes, 1, 18
  elderly patients, 347–348
  fast tracks, 149–150
  frequent users, 349–350
  full-capacity protocols, 150–151
  integrated health care system, 165–167
  legal and regulatory requirements, 100
  Medicaid enrollees, 3
  mental health problem-related, 61
  patient-centered care, 25
  patient characteristics, 2, 3, 39, 349
  patient insurance coverage, 52
  patient leaving before being seen, 41–42
  patterns and trends, 1, 2, 18, 38, 39,
    293, 345–350
  pediatric patients, 348
Advanced life support (ALS) protocols,
  90–91
Advanced practice nurses, 231
Adverse events
  causes, 23–24
  information technology for monitoring,
    173–174
  information technology to prevent,
    184–186
  risk in EDs, 23
  teamwork training to reduce, 244–245
  types of, 23
Agency for Healthcare Research and
  Quality, 112, 115, 264, 299

E

Economics
  barriers to primary care, 45–46
  cost of ED services for Medicaid
    patients, 54
  cost of ED services for Medicare
    patients, 54
  cost of physician liability insurance, 224
  demonstration project grants, 15–16,
    108–110, 124–125
  disincentives to patient flow
    improvement, 99–100, 130,
    157–158
  funding for disaster preparedness, 282,
    283–284, 285
  funding for new national emergency
    care agency, 123
  government support for safety net care,
    44
  health care sector share of GDP, 5
  implementing a national health
    information system, 170
  incentives to reduce ED crowding, 5–6,
    156–157
  information technology investments,
    169, 194–196
  reimbursement trends, 56–58
  research funding, 12, 294–295, 298–
    300, 308–309
  rural health care facilities, 66
  state funding mechanisms for emergency
    care, 59
  See also Costs; Uncompensated care
Effectiveness of ED care, 24–25
Efficiency
  barriers to improvement, 26, 152
  benefits of regionalization, 88
  current inadequacies, 130
  disincentives to improving, 99–100,
    130, 157–158
  hospital leadership for improvement in,
    6, 152–153
  incentives to improve, 5–6, 156–157
  See also Patient flow
Elderly patients
  ED visits, 347–348
  mental health problems, 61
  traumatic injury mortality, 293
Elective surgery schedule, 141, 157, 158

Electronic health records (EHRs), 151–152,
  168, 177
Emergency care system
  current fragmentation, 16, 22, 81, 111
  current reform efforts, 102–107
  definition, 31
  goals, 81–82
  within health care system, 129–131
  historical and conceptual development,
    353–356
  implementation of reform, 110–111
  performance measurement, 94–96
  public perception of performance, 94
  recommendations for new national
    agency, 16, 119–124
  scope, 31, 81
EMERGency ID NET, 280, 304
*Emergency Medical Services Agenda for the
  Future*, 29, 82–83, 112, 117
Emergency medical services (EMS). *See*
  Prehospital emergency medical
  services
Emergency Medical Services for Children,
  27, 92
Emergency Medical Services Systems Act
  (1973), 83, 355
Emergency Medical Treatment and Active
  Labor Act (EMTALA) (1996), 3, 10,
  26–27, 100–101, 157, 218–219, 346
  effects on physician supply, 226–227
  hospital staffing and, 226
  recommendations for changes in, 102,
    124
  violations of, 158
Emergency Medicine Foundation, 296
Emergency Severity Index, 182–184
EMS Performance Measures Project, 95
Ethical practice in human subjects research,
  313–314
eTRIAGE, 184

F

Failure modes and effects analysis, 132
Fast tracks, 149–150
Federal Emergency Management Agency
  (FEMA), 112
Federal government
  disaster preparedness policies and
    practices, 261–262, 264–265, 270,
    283–284, 285

recommendations for research, 237,
251
in rural areas, 11, 68–69, 237, 247–250
social and psychological care, 236
stresses of ED environment, 209,
240–241, 243
supply challenges, 236–237

See also Nursing staff; On-call
specialists; Physicians; Specialized
medical services

Z

Zone nursing, 150